1100

*BEHAVIOR
DISORDERS IN
SCHOOL-AGED
CHILDREN*

CHANDLER PUBLICATIONS IN EDUCATIONAL PSYCHOLOGY
David G. Ryans, *Advisory Editor*

BEHAVIOR DISORDERS IN SCHOOL-AGED CHILDREN

Harvey F. Clarizio
Michigan State University

AND

George F. McCoy
Illinois State University

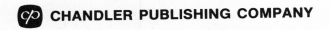 **CHANDLER PUBLISHING COMPANY**

Book and Cover Designed by Joseph M. Roter

Cover Photo by R. Keith Richardson

CHANDLER PUBLISHING COMPANY
666 FIFTH AVENUE
NEW YORK, N.Y. 10019

To our wives and children

CONTENTS

TABLES

PREFACE

The mental-health problems of children are a matter of national concern. Governmental concern has been reflected in the formation of the Joint Commission on the Mental Health of Children, which is reporting to Congress at the time of this writing. Despite the widespread interest, few mental-health professionals receive adequate preparation for understanding childhood disorders, and university faculty as well as graduates openly deplore this neglect. The lack stems in part from a dearth of suitable texts, especially of books which consider both the psychological and the educational aspects of deviant behavior.

The purpose for writing this book was to gather and evaluate the clinical intuitions, facts, and conclusions about disturbed children and adolescents. It is intended for advanced undergraduates and beginning graduate students who are preparing to become clinical psychologists, school psychologists, school counselors, school social workers, special-education teachers, and, most importantly, regular classroom teachers. While the book is not a "how-to-do-it" manual, there are some practical guides for coping with specific problems. The fundamental aim is to provide an introduction to the field of behavior disorders in children.

The book is organized around three major areas. Part I entails a discussion of the issues associated with normal development together with possible outcomes. Attention is also given to the concept of diagnosis and its current role in childhood disturbances. Finally, the incidence of emotional disturbance in youth is considered as well as the factors influencing these figures.

Part II includes discussion of six "types" of disorders among deviant youth. Attention is addressed to (1) the characteristics of various syndromes, (2) theories of etiology, and (3) various treatment programs. In keeping with the educational orientation of the book, certain topics customarily included in a text on the abnormal psychology of children have been omitted. Notable among such exclusions are habit-training problems and psychosomatic disorders. On the other hand, emphasis has been given to topics closely related to the adjustment of school-aged youth. The chapters on learning disabilities and on the socially disadvantaged are clear-cut examples of the educational point of view.

Part III is concerned with intervention and prevention strategies. Some of the major approaches to therapy are presented. Consonant with the data-oriented nature of the book, psychotherapy as a means of behavioral change is appraised in the first chapter of the part. Behavior-modification approaches are considered in the second chapter and in the one following, where interventions available in the community setting are discussed. A chapter pertaining to classroom discipline has been included for those who must cope with troublesome youth either as teachers or as consultants to teachers. Concluding the book is a chapter on preventive strategies.

No attempt has been made to present a consistent theoretical framework although an eclectic sampling has been made of postulates stemming from psychoanalytic theories and/or learning theories. While the contributions of biological and social forces to deviant behavior are examined, the major focus is on the role played by psychological factors. The most distinctive aspects of the book inhere, perhaps, in its empirical orientation and in its psychoeducational emphasis.

Many people have contributed to the development of this book. We are especially grateful to Robert D. Wirt for his perceptive review of the manuscript. We are also deeply indebted to Myrtle Yoshinaga and Thomas Houle for their careful library research and editorial acumen. Thanks are also extended to Marvin Kaplan for his helpful observations.

Portions of this book have appeared in the *Journal of Special Education* and in *Mental Hygiene,* and to the publishers we extend our gratitude for permission to use the materials.

H. F. C.

G. F. M.

*BEHAVIOR
DISORDERS IN
SCHOOL-AGED
CHILDREN*

Part I

Developmental and
Diagnostic
Considerations

1

Normality: A Developmental Perspective

NORMAL BEHAVIOR PROBLEMS
COMMON GROWTH PROBLEMS
   ● DEPENDENCY ● CONSCIENCE DEVELOPMENT ● SEX-ROLE IDENTITY
   ● ANXIETY ● AGGRESSIVENESS ● ACHIEVEMENT MOTIVATION
   ● PARENTAL INFLUENCE ON BEHAVIOR
ADJUSTMENT MECHANISMS
THE STABILITY OF DEVIANT BEHAVIOR
CRITERIA OF NORMALITY
   ● THE STATISTICAL APPROACH ● THE IDEALISTIC APPROACH
   ● TOWARD A DEFINITION OF NORMALITY
GUIDELINES FOR REFERRAL

In this chapter, the issue of normality will constitute the main theme. What seems especially needed in the assessment of normality is evaluation from a developmental perspective. Such evaluation requires a consideration of normal maladjustment as well as of clinically deviant behaviors. It also requires a knowledge of typical growth problems (for example, dependency) and a discussion of the stability of behavioral traits, especially those assumed to be abnormal. In implementing a developmental framework, we will show that all children have adjustment difficulties, but that having problems cannot necessarily be equated with pathology. Next, we will review socialization pressures to which all children in our society are subjected along with some of the more likely adaptive and maladaptive outcomes of such pressures. Following a brief review of defense mechanisms, we will then, in the section on the chronologic stability of deviant behavior, critically examine the long-held assumption that emotional problems in children become more firmly entrenched with advancing

3

age. Finally, following a consideration of two basic approaches to the issue of normality, a definition of normality will be cited and some guidelines stated for referral to mental-health professionals.

NORMAL BEHAVIOR PROBLEMS

Two points should be recognized at the outset: (1) Every parent, teacher, and clinician carries with him a set of norms and/or standards with which he evaluates the appropriateness of child behavior. (2) Over the years, certain behaviors have come to be seen as abnormal. Corresponding to these two assertions are two questions: (1) How do people acquire the norms against which they render judgmental decisions pertaining to normality or abnormality? (2) How realistically based are their judgments? In an attempt to answer these questions, we will look briefly at some of the major sources from which norms arise and then at studies which raise questions as to how abnormal some behaviors are.

Parents, in addition to their life experiences, rely heavily on accessible literature which describes the mythical "average" child or perhaps confuses them with discussions of individual differences among children. Clinicians, in developing norms with which to evaluate child behavior, rely to a considerable degree on their training in psychopathology and on their clinical experiences with psychiatric populations which might create a tendency within the beginning clinician to exaggerate the severity of many problems found in children. Teachers, like parents, have also been sensitized to emotional problems which children present in the classroom. Heightened teacher sensitization, stemming from college courses in education and psychology, is reflected in the fact that more children are referred to child-guidance clinics by schools than by any other agency.

Because of the current cultural propensity to be anxious about our anxieties, we might well be predisposed to be overconcerned about a good many minor or transient childhood problems. What might not be readily evident is the extent of problem behavior among normal children. The expanding knowledge of children indicates that "abnormal" behavior among children is plentiful. We now recognize that no child is completely free from emotional difficulties. The prevalence of problems is, in fact, so rife that some developmental psychologists doubt that these deviations should be regarded as abnormal. From a strictly statistical concept of normality, it is almost inadmissible to contend that such large numbers of children should be labeled as deviant. We are by no means implying that parents, teachers, and clinicians commonly overestimate the seriousness of childhood problems, nor that we should dismiss problems of a developmental nature. It is our thesis, rather, that in assessing a child's behavior, we need to develop norms based on a more developmental frame of reference. Such norms can best be compiled through the study of problem behavior among fairly representative samples of children who are not preselected on a problem basis. The increasing focus of attention on children demands that more specific information be available regarding the significance of such behaviors so as to plan efficient and effective treatment regimens.

A study with which every student of child adjustment should be familiar is the California Growth Study, beyond a doubt the landmark investigation in developmental problems of normal children (MacFarlane, Allen, & Honzik, 1954). Despite the limitations associated with longitudinal research, the California Growth Study nonetheless provides the best evaluative frame of reference available from a developmental standpoint. The study began in 1929 with the selection of every third child born in Berkeley, California, during an 18-month period from January 1, 1928, through June 30, 1929. The sample consisted of 252 youngsters, half of whom constituted the guidance group, and half of whom served as a control group. The present study concerns itself with the control group whose developmental problems between the ages of 21 months and 14 years were studied through the use of open-ended interviews with mothers. The sample was admittedly biased in favor of the upper-middle-class socioeconomic population. Of the 126 subjects selected in infancy, 86 were still available for study at the age of 14. The 46 problems studied were subsumed under these categories: biological functioning and control (e.g., soiling); motor manifestations (e.g., nailbiting); social standards (e.g., lying); and personality patterns (e.g., shyness). The extensiveness of such problems is revealed in Table 1, which shows behavior problems manifested by one-third or more of this population at various age levels. The data contained in this chart offer us some crude norms for indicating deviant behaviors that are developmentally observed in a randomly selected group of children. Note that both sexes had an average of five or six problems at each age level between 21 months of age and 11 years of age. From a statistical viewpoint

TABLE 1. BEHAVIOR PROBLEMS SHOWN BY ONE-THIRD OR MORE OF NORMAL BOYS AND GIRLS AGED 1¾-14 YEARS [BEHAVIOR PROBLEMS SHOWN BY ONE-THIRD OR MORE OF THE BOYS AND GIRLS AT EACH AGE LEVEL — MACFARLANE, ALLEN, & HONZIK, 1954]

		AGE													
		1¾	3	3½	4	5	6	7	8	9	10	11	12	13	14
Enuresis (diurnal & nocturnal)	B	+													
	G	+													
Soiling	B														
	G														
Disturbing dreams	B										+				
	G						+				+	+			
Restless sleep	B	+													
	G														
Insufficient appetite	B														
	G						+								
Food finickiness	B		+												
	G	+		+	+		+								
Excessive modesty	B														
	G														
Nailbiting	B													+	+
	G									+		+			
Thumbsucking	B														
	G	+	+												
Overactivity	B		+	+	+	+		+	+	+					
	G			+	+	+	+								
Speech	B														
	G														
Lying	B			+	+	+	+		+						
	G				+	+	+	+							
Destructiveness	B														
	G														
Overdependence	B														
	G														
Attention demanding	B														
	G														
Oversensitiveness	B			+	+	+		+	+	+	+	+	+		
	G				+	+	+	+	+	+	+	+	+	+	+
Physical timidity	B														
	G			+		+									
Specific fears	B		+	+	+	+	+	+	+	+		+			
	G	+	+	+	+	+	+	+	+			+			
Mood swings	B							—	—	—	+	+		+	
	G											+			
Shyness*	B	—	—	—	—	—	—	—							
	G											+			
Somberness	B					+									
	G						+								
Negativism	B			+		+									
	G				+										
Irritability	B														
	G														
Tempers	B	+	+	+	+	+	+	+	+	+	+	+	+	+	
	G	+	+	+	+	+	+	+				+			
Jealousy	B					+		+	+	+	+	+	+		
	G			+		+	+		+						
Excessive reserve*	B	—	—	—	—	+	+					+	+		
	G					+	+	+	+	+	+	+	+		+

*——Data not obtained

*—Data not obtained.

Source: J. MacFarlane, L. Allen, & M. Honzik. A developmental study of the behavior problems of normal children between twenty-one months and fourteen years. Berkeley: Univer. of California Press, 1954. Reprinted by permission of The Regents of the University of California.

of normality, these data do not support the contention that the average or normal child can be defined as one who has no problems.

Basically, five developmental patterns were identified among the problems investigated. The problems, which declined with age, were (1) elimination controls (enuresis and soiling), (2) fears, (3) thumbsucking, (4) destructiveness, and (5) temper outbursts. Only one problem, nailbiting, increased with age, although this too was beginning to drop off by age 14. Insufficient appetite and lying were problems which reached a peak and then subsided. Included among problems characterized by twin peaks were restless sleep, disturbing dreams, physical timidity, irritability, and demanding of attention. The first elevation of these bimodal problems often occurred near the age of entrance into school, and the second elevation at the beginning of adolescence. Oversensitiveness was the sole problem which was unrelated to age.

Sex differences were also discovered in relation to certain problems, as shown in Table 2. The incidence for boys was significantly higher for such problems as overactivity, demanding of attention, temper tantrums, and lying. Problems for girls more commonly centered around excessive modesty, shyness, and specific fears.

Another finding of interest deals with differences related to sibling order. For example, withdrawal and internalization patterns of adjustment were more common among first-born boys in contrast to more aggressive and competitive patterns of adjustment among non-first-born boys. Only two problems, thumbsucking and oversensitiveness, differentiated first-born girls from second-born girls. Interestingly, among the four sibling groups, it was the first-born girls who manifested more problems and had the most conflicting modes of adjustment.

Another study which deserves careful consideration in the study of maladjustment among a nonpsychiatric childhood population was conducted by Lapouse and Monk (1958). These investigators conducted structured interviews with mothers of 482 randomly selected children in Buffalo between the ages of 6 and 12. The findings, as shown in Table 3, reinforce the findings of MacFarlane and his associates on the frequency of problems among a run-of-the-mill group of youngsters. Note that almost half of the 482 youngsters were rated as overactive or as having at least 7 or more fears, according to the mothers' reports. These data would certainly suggest that such behav

TABLE 2. DIFFERENCES IN THE INCIDENCE OF BEHAVIOR PROBLEMS BETWEEN NORMAL BOYS AND GIRLS AGED 1¾-13 YEARS [SEX DIFFERENCES IN THE INCIDENCE OF PROBLEM BEHAVIOR—MACFARLANE, ALLEN, & HONZIK, 1954]

| Age in Years | Problems Having a Statistically Significant* Greater Incidence among: | |
	Boys	Girls
1¾	Diurnal enuresis Excessive emotional dependence Irritability	
3		Excessive modesty Specific fears
4		Thumbsucking
5	Temper tantrums	Thumbsucking Physical timidity
6		Food fussiness Oversensitiveness Mood swings
7	Stealing	Excessive emotional dependence Shyness Excessive reserve
8	Hyperactivity Temper tantrums Lying	Excessive modesty Excessive reserve
9	Excessive demanding of attention	Shyness Somberness
10		Excessive reserve
11	Lying Excessive demanding of attention Jealousy Competitiveness	Shyness
12	Overactivity Lying	Disturbing dreams Physical timidity
13	Overactivity Selfishness in sharing	Specific fears

*At the 5 per cent level or better.

Source: J. MacFarlane, L. Allen, & M. Honzik. *A developmental study of the behavior problems of normal children between twenty-one months and fourteen years.* Berkeley: Univer. of California Press, 1954. Reprinted by permission of The Regents of the University of California.

iors typically characterize normal development in children. Lapouse and Monk posed an interesting question: Is there an association between number of fears and worries and other so-called pathological behaviors, such as bedwetting, nightmares, and tension indicators?

TABLE 3. THE FREQUENCY OF SELECTED BEHAVIORS IN A SAMPLE OF CHILDREN AGED 6-12 YEARS AS REPORTED BY MOTHERS [PREVALENCE OF CERTAIN BEHAVIOR CHARACTERISTICS IN A WEIGHTED REPRESENTATIVE SAMPLE OF 482 CHILDREN AGED 6 TO 12, AS REPORTED BY MOTHERS — LAPOUSE & MONK, 1959]

Behavior	*Per Cent of Children*
Fears and worries, 7 or more present	43
Wetting bed within the past year	
All frequencies	17
Once a month or more	8
Nightmares	28
Temper loss	
Once a month or more	80
Twice a week or more	48
Once a day or more	11
Stuttering	4
Unusual movements, twitching or jerking (tics)	12
ᵖⁱring nails	
All intensities	27
Nails bitten down (more severe)	17
Grinding teeth	14
Sucking thumb or fingers	
All frequencies	10
"Almost all the time"	2
Biting, sucking or chewing clothing or other objects	16
Picking nose	26
Picking sores	16
Chewing or sucking lips or tongue or biting inside of mouth	11

Source: R. Lapouse & M. Monk. Fears and worries in a representative sample of children. *Amer. J. Orthopsychiat.*, 1959, 29, 803-818. Copyright ©, the American Orthopsychiatric Association, Inc. Reproduced by permission.

Surprisingly, no significant relationships were found despite the assumptions of some clinicians that fears and worries are symptomatic (or indicative) of other kinds of maladjustment.

In a later analysis, Lapouse and Monk (1964) divided the subjects according to sex, race, social class, and family size in order to disclose the relationships among these variables and the likelihood of behavioral deviations. Their findings may be summarized as follows:

1. Age was clearly the demographic factor most clearly associated with the occurrence of behavioral deviations. With increasing age, the prevalence of behavior deviations declined for school-age children. In other words, the younger children, ages 6 through 8, by far surpass

the older children, ages 9 through 12, in the number of behavior deviations.

2. Boys have a higher incidence of behavior deviations than do girls. Sex differences were most pronounced with respect to management of behavior, for example, overactivity and teachers' complaints about behavior.

3. The frequency of behavior deviations was higher among Negro children than white children. Because of the socioeconomic differences between the two groups, it was not possible to evaluate racial differences adequately.

4. With race held constant, there were extremely few differences in the incidence of behavior deviations among the two white groups of different socioeconomic standings.

5. There seemed to be very little difference in the amount of deviant behavior between only children and children with siblings.

In short, younger elementary-school children, Negro youth, and boys were, in descending order of susceptibility, the most likely to deviate from norms established on the 482 children used in the study.

Additional evidence of behavior problems among normal children is forthcoming in studies on delinquency. In one study dealing with the extent of unrecorded delinquency, adolescents enrolled in institutions and in high school were asked to report anonymously whether or not they had ever engaged in any of a list of 23 acts of delinquency (Short & Nye, 1958). The most striking finding was the sweeping incidence of reported delinquency activities among the legally nondelinquent adolescents. The delinquents could be differentiated from the legally nondelinquent youth in terms of the frequency of reported delinquent acts. Yet 50 per cent or more of the latter group reported skipping school, stealing things worth less than $2, buying or drinking alcoholic beverages, intentionally damaging property, and violating game laws. While the findings of this study should probably be tempered to some extent because of the limitations of the self-report method, the reader need only examine his own conscience relative to commission of similar acts during his high-school period to confirm the extensiveness of antisocial behavior. A certain amount of nose-thumbing is apparently not an uncommon phenomenon among adolescents in our society. Theft, property destruction, and other forms of antisocial behavior should, within limits, probably not be considered as deviant but within the boundaries of normality (Havighurst, 1966).

In sum, we are not implying that certain behaviors, such as stealing and nightmares, cannot be indicative of serious emotional disturbance in children. We have stressed, however, that the heightened concern about the emotional health of our youth, coupled with the sometimes faulty bases on which norms are developed, render us somewhat prone at times to overlook a parsimonious, developmental interpretation. The magnitude of the problem might consequently be exaggerated in certain cases. Also, we do not want to leave the impression that "normal maladjustments" are unimportant and therefore should be left to self-resolution. Though common, these problems are in need of alleviation since they distress both children and the adults who must deal with these disturbances. In keeping with our developmental orientation, we now turn to a consideration of tasks to which all children of our culture are exposed because of their biological, interpersonal, and cultural surroundings.

COMMON GROWTH PROBLEMS

In this section, we will examine in greater detail certain growth problems which are common to all children in our society. These growth problems center around certain personality variables which are believed by personality theorists and clinicians alike to play a central role in the formation of both healthy and disordered personalities: dependency, conscience, anxiety, aggressiveness, and achievement motivation. Attention will be focused on the child-rearing antecedents of these five personality constructs as revealed in representative research studies. Common adaptive and maladaptive outcomes as well as the symptoms and the child-rearing practices will be presented for each of the personality variables under consideration.

1. DEPENDENCY

All children are born in a state of dependency. Because of the child's helplessness, he must learn to depend on his mother for fulfillment of his basic needs. A prolonged period of helplessness sets the stage for the child's associating his mother with the reduction of painful stimulation and the satisfaction of his basic drives. The child comes to depend on her for satisfaction of his emotional needs as well. The genesis of dependency, then, appears to have its roots in early experiences of relatively consistent gratification of dependency needs by the mother (Mussen, Conger, & Kagan, 1969). While the parents are initially very accepting of the child's total reliance on them, it is not long, especially in our society, before the child is expected gradually to forgo some of his dependency and strive toward becoming a more self-reliant individual. In fact, it seems as though the child just begins to unlearn some of his dependency not long after he has originally learned it.

How does dependency manifest itself? For Beller (1955) there are five signs of dependency. The first sign is seeking help. Rather than taking the initiative, the dependent child goes to the adult for help not only when he encounters some obstacle in attempting to perform an assignment but even when the task is of a routine nature. Another sign of dependency is attention-getting behavior. The dependent child habitually wants the adult to watch him or talk with him or look at something he has produced, like a drawing. Seeking physical contact is another behavior suggestive of dependency. The child may want to sit on the parent's lap or cling to his mother tenaciously. Physical proximity or the desire to be close to an adult is a fourth sign of dependency which is closely related to the desire for physical contact. Finally, dependency can also be manifested in the seeking of approval. Some authors believe that seeking attention and wanting approval represent more mature forms of behavior than does seeking physical contact or proximity, since the former are characteristic of older children whereas the latter are more characteristic of younger children. Not only does the nature of the dependent response change with age, but the object of the dependency also shifts with age. As the child matures, emotional dependence on peers increases, while emotional dependence on adults decreases (Heathers, 1955). A partial explanation of this shift might well be attributed to the fact that older children provide their classmates with social reinforcers more frequently than do younger, nursery-school children (Charlesworth & Hartup, 1967).

Frequently, it is not an easy matter to define or classify dependency behaviors (or other social-psychological behaviors, for that matter). The confusion stems in large measure from the judgmental process involved (Walters & Parke, 1964). It is very difficult, for instance, to tell whether a given behavior represents an achievement orientation or approval-seeking behavior, especially if judged apart from the cultural context. Granted the limitations associated with such judgments, most workers agree as to the existence of two varieties of dependency

—instrumental and emotional. In instrumental dependency, the child seeks help in reaching a given goal. The student, for example, might be dependent upon his teacher for completion of a given arithmetic assignment. In emotional dependency, the child seeks the social responses of others, for example, approval as a goal per se. Chronologically, instrumental dependency (the seeking of another as a means of securing assistance) apparently precedes emotional dependency (essentially affiliation or attachment). The sexes probably do not differ appreciably in terms of over-all dependency. Some workers believe, however, that because of cultural forces, the former is typical of boys and the latter typical of girls.

One of the hazards inherent in the socialization process is that either too strong or too weak a dependency drive may interfere with the child's adjustment. Let us look, first of all, at the pattern of strong dependency or "overdependency," for which there are two proposed theories, both of which focus on parent attitudes. One theory, proposed by Levy (1943), suggests that maternal overprotection may lead to overly dependent behavior in children. In his study of 15 cases of overprotective mothers, he found their children to be passive, dependent, and submissive. Heathers (1953) likewise concluded that dependent behavior may stem from maternal overprotection. The mothers in Heathers' study not only permitted dependent behavior but also reinforced it.

In an attempt to understand the role of overprotection in the production of dependency, some authors regard maternal overprotection and excessive indulgence as equivalents. Two other possibilities exist, however, regarding the relationship between this form of child-rearing practice and dependent behavior. First, it is possible that the overprotective mothers directly and typically reinforce the child for such behaviors. Second, overprotection, especially when combined with maternal domination and restrictiveness, may be experienced by the child as a frustration which leads to the compensatory or secondary development of dependent behavior (Hartup, 1963). While the nature of the relationship is not altogether clear, the conclusion that maternal overprotection is one factor in dependent behavior in children seems tentatively justified.

Another theory which is prevalent views dependent behavior in children as a result of maternal rejection. The notion that maternal rejection is an antecedent of dependent behavior in children receives considerable support from empirical research, as is evidenced in Hartup's (1963) review of the literature. According to this view, the child's dependency needs are frustrated, with the result that the child, lacking sufficient support and nurturance, is unable to progress successfully through the experiences culminating in independence. Frustration of basic dependency drives is quite apt to occur in our culture because of the societal emphasis on early independence training. Many parents and teachers, in their eagerness to develop independence in children, fail to recognize that dependency is a prerequisite for independence. Paradoxically, the child can become independent only after he has learned that he can depend on his parents' acceptance, approval, and support.

Stendler (1954) notes that there are two critical periods during which the preschool child might become overly dependent as a consequence of excessive frustration. The first occurs near the end of his first year of life. At this time, the child, who recognizes in a primitive fashion his dependence on the mother, begins to test out the mother to see if he can indeed rely on her. During this period, it is essential that the infant's dependency needs be met. If separated from the mother during this period, the infant is likely to experience anxiety which the child will later attempt to dissipate through excessive demands on the mother when she is available. Such anxiety serves to heighten the dependency drive, with the result that overdependence can ensue. The second critical period comes between the ages of 2 and 3 when a child is expected to relinquish some of his dependency. Disturbances of a serious nature at this time can again arouse anxiety over his dependent relationship with the mother, thereby strengthening the dependency drive. Sears, Maccoby, and Levin (1957) reported that parents who irritably rejected their children's requests for dependency but who eventually succumbed to such demands produced the most dependent children.

What becomes of the dependent child? Will he always remain dependent? The only longitudinal study on dependency underscores the importance of cultural influences on the developmental stability of this drive. Kagan and Moss (1960) studied 27 males and 27 females from birth through adolescence as part of a longitudinal study at the Fels Research Institute. Their results suggest that passive dependent behavior remains stable over time for the dependent female. but not for the dependent male. The results are interpreted in light

of societal pressures for the male to become self-reliant and autonomous and for the female to be passive.

Approval and disapproval afford parents powerful tools for influencing socialization through positive reinforcing or negative anxiety-
arousing consequences. By the use of approval and disapproval, the
parent is able to shape the child's behavior, for the child soon
learns which behaviors bring approval and which ones bring disapproval and subsequent anxiety. Later, as social contacts extend to other
adults, dependency serves as a potent source of the child's learning
the rules of social life. In this sense, dependency underlies much of the
socialization process of children.

Not all youngsters are given the opportunity to learn dependency.
As noted above, the social-learning theorist views dependency as a
consequence of the mother's or caretaker's satisfying of the infant's
needs; that is, the mother's presence is associated with a state of
comfort and well-being, while her absence is associated with anxiety.
When children are deprived of a continuing relationship with a
caretaker, it is difficult for the kind of conditioning process described
above to occur. Furthermore, there is a tendency in our society for
parents and teachers to overlook the importance of originally learned
dependency. Youngsters who have failed to learn dependency are
frequently difficult to socialize since they have not learned to desire
approval from others.

The importance of learning dependency for the socialization process
is suggested in a study by Goldfarb (1945). He compared 15 children
reared in institutions with 15 children who had spent the first three
years of their lives in foster homes under more normal conditions.
Upon followup, around age 12, dramatic differences were noted
between the two groups. In addition to intellectual deficits, the institutionally reared children also differed from the children in foster
homes in other respects. First of all, the investigator noted the absence
of a normal inhibitory pattern. The institutionally reared youngsters
were characterized by hyperactivity and disorganization. They were
unmanageable, and it was difficult for the adults to control the
youngsters' behavior. Second, the youngsters showed what is described
as affect hunger. In other words, they demanded constant affection
and attention. Third, these children tended to develop very shallow
emotional relationships with others despite their strong need for attention from others. Fourth, they manifested a lack of normal guilt and

anxiety. Following transgressions, these youngsters would typically show no signs of remorse. This lack of anxiety was also reflected in their schoolwork, in that they could accept failure with apparently little feeling.

Although prolonged periods of deprivation during the formative years are most likely detrimental to the development of wholesome personality, short periods of deprivation may have a facilitatory effect on socialization. Gewirtz and Baer (1958) report that adult approval becomes a more potent reinforcer after the child has been subjected to a period of social isolation. This finding clearly suggests that youngsters are more eager to secure adult approval following a brief period of social deprivation (a "time-out period") and are thus easier to socialize.[1]

CONSCIENCE DEVELOPMENT

Following the early work of Hartshorne and May (1928-1930) and the work of Piaget (1932), there was a dearth of activity and interest in the development of moral character. In general, psychologists, influenced by the behavioristic approach expounded by Watson, avoided the topic of moral development in children since psychological matters pertaining to moral character were thought to be unverifiable and inappropriate topics for psychology as a science. In so doing, psychologists neglected one of the most significant components of personality makeup. It was not until the late 1950's that there was a renewed interest in the study of moral development in children. Today, psychologists from various schools of thought recognize that the development of moral character is essential if the child is to become socialized in the ways of his particular culture. Children in the course of development must learn to channel aggressive and hedonistic impulses, to establish internal controls for behavior, and to comply to a reasonable extent with societal expectations. If they fail to do so, they and/or society will most likely suffer.

By "conscience" we mean the internalization of standards and

---

[1]Later research by Walters and Parke (1964) suggests that it is not a "social drive" which heightens the child's susceptibility to influence, but emotional arousal brought about by the isolation procedure. According to this interpretation, the child's state of arousal constitutes an important determinant of his susceptibility to influence by reducing perceptual thresholds and modifying the range and nature of cues to which he will respond.

prohibitions which govern one's activity. The preschool child certainly feels bad when he has transgressed, but primarily because he fears external parental disapproval. Later, around age 4 or 5, the locus of anxiety or fear comes from within and the child experiences guilt when he has transgressed. With the onset of an internal censor, the child is no longer as dependent on external sources to regulate his behavior. Research has concentrated more on the negative side of conscience (guilt and resistance to temptation) than on the positive side. We have been more concerned, perhaps regrettably so, with the "thou shalt not's" (prohibitions) than with the "thou shalt's" (standards).

The child is not born with a conscience. How does he eventually acquire internal standards which regulate the expression of his basic urges and determine the goals he sets for himself? The specifics of conscience formation are not fully known, but basically three factors have been found to play a central role in the development of moral character: the child's cognitive level, cultural factors, and child-rearing practices.

Let us look first at cognitive development. Since moral behavior and knowledge have a cognitive component, it is not surprising that they are influenced to some extent by the child's level of intellectual maturity. The use of reasoning has been found to be associated with high conscience development, but assumes only limited relevance to the very young child because of his limited intellectual powers. Once language comprehension develops, it is easier to explain the expected standards to him, and labels ("good," "bad") can be attached to specific behaviors. Anxiety thus becomes attached to certain misdeeds, and the discrimination between what is desirable and what is undesirable is facilitated. Moreover, once the child has developed greater linguistic facility, he can be taught to substitute words and ideas for the physical expression of certain impulses. For example, the parent can encourage the angry child who possesses language to tell mommy what he's angry about, so that he feels less of a need to express his anger through physical means. With more years of experience, the older child not only understands more fully the expectations set for him but also the rationale underlying them. He has both a deeper understanding and appreciation of certain moral concepts as well as a more highly developed facility for self-evaluation and self-criticism. In fact, behavioral changes associated with the development of moral judgment in Piaget's stage theory seem to be indicative of advancing cognitive development on the child's part.[2]

Cultural factors are also known to influence moral development. They determine, in large measure, the *contents* of conscience, that is, the standards and prohibitions the child will learn. Lower-class parents tend to place great emphasis on conformity to external cues or to authority, whereas middle-class parents emphasize internal regulation of behavior. Consistent with this differential emphasis is the finding that lower-class boys behave more aggressively and experience less guilt in the process than do middle-class boys (Mussen, Conger, & Kagan, 1969). In the lower classes, the child's parents and peer group provide different models or behaviors to be imitated from those of the middle class. The subcultural delinquent, for instance, who is a daily witness to aggression and norm violation in his neighborhood, is provided with a value system which in school and other situations involves him in difficulty since it is at odds with the value structure of the middle class.

A third factor in conscience development has to do with child-rearing practices. The study by Sears and his associates (1957) found that love-oriented techniques, such as the use of praise, warmth, reasoning, and the withdrawal of love, were more effective than materialistic techniques as reflected in physical punishment and deprivation of privileges. The effectiveness of love-oriented practices probably stems from four aspects of parental behavior:

1. Warmth makes the child dependent upon adult approval and lessens his need for deviant behavior to secure attention. It is interesting to note in this connection that the Glueck and Glueck (1950) study found that parents of delinquents are typically less accepting, solicitous, and affectionate in contrast to parents of nondelinquents.

2. The presentation of a model of self-restraint results in the imitation of socially acceptable behaviors.

3. The use of reasoning increases the child's understanding of expectations set for him and gives him additional training in making moral judgments.

4. Certain aspects relating to the timing of punishment (for example, punishment upon the initiation of the transgression) also make for the development of more effective controls (Becker, 1964).

---

[2]For a fuller discussion on the role of intelligence in moral development, see Kohlberg (1964).

There are two dangers associated with the development of internal controls. On the one hand, conscience may be too strict; on the other hand, conscience may be too lenient. Both extremes can pose hardships for the individual and for society. In other words, expecting too much and expecting too little of the child can have equally undesirable consequences. If conscience is too strong, it may inhibit behaviors that are not in need of censorship. Such unnecessary restrictions reduce the child's behavioral freedom, adjustive flexibility, and personal spontaneity. In the extreme, a restrictive conscience can create conflicts and produce feelings of guilt, self-dissatisfaction, depression, and inhibition—symptoms commonly associated with neurosis. Though a repressive conscience can lead to the above symptomatology, it should not be automatically assumed, however, that the neurotic youngster is necessarily any more moral than the normal youngster. What limited evidence there is suggests that the relationship between neurosis and moral character is slight. The neurotic child may be personally dissatisfied because he is not living up to what he would really like to be, but he is not necessarily self-critical because of perceived shortcomings regarding moral issues (Kohlberg, 1964). An example would be the neurotic adolescent boy whose compulsive seduction of females failed to generate in him any perceptible moral anxiety. The disturbed youth was quite concerned, however, about realizing his ideals of masculinity.

Since conscience consists of attainment ideals as well as prohibitions, there is a possibility that a child with a demanding conscience will strive for goals which are difficult if not impossible to attain, thus resulting in excessive anxiety and frustration on his part. The reader is perhaps familiar with the student who focuses not on the nineteen problems he had correct but on the one problem he had wrong, or the student who is upset because his straight "A" average was ruined by a "B" grade. Such youngsters tend to be unduly harsh and severe with themselves. Consequently, they enjoy life less. A certain amount of striving, ambition, and self-dissatisfaction seems to be desirable, but too little self-satisfaction can become a definite handicap.

At the other extreme is the child whose conscience is too lenient. This deficiency may manifest itself in such norm-violating behaviors as delinquency and lying. This youngster not uncommonly behaves as though rules were not for him. In the more severe cases of antisocial behavior, the child may not experience appropriate guilt feelings for his misbehavior. Two major investigations dealing with delinquent youth reported that both middle-class and lower-class delinquents are deficient in self-critical guilt reactions (Bandura & Walters, 1959; McCord & McCord, 1956). Similarly, Kohlberg (1964), in his study of lower-class delinquents, noticed that his subjects were functioning at an early stage of premoral judgment. He concluded that "simple developmental arrest" characterized the majority of his subjects. Lacking in sufficient internal controls with which to police their behavior, these youngsters require constant external surveillance. But external supervision is not a feasible means of handling this problem, for one cannot oversee all of the child's activity.

Ideally, the child should have an optimal amount of conscience. On the prohibitive side, he should be able to experience realistic guilt when he has committed a serious transgression. On the self-realization side, conscience should assist in the development of an integrated personality which can seek and achieve culturally congruent goals. Unfortunately, it is difficult to achieve a mature conscience in our society since cultural pressures often discourage one from thinking-through matters of a moral nature for himself.

SEX-ROLE IDENTITY

Identification with the parent results not only in the internalization of social rules but also in the acquisition of an appropriate sex role, that is, in the incorporation of beliefs, attitudes, and behaviors which are consistent with the cultural expectations for one's sex. The sex-appropriate male characteristics include competitiveness, independence, physical aggression, dominance, and achievement. Sex-typed characteristics appropriate for females, on the other hand, include conformity, passivity, and dependency. Three reasons have been advanced to explain the acquisition of sex-appropriate behaviors:

1. Praise, recognition, and acceptance by both parents and peers for engaging in behaviors consistent with one's sex role.
2. Anxiety over rejection by significant others for deviations from appropriate sex-role standards.
3. Identification or imitation of an adequate model of the same sex (Kagan, 1964).

Disturbances in sex-role identifications have been found in families where the father is absent. In such cases, the boy shows less masculine behavior and is apt to be rejected by his peer group. The father's absence, however, seems to have little influence on the fantasy play of young girls. Disturbances in sex behavior have also been associated with difficulties in sexual identification. Adolescent boys with non-masculine interests were found to be more anxious about sexuality and less prone to have erotic associations with the opposite sex than were boys with more typical masculine interests (Kagan & Moss, 1962). In a similar vein, homosexual men were less likely to have engaged in masculine activities, such as competitive games and fighting as children, in comparison with a control group of normals (Bieber et al., 1962).

ANXIETY

Many authors have distinguished between anxiety and fear by postulating that the former is a diffuse and undifferentiated apprehensive response to anticipated threat, whereas the latter is supposedly bound to a specific object or situation. In children, however, it is difficult to differentiate between these two states because the developing personality and intellectual processes do not permit the finer or sharper separations between genuine and fantasied threats that are more characteristic of the mature adult (Erikson, 1950). Further, since the experiential aspects of these two emotional responses do not appear to be appreciably different and since both terms refer to the unpleasant feeling states involving physiological reactions, the two terms will be used interchangeably for the purposes of discussion here.

How does anxiety manifest itself? In its more severe forms, anxiety is most commonly seen in neurotic disorders, for example, the rather total disorganization as seen in school phobia. In its less extreme forms, the individual feels apprehensive, ill at ease, and that some impending danger is imminent. The following list of behavioral manifestations of anxiety has been proposed by Andrus and Horowitz (1938): frequent bad temper and angry outbursts; nervous habits; preference for adult company or that of younger children; rough, bullying behavior such as whining and tattling; overcompliance to adult authority; overreaction to criticism; introversion or withdrawal into fantasy as a means of coping or escape; satisfaction from behavior which leads to unpleasant relationships with peers and adults.

Current research employing anxiety as a central variable has explored its effects on both intellectual and personality functioning. In terms of cognitive functioning, highly anxious children tend to be lower in both intelligence and achievement at the elementary-school and secondary-school levels (Sarason, 1963). Highly anxious students also appear to do more poorly on creativity tests (Reid, King, & Wickwire, 1959). In brief, high anxiety appears to affect adversely complex intellectual tasks such as those typically performed in a classroom setting, whereas the successful accomplishment of easier or simple tasks is facilitated by high anxiety. The evidence further suggests that very anxious children might perform best in a nonthreatening, secure classroom. Classroom observations, for example, showed that highly anxious boys are less task-oriented than are low-anxiety boys. Greater insecurity is also evident in their relationships to the teacher. Curiously, anxiety seems to affect girls differently in that the highly anxious girls, in contrast to those low in anxiety, evidence less distractibility and stronger achievement motivation.

As to the influence of anxiety on personality and social functioning, Ruebush (1963) has noted the following:

1. High-anxiety pupils when compared to those low in anxiety are not as popular with their peers.

2. High-anxiety children are more susceptible to propaganda.

3. High-anxiety children have more negative self-concepts and are more self-disparaging. Body image also seems impaired.

4. Dependency is also characteristic of high-anxiety children, though more so for boys than for girls.

5. Anxiety is inversely related to the open expression of aggression toward others, but positively related to signs of anxiety about one's own aggressive feelings.

6. Diminished behavioral freedom and anxiety tend to go hand in hand, as manifested behaviorally by indecisiveness, cautiousness, and rigidity.

How does anxiety arise? Very little empirical research has been conducted on the parental antecedents of anxiety. Sarason (1960) reports that mothers of high-anxiety children are quite defensive in interviews. Such evasiveness and guardedness, though in themselves clues to the personality makeup of these mothers and their manner of interacting with their children, have nonetheless hampered research on the relationship between child-rearing practices and the development of anxiety. Though experimental evidence concerning parental role in the production of childhood anxiety is sparse, clinical experience with anxious children and their parents has offered us some insights into its development. Cameron (1963) has discussed the various following ways in which children can be given training in anxiety:

1. By having a parental model who is anxious, the children may become habitually apprehensive simply as a result of incidental parent-child associations.

2. Some children are taught to search out every conceivable danger in their everyday lives. We recall the case of a divorcée who was obsessed by the idea that her ex-husband would come and take her only son, as the man had once threatened. The mother alerted the son to this ever-present danger, and taught him to lock all doors at home, to keep the shades drawn, to stay indoors as much as possible, and to be especially careful on his way to and from school. It is little wonder that this youngster became terribly tense and apprehensive.

3. Some children are used as confidants by their parents. In this role, the children are exposed prematurely to difficulties of adult adjustments such as financial burdens and marital problems. Lacking the necessary maturity to understand fully such problems as well as the ability and experience to cope with them, the children become overwhelmed and disillusioned by the uncertainties of life. Consider the boy whose mother continually tells him how bad his father is, how he does not pay the bills, how unfair he is to her, how she could have married a better man. This child's parental loyalties thus become divided, and a fundamental source of his personal security thereby undermined. Such a child is obviously vulnerable to strong feelings of personal anxiety.

4. Parental perfectionism can also make for anxious children. The parent who is never satisfied with his child's performance, who habitually tells him that he could do better, who sets standards above the child's ability level, produces a child who is self-dissatisfied and open to feelings of anxiety over his failure to live up to expectations.

5. Overpermissive parents are also likely to have highly anxious children because children need definite limits set for them in order to feel secure. Without such limits, the child is not sure of the boundaries of his behavioral freedom. Consequently, environmental predictability is lessened and uncertainty heightened.

Anxiety is most likely a universal phenomenon in children and is clearly exhibited by age 3 (Temple & Amen, 1944). Major sources of anxiety in children center around the possibility of physical harm, the loss of parental love, feelings of guilt, cultural deviation, and feelings of inadequacy as reflected in an inability to master the environment (Mussen, Conger, & Kagan, 1969). In adolescence, the search for ego identity is added to this list of anxiety sources as a teenager attempts to discover where he is going in life, what his assets and weaknesses are, and how he fits into his newly found roles.

While anxiety does sometimes become a crippling force, we should not regard it as necessarily undesirable and therefore try to shelter youngsters from it. In all probability, youngsters of this generation will have to learn to live with more anxiety as adults than we do. Obviously, youngsters should not be exposed to needless anxiety-producing experiences; yet, it is equally undesirable to eliminate anxiety entirely or to reduce it to an absolute minimum since adequate socialization requires some feelings of anxiety on the child's part. Somewhere between the extremes, there is an optimal level of anxiety. If anxiety deviates markedly from this level in either direction, the socialization process is hindered.

AGGRESSIVENESS

The best-known theory advanced to explain aggressive behavior in children is the frustration-aggression hypothesis developed by Dollard and his associates at Yale (1939). According to this view, frustration is the primary and natural antecedent of aggression. Where one encounters aggressive behavior, one can assume that it has been initiated by frustration. There is some evidence to support this assumption. One study found that aggressive male pupils, as rated by their classmates, had fathers who severely punished aggression in the home (Eron et al., 1961). In comparing a group of delinquents with non-delinquents, Glueck and Glueck (1950) reported a higher use of physical punishment and lower usage of reasoning among parents of delinquents. The existence of a family milieu characterized by punitiveness, threat, and parental rejection was found to be, through direct observation, one major factor among familial correlates of aggression in male children (McCord, McCord, & Howard, 1961). Thus, various investigators have consistently reported that in some manner the punishment of aggression, which frustrates the child, is related to heightened aggressiveness in the child. The authors view this reasonable finding as supporting the position that aggressive behavior is learned as a consequence of early childhood interactions within the family setting. It has become increasingly evident, however, that the frustration-aggression hypothesis is inadequate in accounting for all aggressive behavior. Recent evidence leads us to a second theory, which centers around modeling.

Bandura and Walters (1963), who do not regard the evidence for the frustration-aggression hypothesis as substantial, emphasize the role of imitation and reinforcement in the acquisition and maintenance of aggressive behavior in children. According to this social-learning-theory viewpoint, exposure to aggressive models should lead to aggressive behavior on the part of the child. This view is well substantiated by several experimental studies which show that even though the subject may not have been frustrated, increases in aggression follow exposure to aggressive models. In keeping with this theory, lower-class children manifest more overt physical aggression than do middle-class children, presumably because the lower-class model is typically more overtly aggressive. McCord, McCord, and Zola (1959) noted that boys who had deviant parental models were more apt to engage in antisocial activities. In brief, both laboratory and real-life field studies buttress the notion that imitation plays an important role in the genesis and maintenance of aggressive behavior.

Aggression is very common in children. Sears and his associates (1957) reported that almost all mothers had to handle instances of intense aggression directed against the parents by the preschool child. Childhood aggression is so common as to be thought almost universal.

Yet, if the child is to become a socialized adult, he must relinquish aggression or learn new modes of expressing it. There are dangers involved in the socialization of aggressive behavior, however. Socialization processes must not be so harsh as to inhibit severely the expression of aggressive behaviors, for these are necessary for a successful adjustment both in childhood and in later life. Without assertiveness, competitiveness, and self-confidence, the child is placed at a distinct disadvantage in coping with the demands of life, for it is not the meek or submissive who inherit the earth in our success-oriented culture. Rather, in our society as in many others, training in self-reliance and encouragement of achievement-striving represent particularly important aspects of the socialization process, especially for males. Training in aggression is necessary not only for fulfillment of the male's economic role, but for other aspects of psychosocial functioning as well. Unless children are responsive to socialization pressures in this area, societal punishment of either an overt or a covert nature is likely to be their fate.

Repeated severe punishment of aggression during the preschool years has been found to increase the child's aggression anxiety. Consequently, the youngster comes to feel uncomfortable and ill at ease in situations which arouse his aggressive impulses and he commonly responds with feelings of guilt, fear, self-deprecation, or embarrassment. Yet, because punishment itself is a frustration, the aggressive drives do not decrease, but increase, leaving the child in an ambivalent and conflict-laden status. In brief, the aggression has increased in strength, but this only serves to intensify his anxiety since he has no suitable means of expression. A vicious circle is thereby established.

A certain amount of aggression is a sign of a robust and well-balanced personality. We consider it both normal and desirable for the child to defend his rights and to fight back if the situation warrants. The child should not be made to feel guilty or fearful in exercising his right to justified anger. On the other hand, aggressive impulses cannot be allowed a free rein, for such license too can have an equally undesirable socialization consequence. The aggressive child is not at peace with himself or with his peer group. Since aggressive attacks elicit aggressive responses, it is not surprising to find a negative correlation between popularity and aggression (Winder & Rau, 1962).

Athough still widely accepted, the catharsis theory of aggression has received surprisingly little empirical support. According to this view, the release of aggressive behavior should produce a diminution of such behavior; that is, aggressive behavior should extinguish itself if allowed unrestricted expression. In actuality, it appears that a permissive approach to the treatment of acting-out behavior in children achieves the opposite effect. In a permissive atmosphere, the child is less fearful of punishment and his inhibitions decrease. Cathartic release may be appropriate for withdrawn youngsters, but its use with aggressive children certainly seems contraindicated. Despite the negative evidence to date, however, the catharsis theory continues to receive wide acceptance among professionals in the field.

Whereas the combination of parental restrictiveness and hostility not uncommonly produces neurotic-like problems in children, the combination of parental permissiveness and hostility is commonly found in cases of maximal aggression and delinquency (Becker, 1964). In other words, the highest level of aggressive behavior occurs when the child is reared under conditions which promote feelings of hostility in him, and which at the same time fail to impose limits on his acting-out behavior when hostility does occur.

How should aggressive behavior in children be handled? Very permissive handling of outbursts leads to increased aggressive activities on the child's part. If the mother is both permissive and punitive, the child is apt to become even more highly aggressive, and perhaps even delinquent. And if the mother is restrictive and punitive, the probability that the child will become socially withdrawn and intra-punitive is increased. So neither overly strict nor overly permissive treatment seems to be the desirable way of coping with this kind of behavior. A major study of child-rearing practices of preschool children (Sears et al., 1957) found that the most effective technique consisted in stopping the behavior but through techniques other than physical punishment. The child must know that the parent or teacher disapproves of such noncompliant behavior, but the generation of additional frustration and anger must be avoided in the management process. A warm, self-controlled parent capable of setting firm and clear-cut limits in a consistent and nonpunitive manner is apt to have minimal difficulty in guiding the development of aggressive behaviors. Adequate socialization is maximized through reasoning, affection, and appropriate models.

ACHIEVEMENT MOTIVATION — *desire to do something well*

The notion of personal competence has assumed a central status in recent years among many mental-health professionals. The concept of competence is to some extent replacing that of contentment as a yardstick of mental health. The ability to handle the stresses and strains associated with one's roles in life is assuming greater significance as an index of one's mental health than is intrapsychic freedom from anxiety. To be considered competent in our culture, an individual must be able to sustain himself in coping with the demands of reality. In the case of the child, the demands of reality in large measure center around the demands of our educational system, for school is the child's main job and success in this training is a necessary if not sufficient condition for effective functioning as an adult. In our society, youth must achieve, and to do this they need some degree of achievement motivation.

What is achievement motivation? Stated most simply, it is the child's desire or attempt to do something well. He might want to perfect a skill such as jumping rope, to run a mile more quickly, or to perform a task more efficiently. The child comes to judge his own performance in terms of certain standards of excellence. In addition, he comes to experience unpleasant or pleasant feelings about achieving these standards.

How does achievement motivation develop? Certainly, children are not born with standards of excellence. When and how does the desire to achieve arise? There appears to be no research which has investigated the age or conditions surrounding the emergence of achievement behavior. We do know, however, that individual differences in achievement motivation exist among 4- and 5-year-olds. Students in the primary grades also differ from one another with respect to the degree and area of achievement motivation. Crandall (1961) found, for instance, that some pupils spent more time and worked more intensely on intellectual pursuits, while others concentrated on artistic or mechanical pursuits. The desire for excellence in achievement not only arises early, but also tends to persist into adulthood. In one major longitudinal study (Moss & Kagan, 1961), it was reported that intellectual and recognition strivings were stable from childhood (grades 1 through 4) to young adulthood. Moreover, such strivings were equally stable for both sexes.

Though one must consider seriously the contribution of the peer group to achievement motivation among older youth, it would seem that parental interaction is a crucial determinant of achievement motivation in the young child. What parental behaviors are associated with the development of intellectual striving in young children? The pioneering study in this area was conducted by Winterbottom (1958). It was reported that mothers of boys rated high in achievement motivation expected self-reliant behavior relatively early and gave a freer rein to the child's spontaneous desire to be independent. In addition, these mothers directly reinforced independent behavior when it occurred. Moss and Kagan (1961) also noted that maternal "pushing" of the developmental timetable was a moderately successful predictor of intellectual competence in adulthood. Bandura and Kupers (1964) demonstrated that preschoolers, merely by observing the achievement behavior of others, may develop similar standards of excellence. It appears that high levels of parental involvement provide a basis for achievement motivation, although the impact of parental attitudes and child-rearing practices on achievement motivation will vary with the sex of the parent and child and the kind of achievement motivation.

What happens when the student has too much achievement motivation? Are the schools and parents of today pressuring students too much? One way of attempting to answer this question is to examine the personality characteristics of achieving students. Virginia Crandall (1967), an active researcher in this area, had the following to say:

It would appear ... that achieving children, in contrast to peers who perform less well, do not need to depend upon adults but are somewhat compliant and conforming to their demands and accept and incorporate adults' high evaluations of the importance of achievement. They are also able to work without being immediately rewarded for their efforts, show initiative, self-reliance, and emotional control. While achieving children of preschool and early elementary age are somewhat aggressive and competitive, their social relationships are generally good. Achievement, however, seems to be exacting in its toll. By later elementary school or junior high age, aggression and competition have become accentuated, relationships with siblings, peers, and adults show some disruption, and the children are less creative, more anxious, and less able to resist the temptation to cheat. Research on high school students ... indicates that these attributes become increasingly pronounced at later ages. Does this mean that the effort to achieve "produces" the less desirable personality attributes? Or does it mean that only if children have acquired such a personality constellation will they then be able to achieve in our highly competitive, post-Sputnik educational system? Cause and effect relations cannot be determined from these data, but it is obvious that our "education for excellence" is accompanied by certain psychological costs.

Findings such as these most naturally raise questions about the impact on the student's emotional well-being of the knowledge explosion and the current emphasis on increased academic excellence. Debate will most likely continue as to whether academic competition is beneficial or detrimental to later adult coping. Some of the questions which require further investigation have been formulated by Rogers (1969): Should girls, as well as boys, be encouraged to achieve? or does an achievement orientation prove maladaptive for those females who will have to perform routine domestic duties in later life? Do such women project their strivings onto their husbands, thereby imposing additional stress? What goals should we have adolescents seek to achieve? Do some individuals suffer because of a too persistent need to achieve? Is achievement stress a factor in the high incidence of teenage schizophrenia? Are we apt to develop students who achieve out of a fear of failure?

The current stress on achievement is even having a potent impact at the preschool level. It seems especially fashionable today for a parent to have a preschooler who can read. The parents rarely ask if such instruction could be accomplished more readily at a later age. Nor can they verbalize the potential advantages to the child able to read early. Yet, this precocity is something middle-class and upper-middle-class mothers value. The authors are not opposed to early instruction or academic competency in students. We do want to point out, however, that the intense parental involvement which helps to form the basis for achievement motivation also entails some undesirable attitudes and behaviors—rejection, hypercriticism, hostility, and demands for accomplishment beyond individual readiness—which could do more harm than good. Though there might well be dangers associated with too great an emphasis on the child's doing well, it is likely, given our achievement-oriented society, that we will have little choice other than to prepare students to cope with increasing demands for accomplishment.

So far we have discussed the dangers associated with too much press for achievement. What is the child like who possesses too little achievement motivation and low levels of accomplishment? A partial answer to this question is provided in Gallagher's (1964) portrait of the underachiever:

1. The underachieving child grows up in, or belongs to, a cultural group which does not value education, independence, or individual achievement.
2. He has poor parental relationships, in which the parents, especially the father, either show limited interest in academic matters or try to put undue pressure on their children to succeed.
3. The child, unable to obtain satisfaction from parental contacts, seeks out his peer group for satisfying human relationships. Since he searches for others of the same interests as himself, he will often find himself allied with other rebellious and angry children.
4. These children will be faced by teachers and other school officials who ask them to meet standards of behavior which are not possible for them, and who treat these children, in many ways, as their parents do. The children thus place the teachers and the school in the same authority category as parents and reject them and their program.
5. The school, in its attempt to deal with these nonconforming and angry children, is likely to take more strict and repressive measures which will turn the children even more emphatically against the school.

Further, Douvan and Adelson (1958) have pointed out that upwardly mobile boys are characterized by effective, autonomous ego functioning; downwardly mobile adolescents, by demoralization. What are the effects of such demoralization? Among urban ghetto youth,

Smith (1968) notes that deviant behavior may result as a consequence of the feelings of powerlessness and hopelessness associated
with their incompetence:

> ... much deviant and problematic behavior can be interpreted as an attempt to
> seek escape from self and world, or to gain a short-circuited, illusory sense of
> efficacy—thus drug use and the search for kicks. Much, but not all. Some anti-
> social behavior, deviant from the point of view of the environing and super-
> ordinate society, may in part be directed toward alternative modes of com-
> petence that remain available and indeed become normative in the ghetto
> subculture when legitimate channels of effectance are closed off. The com-
> bative prowess of the gang leader and member, virtuosity in aggressive "mother
> talk," audacity in sexual exploits, and competence in the risky skills of the
> hustler belong under this heading, though these directions of activity ob-
> viously also yield extrinsic rewards. The larger society will regard these direc-
> tions of activity as bad, but those who plan and direct rehabilitation programs
> will do well to remember that for many slum youth, all of their resources of
> competence motivation get channeled in these deviant directions. A lot of self
> is invested in them.

Thus, even among antisocial individuals, who not uncommonly convey
the impression of being happy-go-lucky and carefree, we note a serious
and intent desire to become competent and achieve recognition from
others.

As with other aspects of socialization, it appears that too much or
too little training can produce adjustment difficulties. We do not want
to produce either extreme—those who are obsessed with achievement or
those who are inclined to follow the pleasure principle. We must
strive to develop those capable of productive accomplishment without
minimizing their capacities for creative leisure. A balance among
work, love, and play is the ideal.

PARENTAL INFLUENCE ON BEHAVIOR

Table 4 presents an overview of parental influence on the adaptive
and maladaptive behaviors of children. It should be noted that the
same parental antecedent often contributes to widely differing maladjustments. Parental permissiveness, for example, is considered a
factor in childhood aggression, anxiety, and dependency. Findings
of this nature highlight the fact that child-rearing practices and
parental attitudes are only two of many factors which determine later
behavioral outcomes. Other factors of significance include the child's
developmental level, his constitutional makeup, and his perception of

TABLE 4. PARENTAL IMPACT ON COMMON GROWTH PROBLEMS AS TO ADAPTIVE AND MALADAPTIVE OUTCOMES

Growth Problem	Behavioral Manifestations	Parental Antecedents	Adaptive Outcomes	Maladaptive Outcomes
Dependency	Commonly seeks assistance, attention, physical proximity or contact, and recognition.	Overpermissiveness; maternal overprotection; maternal rejection; punishment.	Sense of trust; responsive to social reinforcers.	Dependent passivity; submissiveness; inadequacy.
Conscience	Experiences guilt; resists temptation; is able to make moral judgments.	Perfectionism; unrealistic expectations; love-oriented techniques.	Realistic guilt; adaptive, productive conformity; wholesome expression of basic urges.	Chronic sense of failure, guilt, or fear; low self-esteem; personality constriction; inadequate internal controls.
Anxiety	Exhibits feelings of insecurity, inadequacy, and helplessness; has nervous habits.	Apprehensive model; direct training; premature exposure to adult problems; perfectionism; overpermissiveness.	Facilitation of social and intellectual performance if not severe.	Severe conflicts; generalized behavioral constrictions; impaired higher-level cognitive functioning.
Aggressiveness	Fights others physically or verbally; wants to hurt others; is cruel, disruptive, and unruly.	Repeated severe punishment; indulgence; direct reinforcement; aggressive parental models.	Self-assertiveness; competitiveness.	Acting-out hostile behavior; delinquency; anxious compliance; aggression anxiety; neurotic-like problems.
Achievement motivation	Strives to excel; has high standards.	High levels of parental involvement.	Productive accomplishment; delay of gratification; curiosity about environment; persistence.	Demoralization, sense of powerlessness and hopelessness; obsession with achievement.

his parents, the family constellation, extrafamilial circumstances, the severity and duration of the undesirable parent-child relationships. While it has not been possible to delineate specific, direct, and invariant cause-effect relationships between parental psychopathology and childhood disorders (Frank, 1965), there is ample evidence to substantiate the importance of certain parental antecedents and practices (namely, love versus hostility and overpermissiveness versus restrictiveness) as predisposing factors in childhood forms of maladjustment (Becker, 1964).

ADJUSTMENT MECHANISMS

The individual has several methods of enhancing and maintaining his personality organization in response to the personal threats associated with common growth problems. These are often referred to as "defense mechanisms." Discussions making reference to their functions are typically encountered in explanations of psychopathological conditions, especially the neuroses. It must be kept in mind that these processes are available to all persons, although some mechanisms may be more preferred than others by any one individual. A second point is that these ways for meeting demands are not limited to defensive reactions. Probably more often, at least for the normal individual, the coping response has positive and assertive qualities, just the opposite of being negative and defensive. Here are examples of frequently used adjustment mechanisms:

1. *Repression.* This adjustment mechanism was initially proposed by Freud to designate the efforts to protect the ego by pushing into the unconscious those impulses and thoughts which were unacceptable or painful to contemplate. These threatening forces were id instincts of sex and aggression and superego moral standards. More popularly this adjustment is observed in the inability to recall experiences which terminated in failure or humiliation. The individual seeks escape from these unhappy events by forgetting them.

2. *Identification.* In this process, the person allies himself emotionally and in wishful imagination with another person or group of persons. Children identify with their parents, older siblings, with television or literary characters. In this way, power, status, or adventure is obtained. The children also learn to be like the person identified with, to have the same characteristics, mannerisms, and values.

3. *Compensation.* In this adjustment, a person failing in one line of endeavor looks for success in another area. Not chosen for the ball team, a boy then works hard to make an "A" in science. Criticized as

not knowing how to paint, a girl devotes all her efforts to becoming a successful musician. Each person wants to be successful and if he cannot succeed in one way, he will try another.

4. *Rationalization.* In this adjustment, a plausible explanation is offered as an excuse for some failure or shortcoming. The student who makes a low grade on a test may claim that he was coming down with a cold when he took the test. A girl who was not asked to attend the school prom may maintain that the dance was so boring and unexciting that she didn't want to go anyway. This kind of intellectual face-saving is frequently observed.

5. *Displacement.* This "kicking the cat" reaction occurs when a feeling aroused by one person or situation is transferred and directed to some neutral or safe person or object. A child who feels anger toward a parent may aggressively tear up one of his toys. The term "scapegoating" is also used to refer to this technique of handling feelings, usually those involving aggression, by taking them out on some less threatening person.

6. *Regression.* This is an attempt to keep personal integrity by meeting demands in ways typical of a less mature level of development. Unable to solve problems facing him, the adolescent resorts to childish tactics. Baby talk, temper tantrums, or outbursts of crying may be called up as ways of avoiding responsibility or having his own way.

7. *Projection.* One way to get out of owning up to the weaknesses, inadequacies, and faults which we all have is to attribute them to someone else. Putting the blame on others sometimes requires a considerable stretch of possibilities, as, for example, when during recess, Johnny engaged in a heated verbal attack on Billy, a new pupil, claiming that Billy hated the teacher. Billy was puzzled and could not understand the accusations which were rooted in Johnny's deeply repressed, intense dislike for the teacher.

8. *Reaction Formation.* This method for meeting problems entails a type of reversal reaction. A pupil may want to cheat on a test, but he recognizes that this is not acceptable behavior. As a way of controlling his tendency to cheat, he may become extremely concerned about cheating behavior, reporting observations of suspected cheating, offering plans to prevent cheating, and engaging in diatribes about cheating. Tip-offs as to this type of reaction are suggested by extremely emotional and inflexible attitudes associated with the behavior.

Thus far we have discussed the ubiquity of normal adjustment difficulties, some developmental crises which all youngsters must master to some degree, and some of the adjustment mechanisms used to adapt. What happens to youth when their coping abilities and defenses are not adequate to the task and deviancy results? We have already pointed out certain of the potentially adverse outcomes, but we have not explored the course which various disorders run. Will the delinquent youth, for instance, become a wayward adult? What does the future hold for the schizophrenic child? for the neurotic youngster? It is this neglected topic of stability that we will focus on in the next section.

THE STABILITY OF DEVIANT BEHAVIOR[3]

We have seen that most children experience problems in the course of development and that the resolution of these tasks leads to differential modes of adjustment on the child's part. The question arises, however, as to whether childhood problems and maladaptive modes of behavior are transient or permanent in nature. In other words, does a child grow out of his problems with increasing age, or does he become a mentally ill adult? The answer to this question is of interest to theoreticians as well as to practitioners. To the theorist, knowledge pertaining to the stability of deviant behavior furthers understanding of both normal personality development and childhood psychopathology. To the clinician, such knowledge would better enable him not only to predict the course and outcome of various behavior problems but also to focus treatment on the cases most in need of professional intervention.

Clinicians and developmental psychologists have traditionally differed in their answers to this question of stability. The former are more inclined to view childhood problems as being of a chronic nature, whereas the latter view them as being of a nonpersistent nature. The conflicting views may, in large measure, be a function of the populations studied. Studies based on fairly typical samples of children, for example, indicate that developmental problems are not particularly stable over time. MacFarlane and his associates (1954), for example, note that the magnitude of interage correlations of problems suggests

[3]The material in this section has been reprinted, with minor editorial changes, from Harvey Clarizio, "Stability of Deviant Behavior through Time," *Mental Hygiene,* 1968, 52, 288-293, by permission of the National Association of Mental Health.

nonpersistence over a long age span. Lapouse and Monk (1964) found age to be the variable most closely associated, with the number of behavior deviations among young children surpassing that among older children. These authors conclude that behavior deviations in children are an age-bound phenomenon. In brief, studies based on nonpsychiatric populations indicate that normal behavior problems do not tend to be chronic in nature.

The evidence cited above is based on a developmental approach using samples of normal children whose problems may be less numerous and less severe than those typically referred to psychiatric clinics. How about the child whose problems are sufficiently visible to warrant referral to professional agencies? Does the child characterized by clinical maladjustment grow up to be a mentally ill adult, or does he too tend to grow out of his problems? Investigations bearing on this issue have been of two kinds, retrospective studies and followup studies.[4]

In retrospective studies, mentally ill adults are selected as subjects and their childhood histories are reconstructed through the use of case studies, inventories, and interviews with parents, teachers, and other people. Illustrative of this approach is the study by Kasanin and Veo (1932) in which school histories were obtained through teacher interviews on 54 hospitalized adult psychotics. The subjects had a mean age of 20 years and were classified into one of five categories on the basis of their earlier school histories. Of the 54 psychotics, half were placed in the three categories which represented adequate adjustment (fairly well-adjusted, well-adjusted, and school leaders). Of the 54 patients, 15 were the "nobodies," that is, those whom the teachers could not remember. Only 15 of the 54 patents fell into the "peculiar and difficult" category. This latter finding is rather striking since from the standpoint of rater bias, one would have expected the teacher's knowledge of the former student's hospitalized status to have influenced her recall of the deviant aspects of his earlier behavior. Thus, even though the method should have facilitated the finding of a closer relationship between child and adult disorder, only moderate evidence was found to support such a hypothesis.

Despite efforts to control rater bias among teachers, Bower and his associates (1960) found relatively similar results in their retrospective

---

[4]The followup studies reviewed in this section are "long-term" studies; that is, subjects were reevaluated after periods ranging from 5 to 30 years.

studies. While teachers seemingly recognized the onset of schizophrenia among their former students, they did not view those who later became schizophrenic as having been emotionally sick or as having major problems. On the basis of high-school ratings, predictions would not have been accurate as to later adult pathology.

A major methodological difficulty with retrospective studies is that we do not know how many other children showed similar symptoms during the school years and yet grew up to be normal. This limitation is well exemplified in a study by Renaud and Estes (1961), who studied 100 mentally healthy adults and found that a significant proportion of them had had pathogenic childhoods. Traumatic and pathological events were so common that had the subjects been plagued with psychosomatic or neurotic disorders, background factors could easily have been identified, with the erroneous conclusions drawn that disturbed children become disturbed adults. Schofield and Balian (1959), in studying 150 normal adults, also found that nearly one-fourth of their subjects had had traumatic histories.

Another serious limitation in studies of this sort involves reliance on the memories of adults who knew the subject as a child. The memories of informants are, unfortunately, most likely influenced by knowledge of the psychiatric adult status. Informants may thus selectively forget certain incidents or tend to remember the unusual. It would appear that in light of present findings and methodological limitations, retrospective studies offer at best only questionable evidence to support the notion that the maladjusted child grows up to be the maladjusted adult.

The other major approach involves followup studies in which children seen by child-guidance clinics are reevaluated after a period of time has elapsed. The results of this approach vary appreciably with the criterion of mental health or illness used at the time of the followup. When the clinical judgment of the psychiatric interviewer is used as the criterion, the results suggest that subjects who show maladjustment as children will show maladjustment at adult status. In one of the best-known followup studies, Robins (1966) studied 525 children who had been referred to the same St. Louis municipal clinic between 1924 and 1929. Thirty years later the adult psychiatric and social status of these subjects were compared with that of 100 control subjects. In a check of the adult psychiatric status of those subjects available for followup, only 20 per cent of these former patients fell into the "no disease" category whereas 52 per cent of the control group were so classified. As adults, 34 per cent of former child-guidance patients were characterized by seriously disabling symptoms, as compared to 8 per cent of the matched group of control subjects. Differences were markedly higher in the incidence of sociopathic personalities, and somewhat higher for psychotic disorders and alcoholism. There was, however, little difference between the two groups in the rate of neurotic disturbances (see Table 5). Such behaviors as shyness, nervousness, fears, tantrums, seclusiveness, hypersensitiveness, tics, irritability, and speech defects were not related to adult psychiatric outcomes. This finding suggests that neurotic symptoms in childhood are not predictive of adult neurosis. In fact, control-group subjects had a slightly higher rate of neurosis as adults than did the former patients. Interestingly enough, it was not withdrawn behavior that characterized the preschizophrenic group but aggressive acting-out behavior of an antisocial nature.

In general, the findings of this study imply that former childhood patients, especially those who engage in seriously antisocial behavior, contribute more than their share to adult mental disorders. The emphasis on clinical treatment of delinquency in the 1920's, the differences between the groups with respect to socioeconomic status, the question as to how representative the sample is of other clinic populations, and possible contamination of psychiatric judgments through the awareness of the subjects' past history illustrate some of the difficulties associated with this long-term followup study.

Another major followup study which used a more demanding criterion of mental illness, namely, admission to a mental hospital, arrived at a somewhat different conclusion (Morris, Soroker, & Burrus, 1954). The subjects were 54 childhood patients who had been classified as internal reactors at the Dallas Guidance Clinic 16 to 27 years earlier. Upon followup, the majority of these subjects were regarded as having achieved a satisfactory adjustment, one-third of the group was seen as marginally adjusted, and only one subject had been hospitalized. Later analysis of data obtained from this same clinic suggests, as was true in the St. Louis followup study, that withdrawn and introverted youngsters have a low probability of developing schizophrenia. Schizophrenics were found more often among the "ambiverts," the children with both antisocial and non-antisocial complaints, than among the "introverts" and "extoverts." Former child patients at the

TABLE 5. A SUMMARY OF FOLLOWUP STUDIES ON THE STABILITY OF DEVIANT BEHAVIOR

Investigator(s)	Length of Followup in Years	Relatively Transitory	Relatively Permanent
Robins (1966)	30	Tics; seclusiveness; nervousness; fears; tantrums; hypersensitivity; speech defects.	
Michael, Morris, & Soroker (1957)	16–27	Shyness.	
Coolidge, Brodie, & Feeney (1964)	5–10	School phobia (47 cf 49 returned to school).	
Balow & Blomquist (1965)	10–15	Severely disabled readers (most learned to read at or near the average adult level).	
Levitt, Beiser, & Robertson (1959)	5	Neurotic disorders (three-fourths improved).	
Berkowitz (1955)	10	Predelinquent behavior (three-fourths had no record of delinquency).	
Robins (1966)	30	Sociopathic behavior (one-third showed moderate improvement).	Sociopathic behavior (two-thirds were unimproved).
Eisenberg (1956)	9	Autistic behavior (if useful speech was present by age 5).	Autistic behavior (if mute by age 5).
Eisenberg (1957)	4–5	Childhood schizophrenia (one-fourth achieved a moderately good social adjustment).	Childhood schizophrenia (three-fourths either attained a marginal adjustment or required continuous institutional care).

Judge Baker Clinic who later became hospitalized as schizophrenics also had histories characterized by theft, truancy, running away, and antisocial sexual activity (Nameche, Waring, & Ricks, 1964).

What can we conclude in the light of available evidence? It should be noted that conclusions must be tentative because there has been no study specifically designed to measure the stability of deviant behavior over time and because of the methodological shortcomings of past studies. Bearing the above limitations in mind, we can advance the following tentative conclusions:

1. It appears that certain "types" of disturbed children do contribute more than their share to the population of adult psychiatric disability. However, the extent of overlap between childhood and adult disturbance remains uncertain. This is an area badly in need of additional extensive longitudinal research, for it is neither judicious nor pragmatic, especially in view of the shortage of mental-health specialists, to treat all disturbed children if, for example, only 25 per cent will become significantly maladjusted as adults.

2. While it is commonly assumed that adult behaviors and personality are established in early life experiences and while there is a body of empirical research demonstrating the stability of personality over time, there is nonetheless a real danger in overgeneralization. The possibility of this type of error is well illustrated in Robins' (1966) finding that more than one-third of diagnosed sociopaths showed a marked decrease in antisocial behavior in later life. Though these improved sociopaths by no means became ideal citizens, the fact that more than one-third of this seriously antisocial population did improve noticeably challenges the notion of incorrigibility commonly associated with this diagnosis.

3. In large measure, the stability of the behavior deviation depends on the nature of the problem in question as well as the child's environment. Normal problem behavior which occurs as a developmental phenomenon seems to have a very high probability of being resolved with increasing age. Clinical problems, though having a lower probability of improvement than those of a developmental nature, also seem to have a reasonably high probability of spontaneous remission. Since it is obviously misleading to speak of clinical problems as a homogeneous entity, we have in Table 5 categorized specific clinical problems on the basis of followup studies as tending to be either chronic or transitory in nature. We must not lose sight of the environment in which the individual must function as a major factor in his total adjustment. A dependent adult, for instance, may achieve an adequate adjustment if he has a supportive employer who will take time to give him the attention and direction he needs. Similarly, an individual with strong oppositional tendencies may not experience adjustment difficulties if he has a job in which he is able to work

under conditions of minimal supervision and has an easygoing, submissive wife. Thus, even if personality characteristics remained perfectly constant, we could expect some change in the individual behavior as a consequence of environmental contingencies.

4. Somewhat contrary to prevailing clinical belief, it is aggressive, antisocial, acting-out behavior of a *severe* nature that is most predictive of later significant adult disturbance and most deserving of treatment efforts. In addition to evidence cited earlier, Roff (1961) found that reliable group predictions of military adjustment could be made on the basis of earlier social adjustment in school. Children who were mean and disliked by their classmates commonly had bad-conduct records in military service.

5. Although 2 out of 3 unsocialized aggressive youngsters continue in their antisocial ways, it must not be assumed that the majority of young norm-violators become adult criminals. As Kvaraceus (1966) points out, it is widely agreed that much juvenile delinquency does not inevitably terminate in adult criminal activity. There appears to be a curvilinear relationship between delinquent activity and age. After reaching a peak at age 16, the "delinquency curve" begins to level off (W. Miller, quoted in Kvaraceus).

6. Shyness and withdrawn behavior tend to disappear with advancing age. At worst, these problems are less incapacitating and socially disruptive than those of the antisocial child. Moreover, there is little evidence to suggest that shyness is predictive of later schizophrenia, despite the fact that introverted behavior is often viewed as having dire consequences for mental health. There is a vast difference between the child who can relate and does not, or who wants to relate and lacks the necessary social skills, and the child who cannot relate because of a severe basic incapacity. The best evidence to date suggests that the preschizophrenic child is characterized by both antisocial behavior and serious non-antisocial symptoms (Nameche et al., 1964; Robins, 1966).

7. Neurotic symptoms (fears, hypersensitiveness, tics) often presumed to be the precursors of adult neurotic disturbances have also been found lacking in prognostic power. The findings of current empirical research challenge the long-held assumptions that adult neurotic behaviors result from disturbances in parent-child relations or from parental loss in childhood (Robins, 1966).

8. The probabilities of remission characterizing childhood schizo-

phrenia and infantile autism are indeed low. Yet, although these severe disabilities definitely tend to persist through time, perhaps as many as 1 in 4 of those so diagnosed apparently achieve a reasonably adequate adjustment (Eisenberg, 1957).

9. Generally speaking, it is very difficult to postulate any direct causal relationship between early childhood maladjustment and later specific psychiatric disability. We do know that a goodly number of disturbed children will grow up to attain a reasonably adequate adult adjustment. The truth of the matter is, however, that we still do not fully understand the role of later experiences on personality adjustment. Also, we must not overlook the possibility that some adult disturbances arise independently of childhood problems.

In our present state of knowledge, we can conclude that there is at best only mild or moderate evidence to support the notion that disturbed children turn into seriously disturbed adults.[5] Since the less noxious childhood disorders, say, shyness, are more common than the more severe disorders, say, childhood schizophrenia, it would seem that, all in all, change appears to characterize the course of behavior deviations in children as much as or more than chronicity or stability. The conception of emotional disturbance in children as a progressively deteriorating condition is thus called into question.[6]

---

[5]Undoubtedly, some of the improvement can be attributed to the differential standards of adjustment for children and adults. In the case of children, the ability to learn academic tasks constitutes a primary yardstick for normality. If the child is unteachable, he is considered maladjusted. In the case of adults, however, the ability to learn academic tasks no longer constitutes a basic criterion of adjustment. The basic yardstick has become vocational and social adequacy. If the adult can adapt reasonably well to his environment, he is apt to be seen as normal. Also we must bear in mind that the adult has much greater choice in selecting suitable or more psychologically comfortable surroundings than does the child. The child cannot change his home, his teacher, his school, or his neighborhood. The adult can change his job, his wife, his boss, his friends, and his residence. In other words, the adult is freer than the child to select a setting which is compatible with his style of life. In a sense, he can choose his own norm group, while for a child, there is essentially one set of norms—the school's.

[6]In contrast to long-term followup studies on clinic populations (clinical maladjustment), followup studies of behavior disorders among school children suggest that *school maladjustment* does persist. Balow (1965), for instance, reported that severe reading disability is best considered a relatively chronic problem requiring long-term treatment. Severely disabled readers did benefit from intensive short-term treatment, but their rate of progress dropped below the normal growth rate under less intensive

CRITERIA OF NORMALITY

If all children have problems, what is normal behavior in children? How long must a child manifest abnormal behavior to warrant the appellation "emotionally disturbed"? What criteria are to be used in deciding what is abnormal and what is normal? How does one distinguish between the child who has problems and the child who is maladjusted? Various approaches have been made to the definition of normality in children, although none has proven entirely satisfactory. The issue of normality in children is more than an academic question to those who must render judgments regarding the behavior of children. This question also has ethical and practical ramifications, for the child does not refer himself for treatment but is referred for treatment by the adults in his life. The child may not be in need of treatment even though his parents and teachers believe so. His referral may be simply a result of the parents' or teacher's low annoyance threshold. Shepard, Oppenhein, and Mitchell (1966) found, for instance, that referral to a child-guidance clinic is as closely related to parental reactions (anxious, easily upset, lacking in ability to cope with children) as it is to the child's morbidity. Similarly, teachers with 3-10 years of experience tend to view undesirable acts as being more serious than those teachers with 10 years of experience (Dobson, 1967).

---

assistance conditions. Another followup study (Zax et al., 1968) reported that students identified early in their school careers as emotionally disturbed were as seventh-graders more negatively perceived by teachers and peers, required more attention from the school nurse, and achieved less well in comparison with a group of normal youngsters. Stringer and Glidewell (1967) likewise reported that 87 per cent of students markedly deficient in both achievement and mental health during the early grades maintained the same status throughout elementary school. The research by Stennet (1966) and Westman, Ferguson, and Wolman (1968) also indicates that school maladjustment does not improve with the passage of time. The research literature is not consistent, however. In the Onondaga County studies, for example, it was reported that of 515 students rated as disturbed in 1961 by their teachers, only 160 were so perceived in 1963. In 1965, only 9 of the 480 children were so perceived. Approximately three-fourths of the 515 students were only one-shot affairs in the sense that they were designated as disturbed only once (Mental Health Research Unit, 1964, 1967). Test anxiety, which is also related to school adjustment, does not appear to persist to any appreciable degree over extended periods of time. Test-retest correlations for the Test Anxiety Scale for Children, administered in grades 1 and 5, are only .15 for boys and .20 for girls (Hill & Sarason, 1966). More rigorous research will be needed before we can resolve the issue pertaining to the stability of school maladjustment.

THE STATISTICAL APPROACH

One of the most commonly discussed approaches to normality employs a statistical criterion. According to this standard, normal behavior is defined as what the majority does. The more an individual is like the average, the more normal he is considered to be. For example, the average 5-year-old may be found to have five nightmares a month. If so, this condition would be considered normal. We could also calculate the standard deviation for this distribution which would enable us to know, for example, what percentage of 5-year-olds has as many as ten or as few as two nightmares a month. If a child deviated markedly from the average, he would be considered abnormal in this aspect of his behavior. Similar distributions could be established for other aspects of behavior, such as the number of fears, the frequency of bedwetting, the extent of aggressive attacks, for children of various age levels.

There are some rather noticeable shortcomings in this approach, however. First, the statistical concept of normality implies that what is common is normal. Colds are very common, but are not regarded as desirable or as the absence of illness. Similarly, 95 per cent of boys have masturbated by age 15 or 16, yet masturbation is not necessarily regarded as healthy by the culture at large. Second, abnormality in a statistical sense is not always unhealthy. Take the case of a very creative youngster. On the basis of the normal curve, his creative performance may be statistically infrequent and therefore deviate markedly from the average. Are we to say that this youngster is abnormal when his very talent may lend itself to self-actualization on his part and to benefits for society? A third problem centers around the complexity of personality. It may be possible to gather norms on certain characteristics, for example, the amount of nailbiting, but it is difficult to isolate and quantify many of the subtle or more elusive characteristics of personality. Further, the statistical approach does not lend itself very readily to the study of the integrational or organizational aspects of personality formation. Still another problem exists with this approach, namely, that the norms are frequently based on clinic populations. As noted earlier in the chapter, evidence derived from epidemiological studies strongly suggests that such deviate norm groups provide misleading standards, in that many childhood behaviors, such as fears, are not as pathological as clinicians often assume. Finally, there is the question of cutoff points. Just how many fingernails does a 7-year-old have to bite to be considered abnormal? What percentage of the nailbiting population must he exceed? It is difficult to give definitive answers to such questions.

A variation or subtype of the statistical approach is the use of adjustment to social norms as the criterion of normality. Normality thus becomes defined relatively, according to a given set of cultural values, which are comprised of both laws and customs. The socialization process itself has as its aim the inculcation of social values and the development of behaviors congruent with environmental expectations. That normality be defined as adherence to social norms and abnormality as violation of these social norms is, therefore, not unexpected. Though it seems reasonable to judge deviancy by comparing behavior against social norms, that is, to take into account environmental circumstances, this approach also has its limitations. For example, to what degree does one have to be different from social norms to be judged as culturally deviant? How many times does one have to steal to be considered maladjusted? Most of us have stolen or cheated at times, but we do not consider ourselves to be delinquent. Cutoff points between the conformer and habitual norm-violater are difficult to determine and would probably have to be at least somewhat arbitrary in nature. Another difficulty occurs if we have a sick society, as some contend. Is compliance, then, a sign of normality or of personal maladjustment? Who were the maladjusted Germans—those who fought the Nazi system or those who went along with it? Also consider the lower-class youngster who rebels against school. Is he sick because of his objections to being forced into a situation in which he experiences demands and expectations he does not value, or are some of the institutions in the society sick?

Children and adults can also suffer from overconformity. The problem does not seem to be resolved by a strict adherence to conformity for, eventually, conformity reaches a point beyond which normality is apt to be threatened. Compliance to the point that one's personal integrity is sacrificed is conducive neither to personal nor societal harmony. Further, as Havighurst (1966) argues, it is important that a society educate for certain forms of deviancy, for example, creative behavior. On occasion, a good adjustment demands that we rebel and express dissatisfaction with social mores and institutions. The value for the individual and for society of certain expressions of nonconformity is, unfortunately, often overlooked. Finally, we must ask whose values we are going to use in judging normality. One group in society often differs from another group in the same society with regard to what is considered normal. For example, how would ministers, teachers, social workers, doctors, cultural anthropologists, and laborers as separate groups view a child who habitually curses. In all probability, there would be widely differing views regarding the acceptability and desirability of such behavior.

THE IDEALISTIC APPROACH

The other major approach might be termed the idealistic approach. Whereas the statistical approach primarily describes the frequency of given behaviors, the use of the ideal criterion by definition implies evaluation; and whereas the criteria of social norms involve relativity, the ideal criterion is based on absolute standards of normality. According to this approach, an ideal of behavior is posited for each individual, and a determination is made as to whether the individual is functioning at this level. Illustrative of this approach is Maslow's hierarchy of basic human needs. His hierarchy in ascending order lists physiological needs, safety needs, needs for affection and belongingness, esteem needs, cognitive needs such as a search for knowledge, aesthetic needs such as a longing for beauty, and self-actualization needs. When the needs at the lower levels have been met, the needs on the next step in the hierarchic structure seek satisfaction. People whose needs for self-actualization are pressing for satisfaction are seen as operating at an optimal level. According to Maslow (1954), anything that detracts from the course of self-actualization is psychopathological.

The equating of complete normality with perfection has an undeniable positive air to it, but the use of such ideal criteria is also fraught with difficulties. Ideal criteria, for one thing, are lacking in utilitarian value and, therefore, are of limited value to the clinician in his decision-making process. Guidelines derived from such criteria do not aid the practitioner in deciding whether the child is normal or in need of professional help. Second, few people can ever attain such ideal criteria and even among those whom we do locate, we find human frailties and weaknesses. (Even Peter denied Christ three times.) Finally, the concept of ideal criteria which is concerned with an abstraction tells us what ought to be. It is thus assumed that we know what the ideal attributes to be striven for are and that these are supracultural in character.

Toward a Definition of Normality

While there is no acceptable definition of normality, there are certain ingredients which a suitable definition must include. It should take into account the child's developmental level, for what is regarded as normal at one age might well be viewed as abnormal at a later age, for example, physical aggressiveness or chewing on the carpet. Consideration must also be extended to a child's particular culture or subculture. Since judgments concerning the desirability of a specific behavior vary from one group to another, the relativity of deviancy becomes an important consideration (Havighurst, 1966). Certainly, allowances for individuality must be made. Finally, the definition of normality must be multidimensional in nature; that is, it must take into account how the child functions in various representative areas of development.

The difficulty associated with the definition of deviancy is reflected in Kanner's (1962) observation that it is impossible to locate a definition of the term "emotionally disturbed children," despite the fact that this term crept into the literature sometime during the 1930's. Kanner stresses the fact that this term is too encompassing and diffuse to be of scientific value and points out that scientists generally proceed by analyzing global and nebulous concepts into more specific categories or components. One recent definition which is widely quoted was advanced by Bower (1961), who notes that the emotionally handicapped child has one or more of the following characteristics:

1. An unexplained inability to learn. In other words, the child's difficulty cannot be explained adequately or primarily by intellectual deficits, specific learning disabilities, or by differences in cultural or ethnic background. It should be noted that the inability to use one's intelligence efficiently as manifested by an appreciable discrepancy between actual and expected academic performance carries considerable importance as a criterion of emotional disturbance in children but not in adults. This change in adjustment yardsticks might well be a major factor in explaining the instability of deviant behavior over time.

2. An inability to achieve satisfactory social relationships with children or adults.

3. An inability to behave at a level commensurate with one's developmental status; that is, the child operates at a more immature

level, in terms of his interests and behavior, than do most youngsters his age.

4. An inability to display confidence and belief in one's self or to overcome feelings of sadness.

5. An inability to cope with stressful situations in school without developing psychosomatic reactions, such as headaches or stomachaches.

While all children may at some point in life exhibit some of the inabilities listed above, Bower argues that a child, in order to be considered emotionally handicapped, must exhibit these characteristics to a marked extent and over a prolonged period of time, before the designation of "emotionally handicapped" is justified. In other words, we must also consider the frequency, intensity, and duration of the behavior in determining whether or not maladjustment exists.

GUIDELINES FOR REFERRAL

Many parents and teachers are not sure if they should seek professional treatment for certain children. Parents, for instance, not uncommonly show up at child-guidance clinics expressing uncertainty as to whether the problem is serious enough to justify their presence at the clinic. Likewise, teachers are often in doubt about when to request the services of the school psychologist. When should one refer a youngster for professional help? There are no hard-and-fast criteria whose use permits a definite answer to this issue, but Bower's definition should prove helpful in reaching a decision as to whether the child needs professional assistance. Also of value in this regard is the list of questions advanced by Mayer and Hoover (1961) which can serve as guideposts for referral. If the answers to the questions which follow are such to suggest more than the usual amount of adjustment difficulties, consideration should then be given to a search for outside consultation:

1. Is the child's behavior generally appropriate to the circumstances in which he finds himself?

2. Is the child's behavior generally in keeping with his age?

3. Are there real difficulties in the child's environment that may be blamed for his problem?

4. Has there been a radical change in the child's behavior?

5. How long has the symptom lasted?

The teacher with a problem pupil might consider three basic criteria in reaching a decision about referral. He must, first of all, ask himself if the child's social, emotional, and intellectual needs are being reasonably met within the classroom setting. If the child is unable to benefit academically or achieve relatively satisfying interpersonal relations despite individualized adjustments in the school program designed to promote such development, professional consultation might well be indicated.

Consideration for the rights of normal children must also be undertaken. American public education is based on group methods of instruction and has established its goals for normal pupils. Not infrequently, emotionally disturbed youngsters demand so much of the teacher's time and energy that the educational benefits accruing to the group suffer. As any experienced educator will testify, a teacher can spend as much or more time with one emotionally disturbed pupil as he does with the rest of the class. When the teacher believes that the group's needs are being sacrificed for one child's needs, it is time to seek professional assistance.

The teacher must also take his own mental health into account. Behaviorally disordered youth are often quite skillful at irritating other people. They have mastered a variety of techniques and have had years of experience in antagonizing others. One kindergarten pupil so distressed his teacher that the teacher became obsessed with thoughts regarding the daily management of this child and actually dreaded coming to work. As the teacher recognizes that his own mental hygiene is suffering and that his teaching effectiveness is being impaired, he would do well to request an evaluation for the child, so that additional therapeutic or corrective measures may be planned. The teacher should also remember that he can receive advice regarding the desirability of referral from such co-workers as the school counselor, other teachers, and the principal.

SUMMARY

Discussion in this chapter has centered around the concept of normality. Studies of normal children indicate that developmental problems are rather common. Indeed, data from the California Growth Study show that both boys and girls average 5–6 problems at any given time during the preschool and elementary-school years. The frequency of developmental problems (enuresis, speech difficulties, negativism, overactivity, lying) appears to decrease as the child grows older. Of the more common growth problems, five (dependency, conscience formation, anxiety, aggression, and achievement motivation) were discussed with respect to their behavioral manifestations, parental antecedents, and possible adaptive-maladaptive outcomes. The importance of such attitudinal dimensions as love-hostility and permissiveness-restrictiveness on adjustment was noted. Repression, identification, compensation, rationalization, displacement, regression, projection, and reaction formation represent some of the more frequently used defense mechanisms to ward off personal threats associated with common growth problems.

Defining normality is no easy matter. The two most common approaches to the definition of normality, the statistical and the idealistic, were noted along with their respective shortcomings. Studies on the stability of clinical maladjustment over time indicate that the most severe disorders (sociopathy, infantile autism, and childhood schizophrenia) show a strong tendency to persist into adulthood. Fortunately, these disorders are found to be relatively uncommon. The less severe disorders (for example, subcultural delinquency), which account for the large majority of behavior disorders in children, tend to have a much more favorable adult outcome. School maladjustment seems to be stable, but the research is not altogether clear on this point.

SUGGESTED READINGS

Clarizio, H. F. *Mental health and the educative process.* Chicago: Rand McNally, 1969.

Freud, A. *Normality and pathology in childhood.* New York: International Universities Press, 1965.

Mussen, P. H., Conger, J. J., & Kagan, J. *Child development and personality.* (3rd ed.) New York: Harper, 1969.

Roff, M. *Developmental abnormal psychology.* New York: Holt, Rinehart & Winston, 1966.

REFERENCES

Andrus, R., & Horowitz, E. The effect of nursery school training: insecurity feelings. *Child Develpm.,* 1938, **9**, 169-174.

Balow, B. The long-term effect of remedial reading instruction. *Reading Tchr,* 1965, **18**, 581-586.

Balow, B., & Blomquist, M. Young adults 10-15 years after severe reading disability. *Elem. Sch. J.,* 1965, **66**, 44-45.

Bandura, A., & Kupers, C. J. Transmission of patterns of self-reinforcement through modeling. *J. abnorm. soc. Psychol.*, 1964, **69**, 1-9.

Bandura, A., & Walters, R. H. *Adolescent aggression.* New York: Ronald Press, 1959.

Bandura, A., & Walters, R. H. *Social learning and personality development.* New York: Holt, Rinehart & Winston, 1963.

Becker, W. C. Consequences of different kinds of parental discipline. In M. L. Hoffman & L. W. Hoffman (Eds.), *Review of child development research.* Vol. I. New York: Russell Sage Foundation, 1964. Pp. 169-208.

Beller, E. K. Dependency and independence in young children. *J. genet. Psychol.*, 1955, **87**, 23-25.

Berkowitz, B. The juvenile aid bureau of the New York City Police. *Nerv. Child*, 1955, **11**, 42-48.

Bieber, I., Dain, H., Dince, P., Drellich, M., Grand, H., Gundlach, R., Kremer, M., Rifkin, A., Wilbur, C., & Bieber, T. *Homosexuality.* New York: Basic Books, 1962.

Bower, E. M. *The education of emotionally handicapped children.* Sacramento: California State Department of Education, 1961.

Bower, E., Shellhammer, T., Daily, J., & Bower, M. *High school students who later became schizophrenic.* Sacramento: California State Department of Education, 1960.

Cameron, N. *Personality development and psychopathology.* Boston: Houghton Mifflin, 1963.

Charlesworth, R., & Hartup, W. W. Positive social reinforcement in the nursery school peer group. *Child Develpm.*, 1967, **38**, 993-1002.

Coolidge, J. L., Brodie, R. D., & Feeney, B. A ten-year follow-up study of sixty-six school-phobic children. *Amer. J. Orthopsychiat.*, 1964, **34**, 675-684.

Crandall, V. *Parents as identification models and reinforcers of children's achievement behavior.* Progress Report, NIMH Grant M-2238. Washington D.C.: Government Printing Office, 1961.

Crandall, V. C. Achievement behavior in young children. In W. W. Hartup & N. L. Smothergill (Eds.), *The young child.* Washington, D.C.: National Association for the Education of Young Children, 1967. Pp. 165-185.

Dobson, R. L. The perception and treatment by teachers of the behavioral problems of elementary school children in culturally deprived and middle class neighborhoods. Doctoral thesis, Univer. of Oklahoma, 1966. Dissertation Abstracts 27, 1702 A-03 A, No. 6, 1967.

Dollard, J., Miller, N., Doob, L., Mowrer, O., & Sears, R. *Frustration and aggression.* New Haven: Yale Univer. Press, 1939.

Douvan, E., & Adelson, J. The psychodynamics of social mobility in adolescent boys. *J. abnorm. soc. Psychol.*, 1958, **56**, 31-44.

Eisenberg, L. The autistic child in adolescence. *Amer. J. Psychiat.*, 1956, **112**, 607-612.

Eisenberg, L. The course of childhood schizophrenia. *Arch. Neurol. Psychiat.*, 1957, **78**, 69-83.

Erikson, E. H. *Childhood and society.* (Rev. ed.) New York: Norton, 1968. (Orig. pub. 1950)

Eron, L., Banta, T., Walder, L., & Laulicht, J. Comparison of data obtained from fathers and mothers on childrearing practices and their relations to child aggression. *Child Develpm.*, 1961, **32**, 457-472.

Frank, G. H. The role of the family in the development of psychopathology. *Psychol. Bull.*, 1965, **64**, 191-205.

Gallagher, J. *Teaching the gifted child.* Boston: Allyn & Bacon, 1964.

Gewirtz, J. L., & Baer, D. M. Deprivation and satiation of social reinforcers as drive conditions. *J. abnorm. soc. Psychol.*, 1958, **57**, 165-172.

Glueck, S., & Glueck, E. *Unraveling juvenile delinquency.* Cambridge: Harvard Univer. Press, 1950.

Goldfarb, W. Psychological deprivation in infancy and subsequent adjustment. *Amer. J. Orthopsychiat.*, 1945, **15**, 247-255.

Hartshorne, H., & May, M. A. *Studies in the nature of character.* Vol. I, *Studies in deceit;* Vol. II, *Studies in self-control;* Vol. III, *Studies in the organization of character.* New York: Macmillan, 1928-1930.

Hartup, W. W. Dependency and independence. In H. Stevenson (Ed.), Child psychology. *Yearb. nat. Soc. Stud. Educ.*, 1963, **62**, Part I. Pp. 333-363.

Havighurst, R. J. Social deviancy among youth: types and significance. In W. W. Wattenberg (Ed.), Social deviancy among youth. *Yearb. nat. Soc. Stud. Educ.*, 1966, **65**, Part I. Pp. 59-77.

Heathers, E. Emotional dependence and independence in a physical threat situation. *Child. Develpm.*, 1953, **24**, 169-179.

Heathers, G. Emotional dependence and independence in nursery school play. *J. genet. Psychol.*, 1955, **87**, 37-57.

Hill, K. R., & Sarason, S. B. The relation of test anxiety and defensiveness to test and school performance over the elementary-school years: a further longitudinal study. *Monogr. Soc. Res. Child Develpm.*, 1966, **31** (2).

Kagan, J. Acquisition and significance of sex typing and sex role identity. In M. L. Hoffman & L. W. Hoffman (Eds.), *Review of child development research.* Vol. I. New York: Russell Sage Foundation, 1964. Pp. 137-167.

Kagan, J., & Moss, H. A. The stability of passive and dependent behavior from childhood through adulthood. *Child Develpm.*, 1960, **31**, 577-591.

Kagan, J., & Moss, H. A. *Birth to maturity.* New York: Wiley, 1962.

Kanner, L. Emotionally disturbed children: a historical review. *Child Develpm.*, 1962, **33**, 97-102.

Kasanin, J., & Veo, L. A. A study of the school adjustment of children who later in life become psychotic. *Amer. J. Orthopsychiat.*, 1932, **2**, 212-230.

Kohlberg, L. Moral development and identification. In H. Stevenson (Eds.), Child psychology. *Yearb. nat. Soc. Stud. Educ.*, 1963, **62**, Part I. Pp. 277-332.

Kohlberg, L. Development of moral character and moral ideology. In M. L. Hoffman & L. W. Hoffman (Eds.), *Review of child development research.* Vol. I. New York: Russell Sage Foundation, 1964. Pp. 383-432.

Kvaraceus, W. C. Problems of early identification and prevention of delinquency. In W. W. Wattenberg (Ed.), Social deviancy among youth. *Yearb. nat. Soc. Stud. Educ.,* 1966, **65**, Part I. Pp. 189-220.

Lapouse, R., & Monk, M. An epidemiologic study of behavior characteristics in children. *Amer. J. publ. Hlth,* 1958, **48**, 1134-1144.

Lapouse, R., & Monk, M. Fears and worries in a representative sample of children. *Amer. J. Orthopsychiat.,* 1959, **29**, 803-818.

Lapouse, R., & Monk, M. Behavior deviations in a representative sample of children. *Amer. J. Orthopsychiat.,* 1964, **34**, 436-446.

Levitt, E., Beiser, H., & Robertson, R. A follow-up evaluation of cases treated at a community child guidance clinic. *Amer. J. Orthopsychiat.,* 1959, **29**, 337-347.

Levy, D. *Maternal overprotection.* New York: Columbia Univer. Press, 1943.

McCord, W., & McCord, J. *Psychopathy and delinquency.* New York: Grune & Stratton, 1956.

McCord, W., McCord, J., & Howard, A. Familial correlates of aggression in nondelinquent children. *J. abnorm. soc. Psychol.,* 1961, **62**, 79-93.

McCord, W., McCord, J., & Zola, I. *Origins of crime: a new evaluation of the Cambridge-Somerville youth study.* New York: Columbia Univer. Press, 1959.

MacFarlane, J., Allen, L., & Honzik, M. *A developmental study of the behavior problems of normal children between twenty-one months and fourteen years.* Berkeley: Univer. of California Press, 1954.

Maslow, A. *Motivation and personality.* New York: Harper, 1954.

Mayer, G., & Hoover, M. *When children need special help with emotional problems.* New York: Child Study Association of America, 1961. Pp. 120-122.

Mental Health Research Unit. Onondaga County School Studies, Interim No. 1: Persistence of emotional disturbance reported among second and fourth grade children. Syracuse: N.Y. State Department of Mental Hygiene, September, 1964.

Mental Health Research Unit. Behavior patterns associated with persistent emotional disturbance of school children in regular classes of elementary grades. Syracuse: N.Y. State Department of Mental Hygiene, December, 1967.

Michael, C., Morris, D., & Soroker, E. Follow-up studies of shy, withdrawn children. II, Relative incidence of schizophrenia. *Amer. J. Orthopsychiat..* 1957, **27**, 331-337.

Morris, D., Soroker, E., & Burrus, G. Follow-up studies of shy, withdrawn children: evaluation of later adjustment. *Amer. J. Orthopsychiat.,* 1954, **24**, 743-754.

Moss, H. A., & Kagan, J. Stability of achievement and recognition seeking behaviors from early childhood through adulthood. *J. abnorm. soc. Psychol.,* 1961, **62**, 504-513.

Mussen, P. H., Conger, J. J., & Kagan, J. *Child development and personality.* (3rd ed.) New York: Harper, 1969.

Nameche, G., Waring, M., & Ricks, D. Early indicators of outcome in schizophrenia. *J. nerv. ment. Dis.*, 1964, **139**, 232-240.

Piaget, J. *The moral judgment of the child.* Glencoe, Ill.: Free Press, 1948. (Orig. pub. 1932)

Reid, J., King, F., & Wickwire, P. Cognitive and other personality characteristics of creative children. *Psychol. Rep.*, 1959, **5**, 729-737.

Renaud, H., & Estes, F. Life histories of one hundred normal American males: pathogenicity of childhood. *Amer. J. Orthopsychiat.*, 1961, **31**, 786-802.

Robins, L. N. *Deviant children grown up.* Baltimore: Williams & Wilkins, 1966.

Roff, M. Childhood social interactions and young adult bad conduct. *J. abnorm. soc. Psychol.*, 1961, **63**, 333-337.

Rogers, D. *Issues in adolescent psychology.* New York: Appleton-Century-Crofts, 1969.

Ruebush, B. K. Anxiety. In H. Stevenson (Ed.), Child psychology. *Yearb. nat. Soc. Stud. Educ.*, 1963, **62**, Part I. Pp. 460-516.

Sarason, S. B. *Anxiety in elementary school children.* New York: Wiley, 1960.

Sarason, S. Test anxiety and intellectual performance. *J. abnorm. soc. Psychol.*, 1963, **66**, 73-75.

Schofield, W., & Balian, L. A comparative study of the personal histories of schizophrenic and nonpsychiatric patients. *J. abnorm. soc. Psychol.*, 1959, **59**, 216-225.

Sears, R., Maccoby, E., & Levin, H. *Patterns of child rearing.* New York: Row, Peterson, 1957.

Shephard, M., Oppenheim, A. N., & Mitchell, S. Childhood behavior disorders and the child-guidance clinic: an epidemiological study. *J. Child Psychol. Psychiat.*, 1966, **7**, 39-52.

Short, J., & Nye, F. Extent of unrecorded juvenile delinquency: tentative conclusions. *J. crim. Law, Criminol. Police Sci.*, 1958, **49**, 296-302.

Smith, M. B. Competence and socialization. In J. A. Clausen (Ed.), *Socialization and society.* Boston: Little, Brown, 1968. Pp. 270-320.

Stendler, C. B. Possible causes of overdependency in young children. *Child Develpm.*, 1954, **25**, 125-146.

Stennet, R. G. Emotional handicap in the elementary years: phase or disease? *Amer. J. Orthopsychiat.*, 1966, **36**, 444-449.

Stringer, L. A., & Glidewell, J. C. Early detection of emotional illnesses in school children: final report. Clayton, Mo.: St. Louis County Health Department, 1967.

Temple, R., & Amen, E. A study of anxiety in young children by means of a projective technique. *Genet. Psychol. Monogr.*, 1944, **30**, 59-113.

Walters, R. H., & Parke, R. D. Social motivation, dependency, and susceptibility to social influence. In L. Berkowitz (Ed.), *Advances in experimental social psychology.* Vol. I. New York: Academic Press, 1964. Pp. 231-276.

Westman, J., Ferguson, B., & Wolman, R. School career adjustment patterns of children using mental health services. *Amer. J. Orthopsychiat.*, 1968, **38**, 659-665.

Winder, C., & Rau, L. Parental attitudes associated with social deviance in preadolescent boys. *J. abnorm. soc. Psychol.,* 1962, **64**, 418-424.

Winterbottom, M. The relation of need for achievement in learning experiences in independence and mastery. In J. Atkinson (Ed.), *Motives in fantasy, action and society.* Princeton, N.J., Van Nostrand, 1958. Pp. 453-478.

Zax, M., Cowen, E., Rappaport, J., Beach, D., & Laird, J. Follow-up study of children identified early as emotionally disturbed. *J. consult. clin. Psychol.,* 1968, **32**, 369-377.

2

Diagnosis and Incidence of Maladjustment

Certain specific problems involved in the evaluation of children's behavior, such as the vast prevalence of childhood problems, the nonpersistence of many developmental problems, the inappropriateness of many measuring instruments for children, and so forth, have been discussed in Chapter 1. The present chapter will focus on the generic concept of diagnosis and its applicability to psychosocial disorders. Mention will also be made of the typical dimensions around which classification schemes of children's behavior disorders have been organized, and attention given to four of the most recent efforts in nosology. Finally, the topic of incidence will be discussed, and notice taken of major variables related to the frequency of maladjustment in childhood.

THE CONCEPT OF DIAGNOSIS

The concept and the term *diagnosis* come from the field of medicine. Etymologically, the term derives from the Greek and means "thorough knowledge." As used in medicine, diagnosis involves determination of the nature and circumstances of disease. More specifically, diagnosis permits the distinguishing of one disease from another by establishing mutually exclusive categories of illness. Diagnosis is based on a conception of disease as a condition or process which is characterized by (1) a common specific etiology, (2) a common set of observable signs and symptoms, (3) a known course, and (4) a known outcome which, through specific interventions, can be altered. This line of reasoning has proven a reasonably fruitful one for medicine.

Reasoning analogously, psychologists and psychiatrists have carried over the concept of diagnosis to the study of mental disturbances. After all, both medicine and psychology were concerned with phenomena labeled as "illnesses." Hence, it seemed reasonable that the "medical model" would have a beneficial effect in the resolution of mental disturbances. No one seriously questioned whether physical and psychological problems were in actuality alike. Currently, however, several psychiatrists and psychologists are questioning the validity of the analogy, and basic differences between physical and psychological disturbances are now becoming increasingly evident.

As London (1964) notes,

Insofar as he is concerned with the diagnosis and treatment of illness, the modern psychotherapist has grown up in the tradition of medicine. But the nature of the ailments he deals with and the way he treats them set him apart from the physician and in some ways make him function much like a clergyman. He deals with sickness of the soul, as it were, which cannot be cultured in a laboratory, seen through a microscope, or cured by injection. And his methods have little of the concreteness or obvious empiricism of the physician's—he carries no needle, administers no pill, wraps no bandages. He cures by talking and listening. The infections he seeks to expose and destroy are neither bacterial nor viral—they are ideas, memories of experiences, painful and untoward emotions that debilitate the individual and prevent him from functioning effectively and happily.

In a similar vein, Smith (1968) asserts:

Why should medicine, more than religion or education, provide the framework for helping disturbed people to learn to cope with their problems? "Mental illness" is very different from physical illness, even if some physical illnesses produce disturbed behavior. It is not just somebody's private misery. Mental illness usually grows out of—and contributes to—the breakdown of a person's normal sources of support and understanding, especially in his family. It is part of a vicious circle. Not only has he himself faltered, but the social systems on which he depends have failed to sustain him—family, school, job, church, friendship, and the like. The task is not to cure an ailment inside his skin, but to strengthen him to the point where he can once again participate in the interactions that make up the warp and woof of life. It is also one of helping those subsystems function in ways that promote the well-being and effectiveness of all people who take part in them. Of course, genetic and other organic factors may contribute to a troubled person's difficulties. But primarily, . . . his troubles amount to malfunctions of ordinary social participation.

These differences have certain ramifications with respect to the applicability of the concept of diagnosis to children's disorders. The nature of these differences renders it more difficult for a diagnosis to accomplish its traditional objectives—namely, to achieve reliable assignment to a given category on the basis of observable symptoms, to provide some reference to etiology, to offer a differential prognosis, and to suggest treatment procedures. We shall now consider how effectively psychiatric diagnostic categories meet the criteria characteristic of an adequate classification scheme.

First of all, the clinician should be able to make reliable judgments as to diagnostic categories. In other words, different clinicians should agree on the classification of a given patient. Unfortunately, most diagnostic systems have not satisfied the criterion of reliable classification. Regrettably, it is not uncommon for children to receive different diagnoses as they move from clinic to clinic. Thus, the child who has difficulty in school is labeled aphasic in a speech clinic, a passive-aggressive personality at the child-guidance center, and a reading-disability case at the psychoeducational clinic. The diagnosis a child receives is often a function of the clearinghouse through which he is routed. Clinicians have long decried the inadequacy of the American Psychiatric Association's *Diagnostic and Statistical Manual of Mental Disorders* (1952, 1968), the nosology which has been applied to children's disorders since the initiation in 1954 of reporting by psychiatric clinics nationwide. Many adult disorders, clinicians complain, are rarely found in children, and most childhood disorders must be squeezed into a very small number of categories. In short, the most commonly used classification system today fails to take into consideration the differences between child and adult disorders. Anna Freud (1965) points out that symptoms in children do not necessarily assume the same significance which they do for the adult patient.

In addition to the clinicians' complaints, there is ample research evidence to substantiate the shortcomings of this classification system.

The most extensive data available indicate that of children seen at more than 1,200 psychiatric clincs, 32 per cent were undiagnosed and another 40 per cent were labeled simply as "transient personality disorders" without further differentiation (Rosen, Bahn, & Kramer, 1964). Assignment to a diagnostic category thereby conveys little in the way of accurate information about the symptomatology of a child. Thus, according to available data, more than 7 out of 10 child patients seen in outpatient clinics apparently do not receive a detailed diagnosis. Inadequacies inherent in the classification system, difficulties involved in the examination of children, and a reluctance to pin certain diagnostic labels on children (for example, childhood schizophrenia) probably all contribute to this rather unfortunate state of affairs. The unreliability of psychiatric diagnosis with adult patients is notorious, and there is little reason to suspect that reliability is any higher with children. Moreover, recent factor-analytic studies of behavior ratings of children in public schools do not support the present diagnostic classification system. For example, studies by Peterson (1961) and by Quay and Quay (1965) found that there are two major dimensions, conduct disorder and personality disorder, which account for the majority of the variance among behaviorally disordered children in need of clinical services.

Many workers feel that the nature of etiology differs significantly between the two types of disturbances. Unlike physical illnesses, psychological disturbances typically do not have a specific etiological agent. Rather, psychosocial problems are rooted in multiple causes, a fact which forces one to deal with information on more than the physical level. In addition to genetic and constitutional factors, consideration must be given to the interaction between psychological and social forces. Some classifications attempt to assign disorders to such broad etiological groups as organic or functional. The question arises, however, as to how successful this endeavor can be since the etiology is commonly inferred from the symptomatology. After all, if the diagnosis is based on symptoms which cannot be reliably classified, how can inferences as to etiology based on such observations be any more reliable? Furthermore, when and if we do eventually reach the stage at which our judgments permit reliable assignment to various categories, we are still forced to assume that homogeneous behaviors mean homogeneous determinants (Patterson, 1964). Many clinicians suggest that this is not the case. As White (1964) points out:

Because symptoms are surface phenomena their logical classification corresponds scarcely at all to the logic of the underlying disorders. It is a good deal like classifying books according to the material and color of their bindings rather than by what is discussed inside. It is necessary in every case to go behind the symptoms if we are to understand the nature of a patient's trouble. In addition, symptoms do not fit together, even on the surface, in such a way as to provide an intelligible classification.

On the other hand, Jenkins (1953) argues that if discrete classes of disorders exist, they should be characterized by discrete symptom clusters. This assumption cannot be tested, however, until we have reliability of judgment.

Whereas physical illnesses follow basically the same course and have a known outcome, mental disturbances do not. Anna Freud (1965) points out that it is virtually impossible to distinguish between harmless, temporary disturbances and dangerous, permanent regressions in children. We have at present no sure means of telling which disorders are transitory and simply by-products of developmental strains and which are prodromal of later serious problems. We cannot assume, for example, that childhood neuroses are the forerunners of adult neuroses. Also, spontaneous cures are not at all uncommon in children. To further complicate matters, neither symptom formation, intensity of suffering, nor degree of impairment in functioning is a dependable predictor as to course or outcome among behavior disorders in children. Thus, there are wide differences in course and outcome among children within the same diagnostic category. In brief, there is no satisfactory evidence that current classification systems enable us to predict the course or outcome of a given behavior disorder.

The most essential characteristic advantage of a classification system is that it suggests the treatment of choice. Again, however, there is an absence of evidence to indicate that present diagnostic systems enable us to make a direct correspondence between specific treatments and specific disabilities. In practice, the type of therapy one receives depends primarily on the orientation of the therapist and only secondarily on the child's diagnostic classification. Patterson (1959) notes that the choice of therapy is more contingent upon the training, experiences, and preferences of the therapist than upon the diagnosis. Rosenthal (1962) recalls psychotherapy being referred to as an unidentified process for unspecified problems with unpredictable outcomes. In many instances, it seems that the services offered to patients are determined more by clinic policies than by the patient's needs (that is, by the severity of his disorder). Thus, in children's clinics, children presenting psychotic disorders are less apt to be treated than are children presenting neurotic disorders (Bahn, Chandler, & Eisenberg, 1962). As we will see later in this chapter, the greater services afforded whites as opposed to nonwhites clearly suggest that factors related to the child's prognosis play a more important role than do diagnostic needs in determining the availability of clinic service.

Therapists will sometimes state that certain forms of therapy are suitable for certain groups of children, but the criterion for such statements is a subjective one of inner certitude, not an objective one based on empirical evidence. As London (1964) writes,

Now if this plentitude of treatments involved much variety of techniques to apply to different persons under different circumstances by different specialists, there would be no embarrassment of therapeutic riches here, just as there is not within the many specialties of medicine or law or engineering. But this is not the case, and psychotherapeutic "systems" (or "orientations," as they are often glibly called) speak more to epithets than entities, and more to the perspectives and labels of their founders than to the facts of human behavior. One hardly goes to a psychoanalyst to be cured of anxiety and a nondirective therapist to be treated for homosexuality, as he might to a cardiologist for one condition and a radiologist for another. Nor does the same doctor use Freudian therapy for psychogenic ulcers and Rogerian treatment for functional headaches, as a physician might use medicine for one ailment and surgery for another. On the contrary, being a certain kind of psychotherapist has little bearing on treating a certain kind of problem, but refers rather to the likelihood of treating all problems from the vantage of a certain system. And its champion may see his system either as implying something more grand than mere technique, so that he feels no need for technical precision, or alternately as positing a technique comprehensive enough to apply in general rather than particular, so he feels no diagnostic limit on the ailments it can treat.

At our present stage of development, we do not know what kind of therapy is best for what disorder. Furthermore, we cannot test the assumption that differential treatment programs can be developed for different classes of behavior disorders until a reliable classification system is established.

The basic difficulties discussed above have served to underscore the discrepancies existing between the concepts of physical and mental disorders and have prompted mental-health specialists to wonder if it is appropriate to speak of both under the rubric of "illnesses." (See Table 6.) Current thought regarding this semantic error is aptly expressed in the following statement by Adams (1964):

TABLE 6. CONTRASTS BETWEEN THE MEDICAL AND THE PSYCHOSOCIAL MODELS OF ILLNESS

	Medical Illnesses	Psychosocial Illnesses
Cause(s)	Can usually be isolated and identified; tends to be specific, tangible, and singular.	Difficult to isolate and identify; tend to be less definite, less tangible, and multiple.
Classification	Moderate agreement as to what constitutes a given illness.	Diagnostic categories often convey little meaningful information; tend to be unreliable.
Prognosis	Outcome is generally known and predictable for those with same diagnosis.	Outcome is often uncertain and unpredictable; varies considerably within a given diagnostic category.
Treatment	Tends to be specific for specific illnesses.	Not precisely formulated nor based primarily on the diagnosis.

Failure to clarify these distinctions has had unfortunate consequences. Efforts toward understanding and effective alleviation have long been hampered by the semantic confusion which results when the word illness is used to denote both physical disease entities and maladaptive patterns of interpersonal behavior. This ambiguous usage has perpetrated the glib fallacy that mental and physical illnesses are the same thing. It has interfered with the understanding of fundamental psychological phenomena and made for an ineffectual and often harmful approach to some of the most serious recurring problems in human relationship.

Szasz (1960), in a similar vein, contends that mental illness is a myth, pointing out that a person's troubles cannot be explained as a disease of the nervous system. He feels that man's troubles are best viewed as "problems of living."

There are two schools of thought regarding diagnosis. One contends that the concept of diagnosis is of little value and should be discarded because of its limitations. The other school, while recognizing the limitations inherent in current classification systems, nevertheless believes that some form of taxonomy (one aspect of diagnosis) is necessary. This school concurs with Ausubel (1958), who notes that classification is needed to make possible generalization, concept formation and investigation of relationships between important variables impinging upon the phenomena encompassed within the discipline.

Indeed, scientists cannot work effectively unless they have some scheme for ordering the array of facts or observations they encounter. Therefore, the first stage in any theory consists in the classifying of data. Despite imperfections in present schemes, they nevertheless represent the best means available for prediction (Hunt, 1948). Although current classifications are lacking in clarity, abandonment of them would lead only to greater chaos. How can we compare the differential effectiveness of various therapies for certain types of patients if we have no classification system? How can we communicate effectively with one another? How can any hypothesis be developed and then subjected to a crucial test? How can any general laws ever be formulated? Without nosology, we can have no science. It should be noted that classification merely implies that all cases within a given category have certain similarities, not that they are identical. Classification need not, therefore, preclude further description of individual differences in personality within a given category. The nosology we develop must, however, avoid the pitfalls of the medical model by allowing for varied types of etiology and resultant varied approaches to treatment. As noted earlier, biological, psychological, and sociological factors all interact in the development of maladaptive behavior. The current trend is to stress the role of psychosocial factors in our conceptual schemes, with attention being addressed to the reality conditions, such as family and community factors, which adversely influence the behavior of children. The notion of learning thus becomes a central one in the explanation and treatment of behavior disorders in children.

CLASSIFICATION SCHEMES

Having briefly explored the concept of diagnosis, let us turn to a discussion of actual classification schemes which have been applied to children. A review of the literature reveals more than two dozen attempts from 1920 to 1966 at formal classifications of the totality of behavior problems occurring during childhood and adolescence. As the Committee on Child Psychiatry (1966) notes:

These schemes are based upon strictly descriptive or phenomenological points of view in relation to behavior; currently popular concepts of etiology, ranging from somatic origins to psychogensis; chronological or developmental perspectives; considerations regarding total versus partial personality reactions, parent-child relationships and family interactions; the degree of treatability; or more commonly a combination of several of these conceptional viewpoints.

The following examples are given to illustrate some of the dimensions on which classification schemes are based.

Various classification schemes divide behavior disorders on the basis of etiology into the broad categories of somatogenic and psychogenic. Thus, Pacella (1948) speaks of organic disturbances resulting from structural deviations of the brain (for example, intellectual inadequacies), postencephalitic behavior and posttraumatic behavior as one major category with functional disturbances (for example, habit disorders), neurotic traits and delinquency reactions as another major category. Pacella also notes that a mixture of organic and functional disorders may occur with frequency. Beller (1962) likewise divides childhood personality disorders into three broad categories:

1. Functional behavior disorders, which include conduct disturbances, preneurotic and neurotic disturbances, character disorders and psychotic disturbances.

2. Behavior disorders with an organic basis, including, for example, hereditary disorders and neurological disorders.

3. Mental subnormality, which falls somewhere in-between the functional and organic categories.

Obviously, it is difficult for the clinician to tell whether a given behavior disorder results from psychogenic or somatogenic factors because of the interrelatedness of psychological and somatic processes. For example, we often cannot state with any degree of certitude that a child's hyperactivity, distractibility, and extreme overresponsiveness stem from a brain injury or from an emotional disturbance.

Others have tried to classify behavior disorders on the basis of whether the problem results from environmental forces or from intrapsychic forces. Such an approach is exemplified in Louttit's (1947) scheme. He states that direct primary behavior problems (conduct problems) are directly associated with the home, school, or neighborhood; whereas in indirect primary behavior problems (personality problems), the influence of environmental forces on the child is mediated by internalized conflicts. That Louttit was aware of the overlap between these two categories is evidenced by his admission that aggressive behavior, for example, can conceivably fall into either one or both of the categories.

Miller's (1936) approach is illustrative of conceptual schemes based on the "Who suffers?" dimension. Thus, he accordingly divides disorders into eight categories, three of which deal with subjective disorders, objective disorders, and a combination of the two. In subjective disorders (for example, fears, sleepwalking, educational problems, shyness) suffering is experienced only by the child. In objective disorders (for example, nosepicking, temper tantrums, lying, stealing) others suffer and are disturbed by the child's maladaptive behavior. The combined category refers to the neurotic accompaniments of behavior problems. One factor-analytic approach, which will be discussed in greater detail shortly, essentially categorizes disturbed children as "attackers" and "withdrawers," a dichotomy which also tells who suffers (Becker et al., 1959). This approach also might be considered as an example of schemes based on etiology since it relates these two dimensions of disturbance to parental maladjustment.

An example of a classification system based on developmental considerations comes from the work of Rose (1958), who divides patterns of disturbance into four chronological periods:

1. Patterns of childhood disturbances cover disorders occurring from the time of birth to 2½ years of age.

2. The next chronological category encompasses disorders occurring from the preschool period to the beginning of school.

3. The third developmental category covers the school-age child from age 6 to 11.

4. The final developmental period comes with the advent of puberty and adolescence, covering roughly age 11 to 16.

Each of these four categories are further subdivided according to the types of developmental problems characteristic of the particular period. Such a classification does take into account the fact that a child's emotional maturity is related to age and that different behaviors are appropriate for certain age ranges. Bedwetting, for example, is appropriate for the preschooler, but not for the junior-high-school student.

With this brief background on the dimensions around which classification systems have been based, we now review four of the most recent attempts to order behavior deviations in children.

THE PSYCHIATRIC DESCRIPTIVE APPROACH

Despite the existence of numerous diagnostic systems specifically designed for childhood disturbances, the standard nomenclature from the American Psychiatric Association's *Diagnostic and Statistical Manual of Mental Disorders,* as noted earlier, continues to be the one most commonly used with children. In 1966, however, the Committee on Child Psychiatry devised a proposed classification of childhood behavior disorders which retained many of the important aspects of the standard nomenclature and at the same time introduced modifications necessary for more adequate classification of deviant behaviors in children. Since this recent conceptual framework does allow for greater differentiation between adult and childhood disorders and since it maintains many features of the widely applied standard nomenclature, it will be discussed at length.

While recognizing the importance that genetic and dynamic factors should play in nosology, the Committee on Child Psychiatry believes that it is only the clinical-descriptive aspect of classification which lends itself to study at our present state of knowledge. In keeping with this view, the following ten clinical descriptive categories were proposed: (1) healthy responses, (2) reactive disorders, (3) developmental disorders, (4) psychoneurotic disorders, (5) personality disorders, (6) psychotic disorders, (7) psychophysiological disorders, (8) brain syndromes, (9) mental retardation, and (10) other disorders. This list represents an approximate hierarchical arrangement from wholesome responses to more severe psychogenic disturbances to somatogenic disturbances.

1. *Healthy Responses.* The inclusion of the category "healthy responses" represents the first time that such a category has been included in any system. Its inclusion was designed to overcome the tendency of clinicians to overestimate the seriousness of relatively minor problems or to diagnose in the absence of disease. Although reliable and valid indexes of robustness remain to be delineated, attempts at positive assessment can be undertaken through the use of criteria for specific areas of development. Thus, standards are considered for intellectual functioning (for example, reality-testing ability, inquisitiveness); social functioning (for example, ability to empathize with peers, satisfactory balance in dependence-independence strivings); emotional functioning (for example, frustration power, general

mood); and personal and adaptive functioning (for example, flexibility drive toward mastery). Developmental crises of a limited duration arising from a child's efforts to master developmental tasks (for example, the identity crisis in adolescence) are also included in this category. Note that the concept of stage-appropriateness of behavior thus becomes a basic consideration in evaluating the healthiness of behavior.

2. *Reactive Disorders.* This term has replaced the term "transient situational personality disorders" found in the standard nomenclature and emphasizes the fact that certain maladaptive behavior is a reaction to a given external situation. Thus, in such cases, deviant behavior reflects a conscious incompatibility between the child's impulses-emotions and his social situation. Such situations as excessive academic pressures, parental loss, hospitalization, and so forth are illustrative of events capable of producing a reactive disorder, which can assume many forms (acting-out behavior, withdrawal, depression). Reactive disorders do not constitute an age-bound phenomenon, but they do occur more frequently in young children, whose fluidity of personality organization lessens the possibility for the development of internalized conflicts.

3. *Developmental Deviations.* Developmental deviations constitute another new category which is designed to permit classification of certain deviations heretofore unclassifiable. Disorders so classified extend beyond what is regarded as a developmental variation within the normal range. To diagnose such a disorder, the clinician must have a detailed knowledge of what constitutes normal "abnormal" behavior, which would ordinarily be grouped under "developmental crises." Developmental deviations are sometimes phasic, disappearing with time or parental guidance. In any event, such deviations are not regarded as inevitably of a chronic or permanent nature. Hereditary, constitutional, and maturational factors presumably play a major role in the production of such deviations, although consideration is also given to psychosocial factors in their initiation, maintenance, and alleviation. In the grouping of such disorders, consideration is given to how much of the child's functioning is impaired. Thus, one subcategory, "Deviation in Maturation of Patterns," refers to generalized, widespread delays as well as to precocities or unevenness in developmental patterns. A second subcategory deals with the deviations in specific dimensions of development and accordingly includes dis-

turbances in such particular part functions as motor development, sensory development, speech development, cognitive functioning, social development, psychosexual development, affective development, and integrative development.

4. *Psychoneurotic Disorders.* Disorders in children deriving from unconscious, intrapsychic conflicts are subsumed under this class. Such disorders are viewed as stemming from repression of basic drives, such as aggression and sex. Though their origins date back to the preschool years, neuroses usually do not manifest themselves until the early school-age years, when a certain level of personality development has been achieved. Being unconscious and unverbalized, they tend to have a self-perpetuating character. Even at that, however, the prognosis seems favorable with or without professional treatment. The symptoms resulting from partial repression of the conflict may take various forms. The category of psychoneurotic disorders is therefore subdivided on this basis into the anxiety type, phobic type, conversion type, obsessive-compulsive type, and depressive type.

5. *Personality Disorders.* The term "personality disorders" has been retained although the subcategories differ from those used in the standard nomenclature. The term refers to those deeply engrained personality traits which are in harmony with the child's ego. As such, they are not generally a source of anxiety for the child. Although not clearly manifested until the early school ages, they presumably date back to the early childhood conflicts centering about the management of impulses toward aggression, dependency, autonomy, and sexual differentiation. These disorders may run the gamut from positively organized compulsive traits regarded as assets, at one extreme, to destructively organized personality traits which flagrantly clash with social mores, at the other extreme. The following personality traits are subsumed under this disorder: compulsive personality, oppositional personality, overly inhibited personality, overly independent personality, isolated personality, mistrustful personality, tension-discharge disorders (antisocial personality), sociosyntonic personality disorders (subcultural delinquent), and sexual deviations.

6. *Psychotic Disorders.* Psychotic disorders in childhood are seen as severe disturbances in ego functioning which impair, for example, the child's capacity for adequate thought, speech, emotional responsiveness, and self-identity. The behavioral manifestations, not surprisingly, vary with the child's developmental level. This category is therefore

subdivided into psychoses of infancy and early childhood, psychoses of later childhood, and psychoses of adolescence.

7. *Psychophysiological Disorders.* This terms applies to physiological disturbances in which psychological factors together with predisposing biological factors and present precipitating events are operative in varying etiological degrees. Affected by such disorders are the organ systems regulated by the involuntary nervous system. It appears that almost any such organ system can be so afflicted, and such ubiquity is reflected in the classification system. Illustrative of psychophysiological disorders are such subcategories as disorders of the skin, respiration, gastrointestinal tract, cardiovascular system, and nervous system. Whenever a more total or primary personality diagnosis (for example, psychoneurosis) seems indicated, it should be employed. In fact, multiple classification (for example, psychoneurotic and psychophysiologic skin disorder) is recommended in categorizing psychophysiological disorders exhibiting end-organ responses.

8. *Brain Syndromes.* These disturbances arise from diffuse impairment of the brain tissue and typically interfere with intellectual operations, such as memory, judgment, and discrimination, as well as with emotional stability and impulse control. The prospects for rehabilitation seem more favorable in the case of children versus adults. Since cerebral insults adversely influence the emerging functions and those functions not yet developed, it is more difficult to correlate the severity of intellectual functioning to the severity of actual tissue damage. The two subcategories, "Acute Brain Syndrome" and "Chronic Brain Syndrome," reflect the degree of reversibility, not the onset or duration of the illness or the damage to the central nervous system. As is true of psychophysiological disorders and mental retardation, multiple classification is recommended if warranted.

9. *Mental Retardation.* This category is subdivided on the basis of presumed etiology. The three subcategories thus include the biological group, the environmental group, and the intermediate group in which both the biological and environmental agents are operative. The degree of intellectual impairment—mild, moderate, or severe—is also to be included in the diagnosis.

10. *Other Disorders.* This classification is reserved for disorders uncovered in the future or for future differentiation of currently known disorders.

Another new feature of childhood classification systems is the development of a symptom list. Although the standard nomenclature has such a list, it is not geared to childhood disorders as such. The use of this list should enable the clinician to provide a more detailed description in recording a specific symptom associated, either individually or in clusters, with different disorders at a given age or developmental period. This listing, which is to be used in conjunction with the nosological headings, should also prove helpful especially where a given case does not fit neatly under one class. Moreover, use of this list could establish a basis for later followup of specific patterns that occur during development or treatment.

THE EMPIRICAL APPROACH

The classification system proposed by the Committee on Child Psychiatry undoubtedly allows for a more refined differentiation between adult and childhood disorders, thereby affording the clinician a more realistic diagnostic system in which to operate. Yet, the authors cannot help but feel that this proposed system will not allow for reliable assignment except perhaps to broad categories. Use of the standard nomenclature with adults, after which the proposed classification is modeled, has not resulted in satisfactory reliability of psychiatric diagnosis, and there seems to be little reason to believe that use of the proposed classification will yield a more reliable classification system when applied to children's disorders. An alternative approach to psychodynamic or conceptual attempts at classification is the empirical approach. Though more limited in number, factor-analytic approaches are receiving increasing attention.

Dissatisfied with traditional approaches to classification, some psychologists have advocated an empirical approach which, in contrast to the conceptual approach, not only uses a minimum of assumptions and concepts regarding personality development and behavioral disorders but renders dimensions of disturbed behavior more explicit and operational. Moreover, the multivariate statistical techniques employed in this approach permit independent confirmation of dimensions or categories derived from clinical observation. Thus, greater credence is lent to a classification system if clinicians and factor theorists are able to derive similar dimensions of categories despite their having used very divergent methods.

Quay (1965), in discussing the structure of children's behavior disorders, notes that behavior disorders are most profitably viewed as dimensions, in contrast to types or disease entities, along which all children range. A disturbed child, according to this view, is one whose behavior falls at the extreme of one or more of these dimensions. Quay notes that dimensions should satisfy four internal criteria: They should be (1) as mutually exclusive as possible, (2) as objective as possible, (3) specifically demonstrable as a cluster, and (4) derived from more than one kind of data. The dimensions should also be related to meaningful external criteria that would hopefully be tied to etiology, behavioral correlates, and appropriate differential treatment. Current research evidence based on factor analysis of case-record data, behavior ratings, or personality questionnaires obtained on populations from public schools, child-guidance clinics, and correctional institutions can be consistently reduced to four dimensions or syndromes: (1) the unsocialized aggressive or conduct disorder; (2) the overinhibited neurotic or personality disorder; (3) a socialized or subcultural conduct disorder; and (4) the inadequacy-immaturity disorder. Symptoms associated with the conduct disorders include restlessness, distractibility, laziness in school, irresponsibility, disobedience, hyperactivity, and impertinence. Behavioral manifestations characteristic of the personality disorders include self-consciousness, feelings of inferiority, daydreaming, distractibility, shyness, and lethargy. Behaviors typical of the inadequacy-immaturity dimension include hyperactivity, impertinence, short attention span, distractibility, feelings of inferiority, and self-consciousness (Quay & Quay, 1965). Note that there is some overlapping of symptoms among the three dimensions. Distractibility, for instance, is common to all three dimensions. Thus, in rendering a decision as to which category a child belongs, the clinician or teacher should consider the general list of symptoms rather than relying solely on a single, specific symptom.

Since these are dimensions rather than types, the practicing clinician must deal with values from these dimensions in diagnosing each case. At this time, the data relating these syndromes to meaningful outside criteria (for example, personality questionnaires, parent and teacher ratings) remain meager, although the evidence indicates that there are differential correlates of these behavioral dimensions and that these are consistent with what one would expect.

Though some psychologists may view the empirical approach as doing away with concepts central to advancing the understanding of personality development and psychopathology, the tough-minded clinician would welcome to an area characterized by subjectivity what appears to be a more reliable and objective procedure for the determination of underlying syndromes or dimensions of disturbed behavior.

THE SOCIAL-LEARNING-THEORY APPROACH

Bandura (1968) has outlined a taxonomic schema of behavioral disorders within a social-learning-theory framework. Whereas many of the psychodynamic systems lead one to pursue hypothetical internal determinants of abnormal behavior (for example, Oedipal conflicts), social-learning approaches contend that deviant behavior constitutes "a learned response pattern that often can be directly modified by manipulating the stimulus variables of which both the mediating and terminal behavior are a function" (Bandura, 1968). In other words, once maladaptive behaviors are modified, it is unnecessary to deal with the underlying cause. Whereas many systems focus primarily on the characteristics of persons (for example, passive-aggressive personality), the social-learning approach to taxonomy stresses the *interaction* between the person's characteristics and stimulus situations.

In Bandura's classification system, diverse maladaptive behaviors are reduced to six "relatively distinct" patterns reflecting:

1. *Deficient Repertoires.* The individual, for instance, who simply lacks the social, academic, or vocational skills necessary for an adequate adjustment would score high on this dimension.

2. *Defective Stimulus Control.* The first-grade pupil who, because of insufficient discrimination, behaves in a dependent fashion on his teacher provides an illustration of this dimension of pathology.

3. *Inappropriate Stimulus Control of Behavior.* This situation obtains when formerly innocuous and inappropriate stimuli (for example, the sight of an approaching dog) have acquired the capacity to elicit highly intense emotional reactions.

4. *Defective or Inappropriate Incentive Systems.* Certain maladaptive behaviors (for example, deviant sexual behavior) are acquired and maintained because of the strong positive reinforcing value.

5. *Aversive Behavioral Repertoires.* This category deals primarily with what might be broadly termed aggressive or socially disruptive behaviors, that is, behaviors which generate aversive consequences to others.

6. *Aversive Self-Reinforcing Systems.* Whereas the taxonomy as presented thus far has emphasized the role of *external* reinforcing stimuli in psychopathology, this category provides a place for maladaptive behaviors which are controlled by *self-administered* reinforcers of an aversive nature. Examples include self-generated feelings of misery and self-imposed deprivation, leading to feelings of depression and worthlessness.

Bandura believes that a multidimensional characterization of behavior disorders offers greater predictive and therapeutic utility than does a typological approach. Consistent with a multidimensional approach, each individual is assessed on each of the six dimensions. In addition to providing greater taxonomic flexibility than is inherent in typological systems, the social-learning diagnostic approach also has the advantage of leading to differential treatment procedures.

THE PSYCHOEDUCATIONAL APPROACH

Adopting a social-competency model, Bower (1970) has classified the mental-health problems of children into five levels. In accordance with this model, one is not concerned with the student's anxiety or intrapsychic discomfort but with his inability to handle his anxiety constructively in a school setting. In short, the emphasis is on the student's ability to cope, not on his personal contentment. The five levels, or categories, which might be more accurately construed as a continuum indicating the degree of handicap or social incompetency, are as follows:

Group 1. Those pupils who manifest the ordinary, everyday problems.

Group 2. Those pupils who manifest beginning or minor problems in learning and behavior which exceed normal expectations.

Group 3. Pupils who manifest marked and recurrent difficulties in learning and behavior.

Group 4. Pupils who manifest severe problems in learning and behavior.

Group 5. Pupils who manifest such severe problems that they cannot be maintained in a public-school setting.

For each level, Bower has indicated the most pertinent and beneficial type of school program. An obvious advantage of this system is its facilitation of the psychoeducational decision-making process for deviant youth. For Group 5 youngsters, educational provisions suggested for consideration include a 24-hour residential program, a day-care school program, or home-bound instruction or teaching norms. Children falling into Group 4 can probably still derive some benefit from school attendance if provided with special-class placement. If these youngsters prove unable to maintain some positive contact with the school setting, then placement in a day-school arrangement becomes a possibility. For Group 3 pupils, who are often hanging by their educational bootstraps, educational provisions center around remedial group work, individual tutoring, or mental-health consultation with their teachers. For Group 2 youngsters, the school's role involves early identification in the form of screening programs and early treatment, such as parent-counseling programing. For Group 1 students, the school's job is to provide a wide variety of ego-building experiences. A curriculum broad and flexible enough to encompass individual differences in interest, ability, and cultural background can go far in laying a sound base for a mental-health program.

PROBLEMS IN EVALUATING CHILDREN'S BEHAVIOR

1. *Limited Language of Children.* In addition to the problems which apply generally to the entire field of diagnosis, there are specific problems which are encountered in the evaluation of children's behavior. Children, especially those of preschool age, typically have very limited language in vocabulary and facility. Yet personality-measuring instruments are highly language-oriented. They may require actual skill in reading and interpretation of printed material. In any event, they rely heavily upon the comprehension of oral language by which directions and instructions for making a response are given to the children. In part, because of their language limitation, children are often reported by research investigators as being negative, uncooperative, and refusing to comply. It seems very likely that they simply do not understand what has been asked of them and what is expected of them.

2. *Limited Experiences of Children.* Children also have had limited practice in reporting their own feelings, wishes, or aspirations. This may in part be a function of their limited facility with language, but it is also probably associated with their simply being inexperienced

and thus not being certain of what their feelings and intentions are. A child, for example, may be able to report accurately that he likes something or doesn't like it, but he may be puzzled as to whether he likes something strongly, moderately, very little, or sometimes. He may be totally at a loss when asked to report feelings such as loyalty.

3. *Impact of Sex Differences.* There is growing evidence that there are differential developmental rates, with girls maturing more rapidly than boys. These differences are probably at an optimum at about the time a child ordinarily enters school and continue into early adolescence. There are few measuring scales, however, which present separate normative data for boys and girls throughout this age period. Initially, these differences were thought to be most pronounced with respect to motor responses. Recent evidence suggests that the differences are much more general and probably involve intellectual functioning and other types of performance as well. The existence of such differences in response patterns might be expected to penalize boys while favoring girls.

4. *Relative Instability of Children's Personalities.* Another source of specific problems is that the child is undergoing constant and sometimes rapid developmental growth and change. Failure to take this factor into consideration could result in the erroneous crediting of maturational changes to experimental manipulation efforts. Maturationally induced changes in performance can manifest themselves suddenly within the individual and may be easily masked if the child's performance is represented by the "average" of his group.

INCIDENCE

It is difficult to determine with any degree of accuracy the incidence of emotional disturbance in children since estimates of maladjustment will vary with the definition of disturbance used, the agencies sampled (school, child-guidance clinics, juvenile court, resident hospitals), and the identification methods employed (referrals to professional specialists, rating scales, self-report inventories, and sociograms). Illustrative of some of the above difficulties are the following findings:

1. If mild disturbances are included in the definition of emotional disturbance, the incidence figures may run as high as 1 in every 3 elementary-school pupils (Rogers, 1942).

2. School teachers are apt to overlook the emotionally disturbed

but bright hard-working pupil who is doing well in class (Sarason et al., 1960).

3. On the other hand, school teachers may be more inclined to see maladjustment in lower-class children than in middle-class pupils (Eisenberg, 1960).

4. Rating scales tend to be more valid for boys than for girls, whereas self-report inventories seem to be more valid for girls than for boys (Ullmann, 1952).

5. Incidence figures based on admission to resident hospitals or outpatient clinics are not likely representative of the prevalence of mental disorders because of the many selective factors that determine admission.

6. Court statistics on delinquency must also be interpreted cautiously, in that the quoted figures are affected not only by the types of cases and ages of children over which the juvenile courts in different regions or states have jurisdiction but also by the number and scope of other social agencies available in the community. The great amount of unrecorded delinquency must also not be overlooked.

Bearing in mind these limitations, let us review some of the available statistics in order to gain a rough perspective as to the scope of maladjustment in children.

One of the most wide-ranging studies of public-school youngsters, which was carried out by Bower (1960) in California, indicates that at least 3 youngsters in the average classroom (10 per cent of students) are sufficiently upset as to warrant the label emotionally handicapped. White and Harris (1961), after carefully reviewing six major studies on the incidence of serious maladjustment in public-school children, arrived at a "working estimate" of 4 to 7 per cent. These rates were based on studies conducted between 1927 and 1958 and relied primarily on teachers' judgments. The most recent and thorough review of incidence studies on maladjustment in elementary-school pupils is contained in a report prepared for the Joint Commission on the Mental Health of Children by Glidewell and Swallow (1968). Their data, which are based on 27 studies reported between 1925 and 1967, indicate that 30 per cent of the elementary-school youth show at least mild adjustment problems, 10 per cent are in need of professional clinical assistance, and 4 per cent would be referred to clinical facilities if such services were available (see Table 7). As might be expected, rates based on admissions to out-

TABLE 7. A SUMMARY OF STUDIES ON GENERAL MALADJUSTMENT OF CHILDREN IN GRADES K-12 [PREVALENCE OF GENERAL MALADJUSTMENT OF ELEMENTARY SCHOOL CHILDREN IN THE UNITED STATES (RATE PER 100) — GLIDEWELL & SWALLOW, 1968]

Investigator(s)	School Location	Grade Levels	Race and/or Class	Method	Population at Risk	School Maladjustment	Clinical Maladjustment	Referral
Haggerty (1925)[a]	Minneapolis, Minnesota	1–8	Children from one of the "better industrial districts."	Teachers rated children on 16 "undesirable" behaviors.	801	51.0		
Wickman (1929)	Cleveland, Ohio	1–6	"Representative public school."	Teachers rated children on 51 behaviors.	874	53.0[b]		
				A scale of over-all adjustment.			7.0	
Hildreth (1929)	Lincoln School, New York City	1–12	Unknown.	Teachers used 7 criteria to identify "problem pupils."	500		8.0	
McClure (1929)	Toledo, Ohio	1–8	All children in elementary schools in the city.	Teachers were asked to identify children who "should be referred to the Juvenile Adjustment Agency."	26,364			2.0
Yourman (1932)	New York City, New York	K–8	Children from highest, average, and lowest socioeconomic levels of city; ethnically diverse.	Teachers rated children on a scale of over-all adjustment in school.	13,761		11.0	

[a]For bibliographical citations, see Glidewell and Swallow (1968).
[b]Wickman's 53% and Haggerty's 51% refer to rates for children who gave evidence of one or more of the "undesirable" behaviors rated.
Source: Adapted from J. Glidewell & C. Swallow. The prevalence of maladjustment in elementary schools. Chicago: Univer. of Chicago Press, 1968.

TABLE 7 (*continued*)

Investigator(s)	School Location	Grade Levels	Race and/or Class	Method	Population at Risk	School Maladjustment instrument	Clinical Maladjustment instrument	Referral
Snyder (1934)	Jersey City, New Jersey	K–8	Schools representative of city's population; included children of "native-born," "Polish-born," and "Italian-born" parents; also Negroes.	Teachers identified pupils they considered to be "problems" and gave reasons for their choices.	13,632	6.9		
Young-Masten (1938)	New Haven, Connecticut	K–8	All children in elementary schools in the city.	Teachers were asked to identify children most seriously maladjusted and to give reasons for choice.	11,150	10.0		
Rogers (1942b)	Columbus, Ohio	1 & 2 4–6	Unknown, some variation.	Teachers rated children on modified H-O-W schedule; 9 other criteria, including peer and observer ratings, used.	1,524	42.0	12.0	
Mangus (1949)	Miami County, Ohio	3 & 6	Children, village and rural. County "fairly typical of counties in western Ohio."	Teachers rated children on 7-point scale of adjustment. Combined score from teachers' ratings and from sociometric and personality tests.	1,229	28.1[d]	18.8[e]	
Glidewell et al. (1959)	St. Louis County, Missouri	3	Children, white; all social classes included.	Teachers' ratings on over-all adjustment of the children; 4 categories.	830	28.0	8.2	

Study	Location	Grade	Sample	Method	N	%
Bower et al. (1958)	California	4–6	All social classes; distribution of occupations of parents representative of state as a whole.	Teachers' ratings on over-all adjustment; 3 categories.	5,587	23.9 *[f]
Glidewell (1961)	St. Louis County, Missouri	3	Children, white; all social classes included.	Teachers referred children for professional help.	530	2.0
Morse (1961)	Communities in Michigan, excluding Detroit	K–12	Unknown.	Unknown.		3.0 to 12.0
Turner (1962)	St. Louis, Missouri	3 & 4	Negroes and whites; middle and lower classes.	Teachers were asked to assess adjustment and give reason for judgment.	2,017	32.8
Gordon[g] (1962)	Middlesex County, New Jersey	K–6	Entire range of social classes; about 15% Negro.	Teachers rated children on 5-point scale of adjustment.	53,995	11.3
Cowen et al. (1963)	Rochester, New York	1–3	Upper lower-class, ethnically representative except for substantial underweighting of Jews and Negroes.	Teachers' ratings of ability and their discussions with mental-health team entered into assessment of adjustment based on many criteria.	108	37.0

[c] For an explanation of this schedule, no longer in use, see Rogers (1942b) in Glidewell and Swallow (1968).

[d] Teachers were urged to put 10% of their students in the lowest place on scale.

[e] Had Mangus used "6" as a cut-off on his composite instead of "7," 11.1% of the children would have been judged clinically maladjusted. . . .

[f] Bower et al. suggested that at least 3 children in an average classroom are "emotionally disturbed." Their estimate of clinical maladjustment seems to be about 10%, but which data provide the bases for their estimate are not clear. . . .

[g] Gordon, in a personal communication, supplied race and social-class data for his three studies; he also supplied information about race for the Hunterdon County, New Jersey, and Springfield, New Jersey, studies.

TABLE 7 (*continued*)

Investigator(s)	School Location	Grade Levels	Race and/or Class	Method	Population at Risk	School Maladjustment instrument	Clinical Maladjustment instrument	Referral
Gordon (1963)	Key School, Philadelphia	K–6	Working-class; about 40% Negro.	Teachers rated children on 5-point scale of adjustment.	553		18.6	
				Bower-Lambert screening device.[h]			10.6	
Gordon (1963)	Jamesburg, New Jersey	K–6	Lower middle-class; about 10% Negro.	Teachers rated children on 5-point scale of adjustment.	455		11.8	
				Bower-Lambert screening device.			20.2	
Lichtenstein (1963)	Baltimore, Maryland	1–6	Unknown, some variation.	Teachers identified pupils according to 4 criteria of adjustment.	16,748		9.9	
Woolf (1964)	Hunterdon County, New Jersey	K–8	Sample mostly white.	Teachers used Gordon's 5-point scale of adjustment.	9,618		13.3	
Mental Health Research Unit (1964)	Onondaga County, New York	2–4	Unknown, nonurban, some variation.	Teachers identified "problem" and "emotionally disturbed" children.	6,788	15.3	7.6	

Study	Location	Grade	Sample	Criteria	N			
Springfield Services Department (1965)	Springfield, New Jersey	K–8	Sample mostly white.	Teachers used Gordon's 5-point scale of adjustment.	2,182			12.7
Cowen et al. (1966)	Rochester, New York	1–3	Upper lower-class, ethnically representative except for substantial under-weighting of Jews and Negroes.	Teachers' ratings of ability and their discussion with mental-health team entered into assessment of adjustment based on many criteria.	103	30.0		
Stennett (1966)	Rural northern Minnesota	4–6	Rural, white.	Modified version of Bower screening instrument.	333			22.0
Maes[i] (1966)	Lansing, Michigan	4–6	Unknown.	Mental-health specialists in child-guidance clinic identified children in need of therapy.	588			6.9
White & Charry[j] (1966)	Westchester County, New York	K–12	"Representative of the higher-income, outer rings which encircle many of our large cities."	Children referred to school psychologists by teachers, parents, and others.	49,918			4.8
Kellam & Schiff (1967)	Woodlawn area of Chicago, Illinois	1	Negro, lower-class, "deprived."	Teachers rated children on scale of "global adaptation."	2,010	69.3		
Approximations (weighted means):						30.2	10.5	3.8

[h]This device consists of teacher, peer, and self-report tests.

[i]Because the "referral" children were identified first and then studied with their classmates in this study, this rate is likely to be an overestimate.

[j]In this study, each participating school had a school psychologist on the staff. This degree of availability of school psychologists is unusual and presented an optimum for referral.

patient psychiatric clinics yield a somewhat lower rate. Eisenberg (1960) estimates this rate to be approximately 1 per cent of the childhood population.

Crime statistics for 1962 indicate that there were approximately 478,000 juvenile delinquents handled by juvenile courts in the United States. In terms of percentages, 1.8 per cent of all children in the country between the ages of 7 and 17 were seen in juvenile courts during that year (U.S. Children's Bureau, 1963). If traffic offenses are included, another 312,000 cases, or an additional 1 per cent of the child population in the 7–17 age range, were processed by the juvenile courts. Though it is generally conceded that delinquency has increased over the past decade, there has been much discussion as to whether emotional disturbance is more common today than it was some years ago.

Whether the incidence of childhood disturbance in the United States is on the rise or not is a difficult question to answer since the statistics pertaining to this matter do not lend themselves to unequivocal interpretations. It may well be, however, that the increase in cases seen by child-guidance clinics reflects a heightened concern over childhood disorders rather than an actual increase in such problems. Schofield (1965) suggests that although man through the ages has always experienced anxiety and dealt with stress, current societal attitudes toward man's problems have caused him to "feel anxious about his anxiety." In fact, Glazer (1955), in his analysis of data pertaining to rates of mental disorders in Massachusetts some 100 years ago, contends that the rate of psychosis among the hospitalized population has not changed appreciably except for geriatric populations. Regardless of whether or not mental illness is on the increase, we do know that emotional disturbance in children is not randomly distributed throughout the childhood population. Rather, it is commonly associated with certain variables, the discussion of which follows.

FACTORS RELATED TO INCIDENCE

Age and Sex

That the variables of age and sex are consistently related to both outpatient and inpatient treatment of children has been well established. We know, for example, that referral rates to psychiatric clinics are most commonly highest during the preadolescent and middle-adolescent periods.[1] Thus, Gilbert (1957), in his study of four metropolitan clinics, found that problems occurred most frequently in children aged 6 to 10. Figures based on national records of psychiatric clinics indicate the highest incidence of occurrence in ages 10 to 14 (Rosen, Bahn, & Kramer, 1964). Bower (1961), in studying a public-school population, similarly noted that the highest percentage of emotionally handicapped pupils are in the elementary and junior-high grades, with the lowest percentage of emotionally handicapped children in the early primary grades and later high-school years. In addition, Morse, Cutler, and Fink (1964) reported that approximately two-thirds of classes for emotionally disturbed children in the public schools are at the later elementary and junior-high levels.

We also know that overt pathology in children is largely a male phenomenon. Gilbert (1957), for example, in his study of 2,500 consecutive cases seen at four metropolitan clinics, found that boys outnumbered girls nearly 4 to 1 with respect to aggressive acting-out behavior problems and approximately 3 to 1 for academic difficulties. Contrary to popular belief, he found that the boys even outnumbered the girls with respect to passive withdrawn behaviors. His data, in fact, revealed a sex differential for every major referral problem. Clinic termination rates estimated for the total United States likewise indicate a higher rate of disturbance for boys for every major diagnostic category (Rosen, Bahn, & Kramer, 1964). The sex ratios were almost 3 to 1 for acute and chronic brain disorders, approximately 2 to 1 for psychotic disturbances and transient situational personality disorders, and approximately 3 to 2 for psychoneurotic disturbances and mental deficiencies. The sex ratios were almost identical for psychophysiological disorders, which was the least common diagnosis given in outpatient clinics nationally. A recent large-scale investigation of public-school classes for emotionally disturbed children also revealed a sex ratio of more than 5 to 1 (Morse, Cutler, & Fink, 1964). Juvenile-court records indicate that more than four times as many

---

[1] Glidewell and Swallow (1968) report that age differences per se in the prevalence of *clinical* maladjustment are not great. Data from the Nobles County study also indicate that emotional problems are unrelated to age (Anderson et al., 1959). It might well be that *clinical* maladjustment becomes more difficult for adults to cope with during the preadolescent and adolescent years. Further, teachers and parents are inclined to give the young child a chance to rally and "to grow out of this stage" before seeking professional help. Both of these factors may, in part, account for the higher rate of referrals during the preadolescent and adolescent years of development.

boys as girls are referred for delinquent behavior (U.S. Children's Bureau, 1963).

Admissions to inpatient psychiatric facilities likewise reflect a sex differential for children under the age of 15 (U.S. Department of Health, Education, and Welfare, 1965). Data based on children below the age of 15 in 284 state and county hospitals in the United States indicate that boys outnumbered girls for every major diagnostic category with the exception of psychophysiological disorders, for which the rates were approximately equal. In terms of over-all admission rates, the sex ratio was 2 to 1, with the sex differential being most pronounced in favor of the boys with respect to the diagnosis of personality disorders and transient situational personality disorders. Data based on first admissions to private mental hospitals in the United States similarly reflect a sex differential for children under the age of 15.

Another interesting finding pertaining to the variables of age and sex is the sex ratio after adolescence (Rosen et al., 1964). As shown in Table 8, the rate for clinic termination per 100,000 population for males was 276.5 for patients under 18 years of age in contrast to only 186.5 per 100,000 for male patients 18 years of age or over. In other words, the rate for males dropped approximately one-third after late adolescence. Whereas the rate for males decreased gradually in late adolescence and adulthood, the rate for females increased during these periods. As Table 8 shows, the clinic termination rate per 100,000 for females under 18 years of age was 144.5 in contrast to 176.9 per 100,000 for patients 18 years of age and over. This represents an increase of 22 per cent. With the decrease in disorders for males and the increase in disorders for females, the sex ratios eventually equalize in adulthood. Data based on patients in resident hospitals likewise show an equalization of rates following adolescence (U.S. Department of Health, Education, and Welfare, 1965).

Another curious finding is the greater number of children (especially boys) receiving treatment in comparison to the number of adults receiving treatment. One reason for this differential rate probably has to do with the fact that children are brought to the clinic by others, whereas adults are more likely to bring themselves. The adult might not recognize that he has a problem, or if he does, he may not wish to change himself. These options are not open to the child. If his problem bothers someone else, he is apt to be referred to the clinic even if he is not motivated to modify his attitudes and behavior. Another explanatory factor probably can be sought in clinic admission policies, which may be based on the assumption that early detection of emotional problems results in a favorable response to treatment. The higher childhood rates may also reflect the concern on the part of parents and teachers for the mental health of their children and pupils (Schofield, 1965). Finally, those subscribing to a genetic theory of primary causality for mental illness might attribute the higher incidence of mental disorders in children to "weak protoplasm" which breaks down early in life. In any event, an anticipated increase of 20 per cent in the general population 10 to 14 years of age within the next decade suggests that clinic utilization will likely remain at a higher rate for children than for adults (Rosen, Bahn, & Kramer, 1964). Furthermore, despite the increase in number of psychiatric outpatient clinics from about 500 in 1946 to 1,600 in 1962, a three-fold increment, community mental-health services will ask to be bolstered even further to cope with the increased childhood populations. The trend for treating larger numbers of children as opposed to adults (except perhaps for problems of the elderly) is, therefore, apt to continue for at least the next decade.

Major Disorders

Clinic admission rates vary not only with respect to the age and sex of the patient but also with respect to the type of psychiatric disorders. Gilbert in 1957 studied the data based on 2,500 consecutive cases seen at two metropolitan education clinics and at two metropolitan community clinics (see Table 9). The current emphasis placed on learning disabilities in our society is reflected in the fact that academic difficulties constituted the most frequent referral complaint in the school clinics, followed by mental retardation and aggressive, antisocial behavior. Among the community clinics, aggressive, antisocial behavior was the most frequent referral problem, followed in descending order by anxious behavior, withdrawn behavior, and academic difficulty. Problems of a sexual nature were the least common referred to either type of clinic. These data, in general, suggest that somewhat different types of cases are referred to the different types of clearinghouses available. For example, cases of learning disability and mental retardation tend to be more commonly referred to educational clinics.

TABLE 8. CLINIC TERMINATION RATE FOR MAJOR AND SELECTED PSYCHIATRIC DISORDERS OF MALES AND FEMALES UNDER 18 YEARS OF AGE [CLINIC TERMINATION RATE BY AGE AND SEX, FOR MAJOR AND SELECTED DETAILED PSYCHIATRIC DISORDERS, PATIENTS UNDER 18 YEARS OF AGE, 1961 (ESTIMATED FOR TOTAL UNITED STATES) – ROSEN, BAHN, & KRAMER, 1964]

Rate per 100,000 Population

Major and Selected Detailed Disorders	Males					Females				
	Total under 18 Years	Under 5 Years	5–9 Years	10–14 Years	15–17 Years	Total under 18 Years	Under 5 Years	5–9 Years	10–14 Years	15–17 Years
Total terminated patients	276.5	57.7	324.7	434.5	383.1	144.5	40.2	149.6	205.6	262.0
Total with a diagnosed disorder	186.2	28.8	213.0	303.2	274.3	94.5	18.9	92.1	140.4	191.2
Acute and chronic brain disorders	14.7	7.7	23.9	16.1	8.8	5.5	6.3	10.9	8.0	5.0
Associated with or due to: Diseases and conditions due to prenatal (constitutional) influence	2.6	2.4	4.2	1.8	1.1	1.3	2.0	2.6	1.2	.7
Birth and other trauma	1.9	.7	3.3	2.4	1.4	.6	.5	1.2	1.1	.7
Convulsive disorder	2.5	.9	3.3	3.6	3.0	1.2	.8	2.2	2.4	2.0
Unknown or unspecified cause	5.0	1.6	9.7	5.7	2.3	1.4	1.2	3.3	2.0	1.0
Mental deficiencies	20.9	6.9	27.5	29.7	22.8	13.2	4.7	17.5	17.7	15.7
Mild	6.2	1.5	7.6	9.9	7.7	3.3	.6	4.4	5.0	4.3
Moderate	5.5	1.5	7.3	8.0	6.4	3.7	1.2	5.1	5.2	3.7
Severe	3.0	1.9	4.5	3.0	1.8	2.4	1.3	3.7	2.7	1.6
Severity unspecified	6.1	2.0	8.0	8.8	6.9	3.8	1.6	4.3	4.8	6.1

Psychotic disorders	10.0	1.6	10.2	13.3	23.6	5.0	.7	3.3	5.9	17.6
Schizophrenic reaction:										
Childhood type	5.7	1.5	8.9	8.0	3.4	2.0	.6	3.0	2.9	1.9
Other types	3.9	—	.9	4.6	19.4	2.7	.1	.2	2.7	14.8
Psychoneurotic disorders	19.5	1.0	23.4	35.2	24.2	12.6	.9	11.0	20.4	28.5
Anxiety reaction	8.8	.5	12.2	15.0	9.0	4.3	.4	4.5	6.6	8.9
Conversion reaction	.7	.1	.5	1.5	1.2	1.2	.1	.7	1.8	4.0
Depressive reaction	2.1	.1	1.4	4.0	4.6	2.0	.1	.8	2.9	7.6
Personality disorders	45.5	2.4	34.9	83.4	97.6	17.6	1.0	10.7	28.5	51.4
Inadequate personality	2.2	.1	1.4	3.8	6.0	1.0	*	.4	1.5	3.5
Schizoid personality	5.5	.1	2.8	9.9	15.5	2.2	*	.8	6.4	7.1
Emotionally unstable personality	2.9	.1	2.2	5.1	6.9	2.0	*	.8	3.2	7.3
Passive-aggressive personality	18.6	.3	12.2	37.2	39.6	5.7	.1	3.3	10.1	16.1
Antisocial reaction	3.0	.1	1.1	5.4	9.9	1.0	—	.1	1.3	5.1
Learning or speech disturbance	4.3	1.2	6.3	6.8	2.4	1.2	.5	2.0	1.5	.5
Psychophysiologic autonomic and visceral disorders	1.4	.2	1.7	2.4	1.6	1.3	.1	1.2	2.1	2.7
Transient situational personality disorders	74.2	9.0	91.4	123.1	95.7	36.9	5.2	37.5	57.8	70.3
Without mental disorder	3.6	4.9	3.1	2.5	3.6	2.6	4.2	2.3	1.4	1.4
Undiagnosed	86.6	24.0	108.6	128.7	105.2	47.3	17.1	55.3	63.7	69.6

*Less than 0.05.

Source: B. M. Rosen, A. K. Bahn, & M. Kramer, Demographic and diagnostic characteristics of psychiatric clinic outpatients in the U.S.A., 1961. *Amer. J. Orthopsychiat.*, 1964, 34, 455-468. Copyright ©, the American Orthopsychiatric Association. Reproduced by permission.

TABLE 9. REFERRAL PROBLEMS OF OUTPATIENT BOYS AND GIRLS UNDER 18 YEARS OF AGE [COMPOSITE DISTRIBUTION OF "REFERRAL PROBLEMS" IN FOUR METROPOLITAN CHILD GUIDANCE CENTERS (N = 2,500 CHILDREN; AVERAGE 1.9 COMPLAINTS PER CHILD) – GILBERT, 1957]

Referral Problems	Under 6		6 to 10		10 to 14		14 to 18		All Ages			Total as % of N	Percent of All Cases	
													in 2 Community Clinics	in 2 School Clinics
	M	F	M	F	M	F	M	F	M	F	Total			
Academic Difficulties	3	0	358	126	322	117	146	54	829	297	1,126	45	27	56
Mental Retardation	16	9	166	94	180	123	50	35	412	261	673	27	6	40
Aggressive and Anti-Social Behavior	45	12	242	65	192	39	115	45	594	161	755	30	45	20
Passive, Withdrawn, Asocial Behavior	38	15	174	74	110	50	60	25	382	164	546	22	32	14
Emotional Instability and Anxiety Symptoms	45	16	205	86	108	46	49	25	407	173	580	23	34	16
Hyperactivity and Motor Symptoms	24	12	139	59	69	24	20	5	252	100	352	14	22	8
Sexual Behavior Problems	6	1	12	10	13	6	6	6	37	23	60	2½	4	1
Toilet Training	27	7	50	25	36	14	0	2	113	48	161	6½	12	1
Speech Defects	25	9	62	19	26	9	10	1	123	38	161	6½	6	7
Miscellaneous	14	17	90	38	71	51	34	29	209	135	344	14	20	9

Source: G. M. Gilbert. A survey of "referral problems" in metropolitan child guidance centers. *J. clin. Psychol.*, 1957, 13, 37-42.

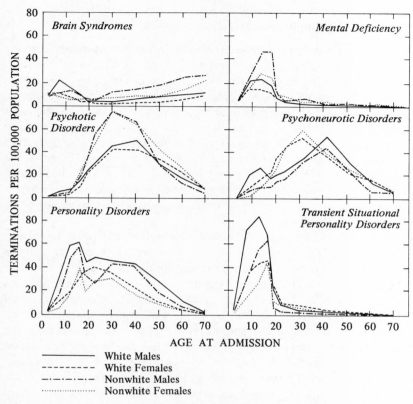

FIGURE 1. *Clinic termination rate by color, age, and sex for each major psychiatric disorder, 1961, data for 579 of 682 clinics in 25 states. (Source:* B. M. Rosen, A. K. Bahn, & M. Kramer. Demographic and diagnostic characteristics of psychiatric clinic outpatients in the U.S.A., 1961. *Amer. J. Orthopsychiat.,* 1964, **34**, 455-468. Copyright ©, the American Orthopsychiatric Association. Reproduced by permission.)

The most comprehensive data on type of disorder as it relates to incidence come from the national reporting program on outpatient psychiatric clinics (Rosen, Bahn, & Kramer, 1964). The data contained in Figure 1 pertain to both major and detailed diagnostic categories and are based on clinic termination rates. While the data are presented in the form of termination rates, they nonetheless provide an accurate estimate of admission rates because of the limited clinic stay for the majority of patients. The major findings of this study can be summarized as follows:

1. During the first decade of life, brain syndromes were relatively high but then declined, with prenatal factors constituting the most common disease entity associated with the brain syndromes in children. During the school years, however, mental deficiencies without organic basis were higher than the brain syndromes. After age 18 the rates for mental deficiency dropped to a low level—a finding consistent with followup studies of the mentally retarded which suggest that certain signs of mental retardation are more evident in academic situations than in nonacademic adulthood situations. Severely retarded children seen at the clinics were more commonly aged 5 to 9, whereas both mildly and moderately retarded youngsters were most apt to be 10 to 14 years of age.

2. Psychotic disorders were relatively infrequent prior to adolescence, according to these data; however, the rates rose sharply in adolescence. Interestingly, the rates for childhood schizophrenia were about 8 or 9 per 100,000 for boys and about 3 per 100,000 for girls at ages 5 through 14. A chronic, undifferentiated type of schizophrenia is the most commonly identified psychosis during the adolescent years.

3. The psychoneurotic rate increased somewhat earlier than the psychotic rate, with a slightly more steady rate for females than males. Anxiety reaction was the predominant neurosis for both sexes, although depressive reactions increased for girls during adolescence.

4. Personality disorders constituted the second most frequent diagnosis for children over 5. Among the personality disorders, the passive-aggressive personality was predominant.

5. Transient situational personality disorders were the most common reported diagnostic category until age 18, at which time the rate dropped abruptly.

6. Psychophysiological disorders constituted the least frequent diagnosis rendered, accounting for only slightly more than 1 per cent of cases with a diagnosed disorder. Perhaps the youngsters suffering from psychosomatic illnesses are more commonly treated by a pediatrician or a general practitioner in a regular medical setting.

These data are interesting but probably should not be accepted at face value. Because of the inadequacies associated with psychiatric diagnoses, noted earlier, it is difficult to state with certitude the types of psychiatric problems with which children of a given age range are afflicted. In interpreting these data, the reader would do well to remember the reluctance to "label" children as well as the inadequacies associated with psychiatric diagnoses.

Educational Maladjustment

There is considerable evidence to show that educational maladjustment is associated with personal maladjustment in school-age children. Burke and Simons (1965), using a questionnaire technique with institutionalized delinquents, reported that more than 90 per cent of the sample had records of truancy and poor school adjustment, nearly three-fourths had failed two or more grades, more than 75 per cent had left school at or before the legal age of 16, two-thirds were reading below the sixth-grade level, and 60 per cent had I.Q. scores in the average range. A recent large-scale investigation of public-school classes for emotionally disturbed children of normal intellectual ability revealed that a significant degree of academic retardation accompanied the emotional maladjustment characteristic of this population (Morse, Cutler, & Fink, 1964). Evidence of the relationship between academic and emotional disturbance was also forthcoming from Gilbert's (1957) findings that academic difficulty constituted a very frequent reason for referral to metropolitan community clinics. Recent data on hospitalized emotionally disturbed pupils indicated that female students were 1 year retarded and male students 2 years retarded in reading and arithmetic achievement when mental age was used as the expectancy criterion (Motto & Lathan, 1966).

Not uncommonly, it is very difficult to distinguish between educational maladjustment and personal maladjustment in school-age youth. The finding of a close relationship between the two is not unexpected since accomplishment in school-related activities constitutes perhaps the major developmental task of youth in our society. Hence, if something interferes with the achievement of a reasonable mastery of this developmental task, it is difficult to conceive that such failure would not adversely influence other aspects of the child's personal adjustment. By definition, developmental tasks are interrelated, so that success or failure in one task tends to increase the likelihood of success or failure in others. We are not by any means equating educational and personal maladjustment. It is obvious that broader and more nonacademic criteria must be considered or applied in arriving at a definition of emotional disturbance in children. We are, however, stressing the notion that adjustment to schoolwork must exercise a pervasive influence on the child's mental health.

Typical findings illustrating the relationship between educational and personal maladjustment are those of Bedoian (1954), who reported that overage children receive significantly lower scores upon sociometric testing than do pupils who are underage or at-age for their grade level. To gain a fuller appreciation of the potential impact school can have on personality formation, the reader has only to reflect on Miller's (1936) estimate that a pupil will spend approximately 12,000 hours in a classroom setting during the course of his 12 years of schooling. One can imagine the number of positive and negative social reinforcers a child receives over such an extended period of time. If the psychology of learning has taught us anything, it is that overlearned activities become a part of us, for better or for worse.

Socioeconomic Status and Race

Mental-health specialists are becoming increasingly aware of and concerned about the role played by social and cultural factors in childhood psychopathology. Clinic termination rates based on data for 579 of 682 clinics in 25 states indicate that nonwhite rates are higher during most of adolescence and adulthood, although lower in early childhood (ages 3 to 11) except for mental deficiency. Moreover, nonwhites tend to be seen for disorders with the greatest impairment (brain syndromes, psychotic disturbances) in contrast to whites (Rosen, Bahn, & Kramer, 1964). Data based on a broader coverage of psychiatric facilities, such as hospitals, private practitioners, and emergency departments, similarly reflect these racial differences (Gardner, Miles, & Bahn, 1963). State-hospital admission rates likewise show considerably higher incidence for nonwhites than for whites (Pugh & MacMahon, 1962). Racial differences at the elementary-school level have not been carefully studied, although problems of classroom management do tend to be more common in the Negro slum school (Glidewell & Swallow, 1968).

The higher incidence of behavior disorders in Negroes than in whites can be attributed to the debilitating influence of such factors as prejudice, discrimination, segregation, an unstable and matriarchal family structure, restricted educational and vocational opportunities, and a deeply rooted negative self-image (Ausubel & Ausubel, 1963).

According to Douglas (1959), externalization of frustrations resulting from such conditions has resulted in a juvenile-delinquency rate in Negroes that surpasses that of whites by at least 2 to 1. Not surprisingly, suppressed feelings of aggression (Karon, 1958) and a high level of anxiety (Palermo, 1959) have been identified as salient features of Negro maladjustment. Though the need for mental-health services appears to be greater for Negroes than for whites, clients from impoverished backgrounds have a relatively shorter length of clinic stay (Bahn, Chandler, & Eisenberg, 1962). As noted earlier in the chapter, psychiatric services are not necessarily correlated with the needs of the clientele.

When socioeconomic status, irrespective of race, is examined, the picture remains basically unchanged. Bower (1961), in his California study, reported a higher incidence of disturbed children among certain occupational groups. The group whose fathers' occupations were categorized as "service" or "semiskilled" produced more than twice as many emotionally handicapped pupils as would be anticipated on the basis of their percentage of the state's total population. Fathers in the "unskilled" occupation category also produced more than their share of emotionally disturbed children. Pupils of fathers who were employed in professional or managerial positions, on the other hand, produced far fewer emotionally disturbed children than was expected. In another study (McDermott et al., 1965), psychiatric evaluation of 263 children of blue-collar workers indicated a significantly higher incidence of personality and borderline states among children in the "unskilled" group than in the "skilled" group. Further, there were noticeable differences in school performance in favor of the "skilled" group. Yet, somewhat paradoxically, referrals to clinics for professional treatment nonetheless were made relatively later for the unskilled group. Additional evidence regarding the influence of socioeconomic variables on mental health is found in Hollingshead and Redlich's (1958) classical study which reported families of unskilled laborers and semiskilled factory workers contributing almost twice their expected share of both disturbed boys and girls for the age group 15 years and under. Conversely, families occupying positions of high social prestige contributed only their expected share of disturbed boys and none at all to their expected share of disturbed girls. In sum, such studies indicate that maladjustment in children is not randomly distributed throughout the social classes. On the contrary, teachers tend to view maladjustment as more prevalent in the lower strata of society. It should be noted, however, that the findings relative to social-class differences are not as consistent and clear-cut as those associated with sex. White and Charry (1966), for instance, found no significant social-class differences between referred and nonreferred children in Westchester County, New York.

As was noted earlier, clinic services appear to be inversely related to the needs of the patients; that is, those patients or groups of patients who need the services most are least apt to get them, while treatment is extended to those who are thought to have a higher improvement rate. Although there is no deliberate policy designed to limit acceptance of the less-advantaged classes (who tend to have the most severe prognoses for treatment), there is considerable evidence to suggest the culture-bound nature of our treatment agencies (Schneiderman, 1965). The notion that social-class status is correlated with acceptance or rejection for psychiatric treatment is given support in a study completed by the Family Service Association of America, showing that a client from the lower classes has only a 30 per cent chance of continuing service in contrast to a 60 per cent chance for middle-class clients. It was also discovered that termination of service by the social worker as opposed to termination by the client himself increases sharply as the social class decreases (Cloward, 1963). Data gathered on public, tax-supported agencies yield essentially similar results. Applying for psychiatric service is apparently like applying for a loan. If you can demonstrate that you really don't need the money, you can get it. On the other hand, if you demonstrate that you really do need it, you are considered a poor risk and you do not get it. Analogously speaking, if the client can demonstrate that he has a stable family, reasonable ego strength, a capacity for insight, adequate verbal facility, and so on, he can get treatment. On the other hand, if he is lacking in these, he is regarded as not ready for treatment and therefore cannot get help. Further, there is evidence to suggest that the mere addition of services per se will not change this state of affairs (Rudolph & Cumming, 1962). It was found, for example, that the higher the status of the community agency, the more rigid or fixed it becomes in technique and in the problems it considers suitable for treatment. Also, the more highly trained the staff, the more efficient they become at rejecting clients who are not yet ready for service. The study concluded that the role of the agency workers is defined not so much in terms of the needs to be met as in terms of the special skill of the workers. Evidence thus suggests that the more professional services improve, the more they are geared to a middle-class clientele.[2]

SUMMARY

In this chapter the concept of diagnosis has been critically examined. Special attention was devoted to the difficulties associated with this concept. Controversy continues as to whether a medical or a psychosocial diagnostic model is more appropriate for dealing with emotional disturbances. Various classification schemes were presented following the discussion on diagnosis. Some mental-health specialists classify according to such factors as etiology, developmental considerations, and "Who suffers?" Foremost among more recent classification approaches are the clinical descriptive approach advanced by the Committee on Child Psychiatry, the empirical approach advanced by Quay, a social-learning-theory approach outlined by Bandura, and the psychoeducational approach proposed by Bower. The need for further research in this area is quite evident. In addition to the general problems associated with diagnosis, there are certain specific problems which complicate assessment of the child's behavior, for example, the child's limited linguistic facility.

The best evidence to date suggests that among elementary-school students approximately 30 per cent show at least mild, subclinical problems of adjustment. There are 10 per cent who need professional attention and 4 per cent who would actually be referred to clinical facilities if the services were available (Glidewell & Swallow, 1968).

---

[2]Although deplorable, clinic policies are not without some reasonable basis in reality. Because the prognostic criteria for successful treatment such as sufficient motivation, verbal facility, adequate education, reasonable insight, and parental support for therapy are often lacking among poor people, limiting their acceptance has some rational basis. It is understandable that mental-health specialists work with clients for whom their techniques are beneficial and shy away from clients for whom their techniques are ineffective. The basic problem is not one of discrimination. Rather, mental-health professionals have not, for the most part, found ways to work with clients from the lower socioeconomic brackets. While we have become increasingly aware of the mental-health needs of the lower socioeconomic segments of our society, we have also lacked the knowledge and skills to treat their problems effectively. We will need to pursue additional research and practice which will expand our competence to treat those vast numbers whose needs are now neglected. Merely changing admission policies will not improve people's mental health. There must also be advances in therapeutic practices.

The relationship is reported between incidence figures and such variables as age, sex, educational achievement, socioeconomic status, and race. Referral rates to clinics tend to be highest during the preadolescent and adolescent years, although it is not altogether clear from data gathered on public-school populations that the actual incidence of *clinical* maladjustment varies greatly with age during the school years. Sex differences in the prevalence of maladjustment have been clearly documented at an approximate ratio of 3 boys to 1 girl. Educational retardation is commonly found among maladjusted youth. Educational maladjustment and personal maladjustment are not interchangeable terms, however. The incidence of maladjustment is reportedly higher among lower socioeconomic groups, but there is less consistency for social-class differences than for sex differences. Data from community clinics do not suggest a higher rate of disorder (except for mental retardation) for nonwhites than for whites until the adolescent years. More careful research will be needed before any definitive statements can be made regarding racial differences and emotional disturbance among elementary-school pupils.

SUGGESTED READINGS

Committee on Child Psychiatry. *Psychopathological disorders in childhood: theoretical considerations and a proposed classification.* New York: Group for the Advancement of Psychiatry, 1966.

Glidewell, J., & Swallow, C. *The prevalence of maladjustment in elementary schools.* Chicago: Univer. of Chicago Press, 1968.

Milton, O. *Behavior disorders: perspectives and trends.* New York: Lippincott. 1965.

Schofield, W. *Psychotherapy: the purchase of friendship.* Englewood Cliffs, N.J.: Prentice-Hall, 1965.

REFERENCES

Adams, H. Mental illness or interpersonal behavior. *Amer. Psychologist,* 1964, **19**, 191-197.

American Psychiatric Association. *Diagnostic and statistical manual of mental disorders.* Washington, D.C.: Mental Hospital Services, 1952, 1968.

Anderson, J. E., Harris, D. B., Werner, E., Gallistel, E. *A survey of children's adjustment over time: a report to the people of Nobles County.* Minneapolis: Univer. of Minnesota Press, 1959.

Ausubel, D. *Theory and problems of child development.* New York, Grune & Stratton, 1958.

Ausubel, D., & Ausubel, P. Ego development among segregated Negro children. In A. H. Passow (Ed.), *Education in depressed areas.* New York: Teachers College Press, 1963. Pp. 109-141.

Bahn, A., Chandler, C. A., & Eisenberg, L. Diagnostic characteristics related to services in psychiatric clinics for children. *Milbank mem. Fund Quart.,* 1962, **15**, 289-318.

Bandura, A. A social learning interpretation of psychological dysfunctions. In P. London & D. Rosenhan (Eds.), *Foundations of abnormal psychology.* New York: Holt, Rinehart & Winston, 1968. Pp. 293-344.

Becker, W., Peterson, D., Hellmer, L., Shoemaker, D., & Quay, H. Factors in parental behavior and personality as related to problem behavior in children. *J. consult. Psychol.,* 1959, **23**, 107-118.

Bedoian, U. H. Social acceptability and social rejection of underage, at-age, and overage pupils in the sixth grade. *J. educ. Res.,* 1954, **47**, 513-520.

Beller, E. K. *Clinical process: a new approach to the organization and assessment of clinical data.* Glencoe, Ill.: Free Press, 1962.

Bower, E. M. *The early identification of emotionally handicapped children in school.* Springfield, Ill.: Thomas, 1960.

Bower, E. M. *The education of emotionally handicapped children.* Sacramento: California State Department of Education, 1961.

Bower, E. M. Mental health. In R. Ebel (Ed.), *Encyclopedia of educational research.* (4th ed.) New York: Macmillan, 1970. Pp. 811-828.

Burke, N. S., & Simons, A. E. Factors which precipitate dropouts and delinquency. *Fed. Probation,* 1965, **29**, 28-32.

Cloward, R. Social class and private social agencies. *Proc. of annual meeting of Council on Social Work Education,* Boston, 1963.

Committee on Child Psychiatry. *Psychopathological disorders in childhood: theoretical considerations and a proposed classification.* New York: Group for the Advancement of Psychiatry, 1966.

Douglas, J. H. The extent and characteristics of juvenile delinquency in the United States. *J. Negro Educ.,* 1959, **28**, 214-229.

Eisenberg, L. *Emotionally disturbed children and youth: children and youth in the 1960's.* Survey of papers prepared for 1960 White House Golden Anniversary Conference on Children and Youth. Washington, D.C.: Government Printing Office, 1960.

Freud, A. *Normality and pathology in childhood.* New York: International Universities Press, 1965.

Gardner, E. H., Miles, H. C., & Bahn A. K. A cumulative survey of psychiatric experience in a community: report of the first year's experience. *Arch. gen. Psychiat.,* 1963, **9**, 369-378.

Gilbert, G. M. A survey of "referral problems" in metropolitan child guidance centers. *J. clin. Psychol.,* 1957, **13**, 37-42.

Glazer, N. Trends in mental disorder. In A. M. Rose (Ed.), *Mental health and mental disorder.* New York: Norton, 1955. Pp. 117-122.

Glidewell, J., & Swallow, C. *The prevalence of maladjustment in elementary schools.* Chicago: Univer. of Chicago Press, 1968.

Hollingshead, A. B., & Redlich, F. C. *Social class and mental illness: a community study.* New York: Wiley, 1958.

Hunt, W. A. Diagnosis and non-directive theory. *J. clin. Psychol.,* 1948, **4**, 232-236.

Jenkins, R. Symptomatology and dynamics in diagnosis: a medical perspective. *J. clin. Psychol.,* 1953, **9**, 149-150.

Karon, B. P. *The Negro personality.* New York: Springer, 1958.

London, P. *The modes and morals of psychotherapy.* New York: Holt, Rinehart & Winston, 1964.

Louttit, C. M. *Clinical psychology of children's behavior problems.* (Rev. ed.) New York: Harper, 1947.

McDermott, J., Harrison, S., Schrager, J., & Wilson, P. Social class and mental illness in children: observation of blue-collar families. *Amer. J. Orthopsychiat.,* 1965, **35**, 500-508.

Miller, E. Classification of the disorders of childhood. In Sir Humphrey Rolleston (Ed.), *British encyclopedia of medical practice.* London: Butterworth, 1936.

Morse, W. C., Cutler, R. L., & Fink, A. H. *Public school classes for the emotionally handicapped: a research analysis.* Washington, D.C.: Council for Exceptional Children, 1964.

Motto, J. J., & Lathan, L. An analysis of children's educational achievement and related variables in a state psychiatric hospital. *Except. Child.,* 1966, **32**, 619-623.

Pacella, B. L. *Behavior problems in children.* Medical clinics of North America series. Philadelphia: Saunders, 1948.

Palermo, D. S. Racial comparisons and additional normative data on the children's manifest anxiety scale. *Child Develpm.,* 1959, **30**, 53-57.

Patterson, C. H. *Counseling and psychotherapy: theory and practice.* New York: Harper, 1959.

Patterson, G. R. An empirical approach to the classification of disturbed children. *J. clin. Psychol.,* 1964, **20**, 326-337.

Peterson, D. Behavior problems of middle childhood. *J. consult. Psychol.,* 1961, **25**, 205-209.

Pugh, T. F., & MacMahon, B. *Epidemiologic findings in United States mental hospital data.* Boston: Little, Brown, 1962.

Quay, H. The structure of children's behavior disorders. Paper read at colloquia at the University of Minnesota, 1965.

Quay, H., & Quay, L. Behavior problems in early adolescence. *Child Develpm.,* 1965, **36**, 215-220.

Rogers, C. R. The criteria used in a study of mental health problems. *Educ. Res. Bull.* (Ohio State Univer.), 1942, **21**, 29-40.

Rose, J. A. The emotional problems of children in psychiatry for the general practitioner; abstract from the seminar series. Carrier Clinic, Philadelphia Mental Health Educational Unit of Smith, Kline and French Laboratories, 1958.

Rosen, B. M., Bahn, A. K., & Kramer, M. Demographic and diagnostic characteristics of psychiatric clinic outpatients in the U.S.A., 1961. *Amer. J. Orthopsychiat.,* 1964, **34**, 455-468.

Rosenthal, D. Book reviews. *Psychiat.,* 1962, **61**, 377-380.

Rudolph, C., & Cumming, J. Where are additional psychiatric services most needed? *Soc. Wk,* 1962, **7**, 15-20.

Sarason, S. B., Lighthall, F. F., Davidson, K. S., Waite, R. R., & Ruebush, B. K. *Anxiety in elementary school children.* New York: Wiley, 1960.

Schneiderman, L. Social class diagnosis and treatment. *Amer. J. Orthopsychiat.,* 1965, **35,** 99-105.

Schofield, W. *Psychotherapy: the purchase of friendship.* Englewood Cliffs, N. J.: Prentice-Hall, 1965.

Smith, M. B. The revolution in mental health care—a bold new approach? *Trans-action,* 1968, **5,** 19-23.

Szasz, T. The myth of mental illness. *Amer. Psychologist,* 1960, **15,** 113-118.

Ullmann, C. A. Mental health screening of school children. *Publ. Hlth Rep.,* 1952, **67,** 1219-1223.

U.S. Children's Bureau. *Juvenile court statistics.* Statistical Series No. 73. Washington, D.C.: Government Printing Office, 1963.

U.S. Department of Health, Education, and Welfare. *Patients in mental institutions in U.S.A., 1964.* Washington, D.C.: Government Printing Office, 1965.

White, M. A., & Charry, J. (Eds.) *School disorder, intelligence and social class.* New York: Teachers College Press, 1966.

White, M. A., & Harris, M. *The school psychologist.* New York: Harper, 1961.

White, R. *The abnormal personality.* (3rd ed.) New York: Ronald Press, 1964.

Part II

Behavior Disorders in Children

3

Psychoneurotic Disorders

DEFINITIONS
SOURCES OF DATA ON INCIDENCE
CHARACTERISTICS
CLASSIFICATION
DIFFERENTIAL DIAGNOSTIC CONSIDERATIONS
  • *REACTIVE DISORDERS* • *DEVELOPMENTAL DEVIATIONS*
  • *PERSONALITY DISORDERS*
ETIOLOGICAL CONSIDERATIONS
  • *PSYCHOLOGICAL FACTORS [The Freudian View of Childhood Origin /*
  Learning Theory / Parent-Child Relations] • *CONSTITUTIONAL FACTORS*
  • *SOCIOCULTURAL FACTORS*
TREATMENT AND PROGNOSIS
EXAMPLE: SCHOOL PHOBIA
  • *INCIDENCE* • *ONSET AND COURSE* • *TREATMENT* • *PROGNOSIS*

Adjustment difficulties included in the psychoneurotic-reaction group have been the objects of much interest, even bordering on preoccupation, from behavioral specialists. At one time such problems were thought to be highly prevalent, identifiable in 1 of every 5 persons. Because of the apparent close relationship with anxiety, psychoneurotic reactions were among the first behavior disorders to be studied extensively in the laboratory. The relative ease with which communication can be established with psychoneurotic persons and the seemingly favorable results elicited by a variety of treatment methods undoubtedly served to encourage and reinforce the attention directed to psychoneuroses. Popular acceptance of these disorders has reached the point of investing the appellation "neurotic" with something of the aura of a status symbol.

Even though many of the initial beliefs about the psychoneurotic reactions have had to be altered or discarded, continued explorations of what are more popularly referred to as *neuroses* have generated some of the most useful understandings applicable to all behavior. Situated somewhere between the severe disorders, as represented by the psychoses, and the "normal" personality, the psychoneuroses have bridged a crucial gap. From this springboard has come impetus counteracting attempts to understand the normal person on the basis of the severely pathological and leading to a more wholesome orientation of understanding the disorganized personality in terms of failures in normal personality organization. The shift to understanding the disordered in constructs drawn from the normal has provided much valuable insight into the way in which individuals attempt to deal with stress and how response patterns can be perpetuated. Approaches which are based on conceptions of normal personality development have added greatly to the clinician's skill in evaluating all behaviors. The initially reported high incidence of neuroses (1 in 5 persons), for example, now seems to have been an artifact resulting from impressions gained by dealing predominantly with pathological personalities.

In this chapter, current concepts and points of view about the neuroses will be reviewed with relevance to these disorders as encountered in children and adolescents. Considerations will include types of stresses, techniques for coping with stress, diagnostic problems, and the necessity for the cooperative involvement of several professional specialties in the management of childhood psychoneuroses.

DEFINITIONS

Descriptions of psychoneuroses have centered around two theoretical orientations. From the psychoanalytic viewpoint, neuroses are regarded as the manifestation of an unresolved internal conflict. The handling of such themes as dependency, competency, and aggressiveness becomes the origin for neurotic conflicts. The ego is taxed to maintain a balance among the personality components and must divert increasing amounts of energy to protection from dangers which seem to threaten psychological security. The symptomatology of the neurosis mirrors the ego's struggle to resolve the basic conflict and lower the uncomfortably high anxiety level. An illustration may be found in the pupil who builds a powerful resentment for the teacher who continually criticizes his efforts in writing. The hostility may be expressed as a sudden paralysis of the hand which would be used to strike the teacher.

From a behavioristic or learning-theory perspective, a high level of anxiety is also deemed essential in the formation of psychoneurotic reaction. The source of the anxiety, which may be in such developmental aspects of personality as individuation, role identification, or social integration, is, however, of minor importance. What is crucial is that the anxiety level is uncomfortable and must be lowered. Social outlets are chosen largely on the basis of availability and retained according to their personal suitability as release avenues. An example is provided by a girl who was never very assertive because she doubted her ability to do anything well. On seeing her listlessness, people frequently commented that she must be ill. Gradually the girl withdrew from participation in new events, offering the excuse of being ill. She seemed to find sufficient satisfactions in the role of an invalid.

Extreme anxiety associated with ineffectiveness in meeting life demands, an outcome common to both of the preceding explanations, is the major characteristic defining a neurotic reaction. The impairment involves the total personality organization, but it tends to be more readily observable in one large life area, such as adjustment to work, friendships, marriage, or physical health. Inadequate functioning persists in the face of evidence of adequate intellectual ability, good physical health, and normal family and home background. A disproportionate amount of personal resources must be directed to seeking outlets and channels for discharging anxiety. Behavior becomes inconsistent and overlaid with an orientation of immediacy and with an ensuing decline in efficiency. Complaints of personal unhappiness, discomfort, and distress are common to this cyclic pattern of intense anxiety and compensatory efforts to reduce the anxiety to a more tolerable level.

SOURCES OF DATA ON INCIDENCE

Estimates of the prevalence of psychoneuroses vary considerably. The early clinicians working with emotional disorders apparently saw a disproportionate number of neurotics. In the past, physicians engaged in general practice have estimated that about half of the persons they see as patients are psychoneurotic. The neurotic individual wants others to know that he is having difficulty and seeks someone to listen to his problems. This trait undoubtedly introduces some exaggeration in estimated reports of incidence. Although tangible data reporting on the incidence of any behavior disorder present many problems of interpretation, as was discussed in Chapter 2, they provide the best available source for suggesting the prevalence of a condition.

1. *Outpatient Clinics.* A report presented by Rosen, Bahn, and Kramer (1964) enumerates persons given terminal outpatient service at community mental-health clinics in 1961. Children (persons under 18 years of age) made up 54 per cent of the approximately 350,000 patients reported. Of the total number of children seen, 1 in 10 was diagnosed as psychoneurotic. In the psychoneurotic category, the number of boys was only slightly higher than the number of girls. The incidence rates followed interesting age-trend patterns, however. Boys showed a peak prevalence in the age range from 9 to 14 years, whereas the peak prevalence for girls was in the 14 to 16 age range. The number of boys in the psychoneurotic category at age 10 years was twice that for girls. The incidence rates became equal at about age 14, and by age 20 the picture was reversed, with female outnumbering male psychoneurotics by 2 to 1.

2. *Hospitalized Inpatients.* The report compiled by Rosen, Bahn, and Kramer (1964) enumerates similar data for approximately 270,000 persons admitted to a state, county, or private mental hospital in 1962 with no prior history of hospitalization (first admissions). The data indicate that approximately 1 child (persons under 15 years of age) in 13 children was diagnosed as psychoneurotic. The incidence ratio for psychoneuroses indicated by inpatient data (1 in 13) is not much higher than that for outpatient data (1 in 10). This figure is surprising when it is considered that hospitalization for children is regarded as a drastic measure only to be taken as a last resort. Nevertheless, the many factors influencing the data as reported make it inadvisable to generalize or offer much interpretation of statistical patterns suggested.

3. *Schools.* Data which might be the most helpful for planning programs to alleviate psychoneuroses, detailed analyses of school populations, have been least available. This fact is unquestionably related to the uncertainty which schools have felt about the entire matter of responsibility for the treatment of behavior disorders. The popular procedure has been to refer these children to facilities outside the

school agencies for care and treatment. The few scattered studies which report incidences of psychoneuroses in school populations often do so in gross ways which may raise more questions than are answered. In a study of children seen at a community child-guidance clinic, for example, Kurlander and Colodny (1965) reported that from 25 to 50 per cent of the children were suffering from psychoneuroses. In a survey of the characteristics of public-school pupils in special classes for the socially and emotionally maladjusted, Morse, Cutler, and Fink (1964) concluded that 60 per cent of the children in these classes were psychoneurotic. There were approximately 3 boys for every 2 girls in the student groups studied. One study carried out in a public-school system carefully assessed the prevalence of the psychoneurotic reaction "school phobia." In this study, Leton (1962) stated that the incidence of school phobia was 3 per 1,000 pupils in the primary grades but increased to 1 per 100 students by high school. Pointing out that most mild and moderate cases may go undetected, he estimated that less than half of the cases of school phobia may actually be diagnosed. The peak of incidence occurs in pupils aged 6 to 10. Leton randomly selected 12 pupils for detailed study as representatives of the disorder. It is interesting that in this group of 7 girls and 5 boys, only 1 pupil came from the lower sociocultural level, 3 from the upper, and the other 8 from the middle.

Much of the confusion encountered in interpreting incidence data stems from biases inherent in the diagnostic "rules" prevailing in treatment agencies. Clinics serving outpatients, for example, tend to favor diagnoses emphasizing situational and temporary conditions (personality disorders, transient situational personality disorders). This orientation of immediacy may mask chronic features, an essential element in making a diagnosis of psychoneurosis. Another difficulty is the lack of information as to the developmental relevance of certain behaviors (fears, nailbiting, night terrors, and enuresis) generally seen in the group of symptoms which identify a neurosis.

Nevertheless, such data as are available must be taken as a start in planning the alleviation of psychoneurotic disorders. The data indicate that, although not the most frequent, psychoneurotic disorders are one of the major behavior problems seen in children. The incidence, ranging from 5 per 1,000 to 1 per 100 pupils, reaches a peak at about age 10 for boys and 14 for girls. Initially more commonly seen in males, the incidence equalizes and then becomes more common for females in adulthood. The relationship between incidence rates and sociocultural levels is not clear and needs additional study.

CHARACTERISTICS

Although the accompanying behavioral responses vary from one to another individual, the common problem is that of handling anxiety. This procedure entails the setting up of protective measures which have the object of preventing the buildup of anxiety and the development of methods for reducing anxiety by release through some available channel. Constitutional, personal, and social factors contribute to the choice of ways for handling anxiety which take the form of extreme responses in the following areas:

1. *Motor Characteristics.* Deviations in motor responses are among the most commonly observed of psychoneurotic symptoms. The expressions often are of an active nature and include episodes of running, floor-pacing, restlessness, hand-wringing, temper outbursts, and tearing or throwing objects. Passive activities seem to be effective in releasing anxiety for some persons. Thus immobile freezing and loss of muscle tone and control (as in fainting or paralysis) are also encountered. Motor responses may take on a perseverative quality, such as the repetitious washing of hands or the avoidance of cracks in the sidewalk. These repeated acts are termed *compulsions.* In still other instances, the motor activity may have a pronounced ceremonial quality. Preoccupations with seeing that stacks of books are exactly aligned, clothes are hanging in a fixed arrangement, shoes are placed in an exact line, and a rigid following of stereotyped patterns of going to bed are examples of such ritualistic motor activities. Yet another variety of motor reactions entails the rhythmic contracting of small or specific muscles, frequently facial muscles; such muscle twitches are known as *tics.*

2. *Somatic Characteristics.* Many psychoneurotic symptoms are of a somatic nature and can pose difficulties in differentiating them from actual physical illnesses. Sometimes these physical complaints are of a vague and general nature, such as not feeling well (malaise), loss of pain sensitivity (anesthesia), loss of appetite (anorexia), feeling dizzy (vertigo), or inability to sleep (insomnia). Other somatic complaints are of a specific nature and include headaches, irregularities of breathing, variations in heartbeat, regurgitation of food,

constipation, and loss of vision or audition. A particularly interesting somatic complaint frequently encountered is that of choking and inability to swallow (globus hystericus). Symptoms in the form of somatic complaints are readily accepted as valid excuses and even secure a certain amount of attention and sympathy for the individual.

3. *Intellectual Disturbances.* Certain characteristics seen in psychoneuroses can be regarded as breakdowns in intellectual functions. The more common of these symptoms have obsessive-compulsive qualities. The repetitive counting of seemingly irrelevant objects (lights, telephone poles, tiles in a floor, steps) and persisting thoughts, songs, or sayings are examples. There may be a ritualistic concern with magic and counteractions to avoid the "bad luck" of breaking a mirror or having a black cat cross one's path. More spectacular but less frequently observed disorders of intellectual functions are brief memory lapses (amnesias); longer periods of losses are known as *fugues.* More difficult to detect are changes to rigid and inflexible ways of thinking.

4. *Emotional Deviations.* The most common emotional reaction associated with neuroses is that of depression and unhappiness. Inhibitory and excessive control of impulses, seen as a feature in some forms of neurotic adjustment, results in a sober and overly serious emotional tone. Other neurotic individuals can become excitedly "charged-up" for brief periods of time, but emotional outbursts of anger and episodes of uncontrollable laughing or crying are more typically observed. With these emotional episodes, the person may appear distraught and apprehensive. If anxiety is considered as an emotion, then anxiety is a basic feature of all neurotic reactions.

5. *Language Characteristics.* Distortions in speech are not commonly observed with neuroses. Some speech pathologists have attempted to relate such a speech impairment as stuttering to a psychoneurotic reaction, but the connection has not thus far been convincingly demonstrated. The voice volume is often low for persons with a neurosis, giving a kind of weak voice. There are also episodes of the other extreme, with shouting and ranting, usually in conjunction with some hypermotor activity. Although rarely encountered, undoubtedly the most dramatic language disability is that of a sudden loss of speech (aphasia). The recovery of usual speech facility is usually spontaneous.

6. *Social Characteristics.* Behaviors symptomatic of psychoneurotic

reactions are distinguished by a social relevance perhaps more than for any other behavior disorder. Pacing the floor, restlessness, and episodes of intense grief or joy are all normal reactions. Keeping one's belongings in some orderly arrangement, being neat, and knowing the correct date and time are realistic expectations made of the responsible person. The fear and avoidance of certain objects or situations are taken as indications of intelligence and of the capacity to profit from experience. The paniclike fears of specific situations (closed-in places, high places, elevators) observed as part of some neurotic syndromes and technically referred to as *phobias* may, at least when first acquired, have had some of these same survival qualities.

CLASSIFICATION

All of these symptoms are seen in varying combinations and amounts. Continued efforts to deal with the neurosis, combined with influences from constitutional and social factors, typically lead to the development of rather durable organizations of responses. As the neurosis persists, a particular characteristic (amnesia, restless motor hyperactivity, profuse sweating, and so on) may come to stand out in the pattern. But many times, and especially in the case of children, the symptoms are in a mixed group. These varied possibilities for handling neurotogenic stresses form the basis for diagnostic classification in one of several psychoneurotic reaction types:

1. *Anxiety Type.* In this disorder, manifest anxiety as an intense feeling of apprehension or impending catastrophe is the predominant feature. There is a minimum of other motor, somatic, or language symptoms, and the acute anxiety may be related to any obvious aspects of the situation, such as the simple announcement "Now we are going to study arithmetic." The anxiety level may subside as suddenly and inexplicably as it appeared. This type of neurotic reaction is possibly made difficult to identify in children because of these cyclical changes in anxiety level and the scarcity of other symptoms.

2. *Phobic Type.* In this neurotic reaction, the anxiety has been displaced from the original threatening situation to other objects or events. The relationship between the original and the manifestly feared object or situation becomes distorted but may still be identifiable. For example, a child may fear being separated from his parents, but

he claims to fear going to school. The fear of attending school serves the purpose, hopefully, of keeping him at home with his parents.

3. *Conversion Type.* In this reaction, the emphasis in resolving the conflict follows a pattern of focusing on a disturbance involving bodily structures and organ systems. Paralyses, tics, blindness, deafness, choking, or more vague conditions of malaise and weakness designate this type of neurosis. It is not a purely chance matter that the symptom typically has possibilities for *secondary gains* for the individual. That is, not only is the child with a "paralyzed" arm not required to write his lessons, but in addition he is freely given solicitous attention by teacher and classmates.

4. *Obsessive-Compulsive Type.* The disorders of this type represent an attempt to counteract the arousal of anxiety by deliberate thoughts (obsessions) or acts (compulsions). The overt behavior may be the opposite of the threatening impulse. Repetitious washing of hands, for example, may mask a desire to be messy. The thoughts and acts are carried out even when they are admittedly unreasonable or inappropriate, and the child may in fact actively resist any effort to interfere.

5. *Mixed Type.* This is a kind of "catch-all" category to allow for classification of psychoneurotic reactions which do not clearly meet criteria for inclusion in one of the other types. It is also useful for psychoneurotic reactions in which a combination of several major symptoms is identifiable, as is often the case with children.

DIFFERENTIAL DIAGNOSTIC CONSIDERATIONS

The wide range of behaviors that are observed in psychoneurotic reactions makes it necessary to compare these symptoms with those seen in other behavior disorders. Final diagnosis may be safely arrived at only after consultative collaboration which brings together observations of the teacher, interviews obtained from parents, appraisal by a physician, and examinations carried out by a psychologist. It is of utmost importance to eliminate the possibility of a real physical illness from the diagnostic considerations. The pattern of high level of anxiety directed into familiar social outlets lends a reality orientation and social relevance to neurotic reactions and provides a sharp distinction from the disorientated and bizarre behaviors of a psychosis. Functioning effectiveness can be reduced by a neurosis and result in below-average performance similar to that seen in mental subnormality. The functioning of the mentally subnormal person remains consistently below par, whereas that of the inconsistent psychoneurotic fluctuates from above to below par. Psychoneurotic disorders require a considerable degree of personality structure before they can form and thus are not usually found in the preschool-age child. Neuroses grow out of the common processes of development and personality acquisition, however, and they are easily confused with normal reactions and response patterns.

REACTIVE DISORDERS

There are many events (sickness, accidental injuries, death of a parent or sibling, pressure from a significant failure) which can be expected to precipitate an intense emotional reaction. Such reactions may be especially pronounced in adolescents who are experiencing one of life's traumas (death of a parent or relative) for the first time. The role of environmental factors in these disorders is evident in the category preferred by some workers, "transient situational reaction." The intensity of the response will vary according to the child's developmental stage and his adaptive resources for coping with the situation. Reactive disorders differ from psychoneurotic reactions by being of short but intense duration and by usually showing a spontaneous recovery. These characteristics are generally sufficiently unique to avoid being confused with psychoneurotic disorders, even though the symptomatic behaviors may be temporarily similar. Reactive disorders may be more frequently confused with developmental deviations.

DEVELOPMENTAL DEVIATIONS

The diagnostic category of "developmental deviations" is provided to accommodate behavioral responses which are variations of normal maturational patterns. It is especially useful when working with children. We have previously considered the importance of evaluating adjustment difficulties in the light of developmental norms (see Lapouse & Monk, and MacFarlane et al., in References to Chapter 1). Accumulating data give ample evidence that thumbsucking, enuresis, temper tantrums, and the like follow developmental patterns which are unique for any one individual. Even though there are normative tendencies, the integration and achievement of these behaviors vary as to time of occurrence, sequence, and degree. They are not ordinarily accompanied by anxiety, and the developmental pattern is individually normal for the person in the sense that progression is evident, but at a pace consistent for the individual child. The actual deviation, which may be in the direction of acceleration (precocity), delay (retardation), or mixed (uneven) quality, can include disruptions in motor, sensory, speech, cognitive, social, psychosexual, or emotional development.

PERSONALITY DISORDERS

The most difficult diagnostic problem is that of differentiating personality from psychoneurotic disorders. Even an experienced clinician finds the distinction is not easily made. The similarity of the overt behavior associated with the two conditions may have contributed to impressions that psychoneurotic disorders are highly prevalent and that they are resistant to change.

Personality disorders are conditions in which the personality has become organized about a dominant trend, such as compulsivity, dependency, isolation, or opposition. Passive-aggressive personality, compulsive personality, and schizoid personality are some examples. The predominating trait is so deeply ingrained in the personality makeup that it identifies the prevalent reaction pattern of the individual, or is "characteristic" for the person. This situation is reflected in the term *character disorders,* preferred by some clinicians to designate personality disorders. As is also true for psychoneurotic disorders, personality disorders are not identifiable until the later school-age period, even though they may have origins in problems and conflicts encountered in infancy or early childhood. A certain amount of stability and development of personality is necessary before this type of organization can take place. As the organization assumes more structure, there is the impression of chronicity of the character trait, and personality disorders become highly resistant to change by usual treatment methods. Although ordinarily only mildly incapacitating, over time and in the face of repeated failures to satisfactorily resolve the conflict, another possibility comes into the picture. Such chronic failure with associated cumulative threat to the individual's security can provide the nucleus for the development of a typical psychoneurotic disorder.

Personality disorders differ from psychoneurotic disorders in that there is minimal anxiety. When present, anxiety is not associated with an intrapsychic conflict. The behavior is extreme, but is not clinically pathological. The impairments are of the most consequence in interpersonal relations, where they may contribute to the child's being regarded as a nuisance, as immature, or as just hard to get along with. The incidence of personality disorders is very high, but only a small number of such persons are seen in clinical treatment facilities. They are, in many ways, only slight exaggerations of normal traits.

ETIOLOGICAL CONSIDERATIONS

There is general agreement that anxiety plays an essential role in the development of a neurosis. In a summary of theoretical, experimental, and clinical data pertaining to anxiety, Maher (1966) discussed three ways in which anxiety may influence performance:

1. Anxiety may function as a fundamental distress reaction that occurs automatically in any situation which threatens survival of the individual, including his value system (self-concept).

2. Anxiety may be a condition of overarousal brought on by a prolonged exposure to intense stimulation and resulting in a disabling of the capacity to inhibit any stimulation.

3. Anxiety may function as a conditioned fear response made to stimuli which in the past were associated with painful punishment.

A clearer picture of how anxiety may operate is suggested by studies of reactions to stress. Two types of stress are to be considered. Brief acute stress, popularly designated as "traumatic," is typically experienced in intense emergency situations. By contrast, moderate or mild stress, termed "chronic," is experienced over a prolonged period of time. Possibly because the impact of acute stress is dramatic and obvious, parents and educators have tended to be more concerned with alleviating the consequences of traumatic stress. Relatively little attention, however, has been paid to problems posed by demands of chronic stress. Research by Davis (1956) indicated that different adjustment processes are called upon to handle acute and chronic stresses. Data gained from studies of men in combat during the Korean War showed that recovery to normal physiological functioning after chronic stress required twice as much time as did recovery from acute stress.

In a followup investigation, Funkenstein, King, and Drolette (1957) observed reactions of college undergraduates to an acute stress situation (memorizing a story under conditions of delayed auditory feedback, time limit, and electric shock) and to a chronic stress situation extending over two years (solving computational problems under conditions of razzing, criticism, time pressure, and frustration). Enormous individual differences in subjects' ability to cope with acute and chronic stress were found. But groups of variables differentially related to ability to cope with the two types of stress were also identified. Perceptions of parents, concepts of self, and fantasies were found to be related to the capacity to deal with acute stress but not related to the ability to deal with chronic stress. Variables related to the ability to master chronic stress but unrelated to the capacity to cope with acute stress included interpersonal relationships, assessment of reality, and integration of personality.

It is generally agreed that the factors related to chronic stress are acquired in a later developmental period, whereas the first set of variables is associated with earlier childhood experiences. In view of the observation that neuroses seem to require an extended time to develop, the capacity to cope with chronic stress may be a crucial factor in neurosis formation. Thus experiences of anxiety are essential, but the type of stress and the capacity for dealing with anxiety may be more important in influencing individual outcomes. A variety of factors—preferred individual adjustment techniques, underlying expectations, and acceptable patterns of behavior for males and females— may differentially favor particular adjustment mechanisms. Parsons (1942), for example, sees socialization experiences favoring obsessive-compulsive characteristics as being more typical for males, whereas hysterical traits are more frequently found in females.

It is possible to outline two general types of adjustment, each potentially neurotogenic, which can be used in resolving anxiety. These are more modes or styles for coping rather than actual discharge outlets. In one pattern, the child may be very much aware of the dynamics of the entire conflict. He can be fully aware of the fact that he is unwanted and unappreciated by his parents. He is painfully aware of his searching questions as to his own adequacy and personal worth. He becomes urgently concerned about his competency and acceptance by all other persons. He begins to take measures to "tighten up the ship" and insure that he will remain in charge. He turns to repression and diverts more and more energy into strengthening all controls. Relationships become agonizingly clear and center about the child's sensitive fear of being unable to remain his own master. Isolation, withdrawal, structured control, and ever increasing use of suppression are essential to keeping the lid screwed down tightly. The tighter the lid is held, the more energy that must be given to holding the lid down. All new experiences, and possible chances for making a more satisfactory adjustment, must be avoided. The child can't afford to make a false move or the castle will tumble.

In another possibility, the person may also be aware of anxiety, but the awareness is qualitatively different. His concern is not so much for the source of the anxiety as for the obvious fact that the high level of anxiety impairs his effectiveness and he fears that this will mean loss of face. His conflict then becomes one of being "anxious about being anxious" and he feels pressured to get rid of the anxiety as quickly as possible. Just as the source of the original anxiety was not too important, so the child is not too selective about how to discharge the anxiety; any way will do. There may be little reliance on repression, and no concern for the long-term effectiveness of the various outlets. Immediate satisfaction, prospects for secondary gain, and simple availability influence the choice of release methods. Total capacity for evaluation is more impaired in this situation than in the conflict described in the preceding paragraph. Consequently, there may be more extreme behaviors and more external indications of tumultuous personality disorganization. The methods chosen for release of tension are frequently so immature as to result in greater loss of face, more desperation, and more anxiety. Genuine insight is difficult, even impossible, for these children.

PSYCHOLOGICAL FACTORS

The outlines sketched are very general, but it is hoped that this will serve to make the reader more aware of the obvious: There is no one explanation which can adequately account for the origins of all psychoneurotic disorders. Recognizing this principle may aid in understanding why so many theoretical explanations of the etiology of neuroses are to be found. In this section, we will review briefly the contributions made by psychoanalytic theorists and learning theorists.

The Freudian View of Childhood Origin

Freud (1949) was convinced that the neurotic disorders he saw in adults had origins in unsatisfactorily resolved childhood conflicts. He had provided a classical description of neurosis ensuing from the person's fear that primitive id instincts, especially those of sex and aggression, would overpower the ego. The personality organization would thus be upset and disorganized. Although id impulses constituted the primary source of threat, conflict and resulting disturbance of the personality balance would also occur when excessive guilt from the superego menaced the ego. In either situation, the ego was faced with having to take steps to defend the personality. The protective measures taken entailed a symbolic representation of the unresolved conflict or, put in other terms, the symptoms were expressions of the perceived threat.

Freud's followers have made many additions to his original concepts. Most of the extensions have been in the nature of allowing greater importance for the influence of socialization. Such accounts have been developed by Karen Horney, Harry Stack Sullivan, and more recently by Robert White.

Horney (1937) was primarily concerned with adjustment as the establishing of socially and personally acceptable relationships with other persons. She described three basic approaches for relating to persons as compliance, aggression, and detachment. When any one of these approaches came to be relied on excessively, the conditions for a neurotic conflict were set in operation.

In his interpersonal theories, Sullivan (1953) believed that the nature of the child's relationships with other persons was the basis for conflicts. When the child experienced warm and satisfying relationships, he gained a feeling of personal security and adequacy. Where these satisfactions were not comfortable or satisfying, the child was inclined to feel insecure and to have a chronic high level of anxiety.

White (1964) recognizes two sources of stress in childhood which can set the stage for neurotic conflict: sudden, intense trauma (being in an accident), or chronic threat (years of never being able to please parents). Either of these threats can leave an impairment, a condition which White compares with the residual motor deficit of the cerebral-palsied child. Such a neurotogenic deficit typically is one involving aggression, dependency, or rejection. The child must establish a protective organization to compensate for the deficit. His entire range of responses becomes oriented toward concealment of the defect. In order to maintain this protective organization, the child makes excessive efforts. These overdriven strivings are identifiable on the basis of three criteria:

1. *Indiscriminateness.* A given response is made all the time, as the child who always seeks approval.

2. *Insatiability.* The child is never satisfied no matter how great the reward; given one gold star, he wants two, and so on.

3. *Overreaction.* An increase to an excessive level of frustration, aggression, or desperation.

By this time the neurosis is well defined, and White believes that the overdriven strivings constitute the basis for maintaining the neurotic disorder and its essential trait of chronicity.

Learning Theory

Laboratory explorations of anxiety have clarified many phenomena seen in association with psychoneurotic reactions. Dollard and Miller (1950) found that anxiety does function as a potent drive, facilitating the acquisition of responses and having properties of generalization. Clinicians had long been puzzled by the apparently maladaptive responses of neurotics, such as the child who is "too ill" to attend a party but complains that he has no friends. Reactions of this type, referred to as the *neurotic paradox,* were shown by Mowrer (1950) to be retained on the basis of having immediate reward value, which seemed to outweigh the eventual consequences of punishment and discomfort.

Continued study indicated that any response could serve to release anxiety and be sufficiently rewarding to become a durable reaction. Thus reaction patterns which had previously seemed irrelevant and illogical were understandable as anxiety-reducing conditioned responses. The difficulty encountered in the laboratory in extinguishing these rewarding responses also suggested a basis for the clinically observed characteristics of chronicity and resistance to change associated with neuroses. The pupil who becomes highly worried about how well he will do on an examination may find the worry reinforced if he does poorly *or* if he does well. A situation is then set for his becoming a "worry bird" in response to each new demand.

Kurt Lewin's (1935) investigations have provided a productive frame of reference for understanding how anxiety is generated by everyday activities. We are constantly faced with having to make choices between two sets of relationships, or goals. Sometimes the choice is a very easy one, but other times it can be difficult. The situation may be an attractive one which holds pleasant rewards, or it may be a negative one which holds unpleasant consequences. Different degrees of conflict may arise from decisions made in resolving these four kinds of situations:

1. *Approach–Approach.* In this case, a decision is made between two pleasant prospectives, such as when a child is asked to choose between a cooky or a piece of candy.

2. *Approach–Avoidance.* Here the decision entails selecting a pleasant or an unpleasant outcome. A young adult may want to marry but at the same time be reluctant to forgo the advantages of bachelorhood.

3. *Avoidance–Avoidance.* In this set of affairs, the child finds it necessary to decide between two objectives, both unpleasant. He must choose whether to complete a disliked homework assignment or to face a parent angered by the fact that the homework is not completed.

4. *Double Approach–Avoidance.* This type of conflict is possibly best understood as a complex approach–avoidance situation. Rather than holding only approach or avoidance attractions, the two goals have both approach and avoidance qualities. Other persons have suggested "double bind" to refer to these cases where whatever response is made has both positive and negative consequences.

It is believed that resolutions of approach–approach situations are the least likely to have unfavorable consequences since the outcome in either case is pleasant. Although sometimes presenting clear alternatives and relatively simple choices, approach–avoidance situations can demand exceedingly fine discriminations which delay solution and introduce a state of suspended tension. There are moderate possibilities for a chronic stress state and subsequent maladjustment. Avoidance–avoidance and double approach–avoidance circumstances are regarded as having the greatest potency for fostering pathological behavior. Not only is a high degree of anxiety aroused by the prospect of punishment for whatever response is made, but there is a built-in feature of chronicity as the individual may seek to avoid making any decision and the conflict hangs unresolved.

Consistent with their belief that the important sources of conflict are inherent in socialization processes, Dollard and Miller (1950) and Sears (1951) have described ways in which acculturization demands associated with training in eating, toileting, cleanliness, sex role, competition, and handling aggression are replete with such stress situations.

As will be seen later in this chapter and in the chapters on therapy and classroom managment, there has risen a group of learning theorists known as behavior therapists who deal strictly with behavior change. In practice, behavior therapists deal rather directly with the symptoms or surface behavior of the disturbed child. For them, a neurosis consists only of neurotic behavior. There is no attempt to invoke or treat underlying "causes." Behavior-modification workers use basic laboratory learning concepts and techniques as reward, punishment, and desensitization.

Parent-Child Relations

Research investigations have regarded parent-child relationships as having a prime influence on the origins of neurotic behavior. The study of parent-child relationships correctly recognized the importance of early experiences and the crucial role of initial contacts with significant adult persons in contributing to behavior. There were errors, however, in classifying parent-child relationships as pure types, when most often they are mixtures. It would in fact be highly unusual for a child to be exposed exclusively to rejection or to acceptance, for example. In his experiences, the child ordinarily encounters a variety of relationships (as overindulgence from parents, acceptance from teacher, domination from scoutmaster, and so on). An even more crucial question is how much "rejection" is necessary to convince a child that he is worthless and inadequate.

It must be recognized that there is an inherent logical security to be gained from believing that children in tense, tumultuous, discordant homes will have many frustrations but few satisfactions. One can picture a child in such a situation using any method in the struggle to maintain himself. Extremely maladaptive reactions to excess aggression, servile dependency, or helpless immaturity could be successful in the battle to maintain himself. Any identification with parents would likely favor the acquisition of additional socially inadequate behaviors. Behavior disorders, including neuroses, could thus be inferred as concomitants of lack of warmth, unsatisfying parent-child relationships, and inferior identification models.

Although an interesting hypothesis, the evidence simply does not support a direct correlation between parent-child relationships and consequent behavior disorder. Robins (1966) found that parental rejection or parental deprivation is not a reliable predictor of adult adjustment. Leton (1962) identified sibling rivalry as frequently as parent-child conflicts in the background of his group of school-phobic children. Bronfenbrenner (1967) believes the parental influence is supplanted by that of the peer group by the time the child is 9 years old, long before the peak in incidence of neuroses. After reviewing the studies investigating the relationship between parent-child patterns and behavior problems, Frank (1965) concluded that there was no obvious consistent connection between the two areas.

If there is a relationship between parent-child interaction and behavior disorder, it is likely of a subtle and indirect nature; for example, the parent may exact a driving achievement orientation on the part of the child as the price for acceptance. Parents undoubtedly influence such crucial personality variables as the child's value system, the type of punishment to be avoided, the kinds of rewards to be expected, and the degree of persistence at a task. The child may acquire the maladaptive value system of parents who reject him just because there is no other value system available for incorporation. It is not easy to demonstrate the pathological outcome when a frustrated mother encourages her son to be antisocial as a way of guaranteeing his masculinity.

CONSTITUTIONAL FACTORS

There have been relatively few studies of the relationship of constitutional factors to neurosis. In an investigation of the incidence of neuroses in twins, Shields and Slater (1961) found concordance rates of 53 per cent for monozygotic (MZ, same egg) twins and 25 per cent for dizygotic (DZ, different eggs) twins. Gottesman (1963) studied 34 pairs of MZ and 34 pairs of DZ twins in an attempt to identify neurotic personality traits of high concordance. He concluded that neurotic patterns with hysterical or hypochondriacal themes had little or no genetic basis, whereas those with anxiety, depression, or obsessional features had a substantial genetic component.

There has been a surge of interest in studying the role of hereditary factors in behavior disorders on a less direct level. These investigations try to identify constitutional tendencies, potentials, or traits. Some of the more successful studies of this type have been conducted by Eysenck and Prell (1951), who found evidence for a heritable tendency for neuroticism. Eysenck has also found that level of anxiety follows familial lines. Information from such indirect investigations must be interpreted as to its relevance for psychoneuroses; for example, if a high level of anxiety facilitates the learning of neurotic behavior, then a significant constitutional basis for psychoneuroses is suggested.

Even more subtle are the possibilities for an interplay between the child's inherent abilities or predispositions and the environmental forces which shape these potentials into his own unique personality organization. The outcome may be a healthy or an unhealthy one. In this connection, Fries and Woolf (1953) carried out an ingenious study which explored the differential impact on personality development occurring when a physically active child is born to parents who cherish peace and quiet rather than to parents who are physically energetic and athletic. In the first instance, the stage is set for chronic conflict.

Although there is evidence indicating a constitutional influence in the development of psychoneurotic disorders, the inability to account for all neuroses on a constitutional basis justifies the contention that other factors also make a contribution.

SOCIOCULTURAL FACTORS

Clinicians have implied that psychoneurotic conditions are related to sociocultural background, but they do not agree as to the specifics of the relationship. Some have maintained that essential psychopathological conditions are more prevalent in lower sociocultural levels, and particularly in "borderline" groups (those about to move downward or upward into another group). Answering the question is made difficult by the presumption that persons from higher sociocultural groups would likely be more able to afford treatment. Persons in lower sociocultural groups would be less able to afford treatment and would not be identified for inclusion in reporting data.

In the light of the presumed importance of sociocultural factors in contributing to neuroses, there is a surprising lack of data showing incidence broken down by sociocultural levels, especially data for children. In a timely followup study of persons with behavior problems, Robins (1966) included a group of 50 psychoneurotics. Of the patients in this group, 31 (62 per cent) came from blue-collar homes, 10 (20 per cent) came from homes in which the family head was dependent or chronically unemployed, and 9 (19 per cent) came from white-collar homes.

A report presented by Proctor (1958) deals with a group of 191 continuous serially selected patients seen at the Child Psychiatric Unit, School of Medicine, University of North Carolina. Of the 191 cases, 25 (13 per cent) were diagnosed as hysterical psychoneurotic disorder. Proctor explained what he regarded as a disproportionately high number of such cases as a reflection of sociocultural forces acting upon the population served by the clinic. He described the area as having predominantly rural inhabitants with low educational and economic levels. The ratio of boys to girls in this neurotic group was about equal. By contrast there were nearly twice as many boys as girls in the other 166 cases.

TREATMENT AND PROGNOSIS

Because the psychoneuroses are sometimes regarded as only other manifestations of physical illnesses and other times looked on as purely psychological phenomena, such uncertainty has influenced efforts to correct these disorders. The variety of situations and factors which have been considered as contributing to the development of psychoneuroses is reflected in a corresponding variety of treatment procedures. The choice of treatment invoked has probably been most closely related to the background and orientation of the particular therapist, but falls into one of the following areas:

Medical Approaches. Physicians, who are probably the therapist group most frequently called upon to deal with neuroses, tend to treat psychoneuroses as they would any other illness. Accordingly, recognized medications of a tranquilizing consequence have been used to calm active distress symptoms, and those of a stimulating nature have been given to pep up and revitalize the depressed and melancholic. In conjunction with the medication, the actively distressed patient may be advised to get more rest; the depressed patient, to arrange a program of experiences with the potential for generating new interests. Treatment by a physician generally entails a minimum of contacts with either the child or the parents.

Psychotherapeutic Approaches. Consistent with the differing definitions and etiological conceptions of neurosis, the application of psychotherapy to the treatment of neuroses has followed two theoretical orientations: the psychoanalytic approach and the learning-theory or behavioral approach. (These are discussed in greater detail in Chapter 9.) From a psychoanalytic approach, therapy sessions have concentrated upon searching out the hidden internal conflict which is considered to be the cause of the trouble. Once the conflict has been identified, the child is helped to understand the relationship between his neurotic behavior and the conflict. More effective ways for resolving the conflict may be given the child, or a more equitable balance among the id, ego, and superego personality components may be attempted. The latter may involve releasing repressed id impulses or strengthening the existing ego. Correction entails direct work with the child, and in many instances followup sessions with the parents, who are viewed as having a significant influence upon the maladjustment problem.

Other psychotherapy approaches pay less attention to the possible influences of hidden conflicts and concentrate on changing behavior by direct application of learning principles. Evaluation of the problem first identifies the factors which are rewarding the undesired behavior and then looks for evidences of residual responses which will meet with greater social approval. These desired responses are then systematically rewarded. When appropriate responses are not found, they may be trained by using the child's existing skills. The parents are generally equally involved since their importance as givers of rewards and as reinforcers of the new patterns of behavior are recognized. In some instances, successes have been reported when only the parents are worked with in this framework of supplying cues and rewards for reinforcing new behaviors. (The general features of this approach are presented in Chapter 9 on therapy, and the specific behavior-modification strategies are discussed in Chapter 11 on classroom management.)

The evaluation of effectiveness in treating psychoneuroses suggests the same outcomes described in Chapter 2. Generally speaking, about two-thirds of the cases are improved, and about one-third or one-fourth of the cases are unimproved. These outcomes remain amazingly constant irrespective of the type of treatment applied and, in fact, even when no specific treatment is made available. Hence it is reasonable to expect that from two-thirds to three-fourths of children referred for treatment of a psychoneurosis will be benefited.

As yet, the data reporting on treatment outcomes do not suggest which cases are likely to benefit and which are not. There is insufficient information for indicating whether work with the child, with the parents, or some combination of methods will prove most effective.

More specific data are needed, especially in view of the common necessity for delaying the treatment program until medical evaluations have been completed and in consideration of the fact that neurotic reactions seem to show improvement, at least for a time, in response to even benign treatment.

Supplementary discussions of treatment outcomes are presented in Chapter 9, where attention is particularly focused on findings obtained by Levitt. A detailed outline of the course of treatment, including treatment methods and outcomes, is also given in the present chapter at the conclusion of the following discussion of a typical childhood psychoneurotic reaction, school phobia.

EXAMPLE: SCHOOL PHOBIA

School phobia is a term that has appeared frequently in the last decade in literature dealing with children and their problems. Technically designated as "childhood psychoneurotic disorder, phobic type, evidenced by chronic anxiety reactions toward school and related facilities," the more popular short title, *school phobia,* refers to a neurotic reaction in which the classroom, school building, teacher, janitor, classmates, school bus, cafeteria, principal, or other specific aspects of the school become extremely fear-arousing for the child. Since it is one of the more frequently encountered types of psychoneurotic reactions observed in children, we have selected it for detailed illustration.

INCIDENCE

In the comprehensive investigation carried out by Leton, identifiable school phobia was found to occur at a rate of 3 per 1,000 pupils. An additional 7 in 1,000 pupils also had school phobia, but in a mild or moderate form which was therefore less easily identifiable. As a group, children with psychoneurotic reactions have been found to have average academic achievement, at least for the initial few years. This characteristic holds true for the specific type, school phobia, despite the tumultuous and erratic surface behavior (Leton, 1962; Coolidge, Brodie, & Feeney, 1964). School phobia is one of the few behavior disturbances more frequently observed in girls than in boys. This differential requires the inclusion of cases from the secondary-grade levels, however, where girls begin to contribute heavily to the incidence rate.

A disproportionately greater number of children with school phobia appear to come from higher socioeconomic levels (Leton, 1962; Levison, 1962). This may be an outgrowth of the fact that families at the higher socioeconomic level as a rule have fewer children. The mothers would thus have more time to become involved in the reciprocally dependent relationship with the child which is frequently observed in school phobia. It is also to be considered that costly treatment would be more available to children from such families, with consequent greater likelihood of identification of neuroses in this group.

ONSET AND COURSE

School phobia is characterized by an acute panic state and an aversion to being in school. As observed by the teacher, the onset seems to be sudden. On closer study, it is usually found that the condition has been slowly developing for a year or more. At first there may be reluctance to attend school, voiced dislike for school, or recurrent questioning, "Why do I have to go to school all the time?" The first real indication of a neurotic problem may be suggested by the appearance of complaints of a somatic nature. Parents who are not much impressed with verbal gripes and grumblings are often spurred to action by their child's claims of having a headache or a stomachache. Fainting or vomiting can easily support the child's contention of illness.

Some parents of school-phobic children seem to have a callous indifference toward their children. In this case the child is often driven to greater and greater excess display and demonstration in order to gain even a flicker of attention. Unfortunately, parents become absorbed in the pattern of excess reactions. Other parents of school-phobic children have just the opposite relationship. They are overly sensitive to the child's expressions. Not only do they overrespond, but they preempt. It is their anticipation tendency that may be the most damaging to the child since it denies him all sayso in his affairs. Overreactive parents are quick to put the child to bed when he says he has a headache; they read to him, entertain him. They call the physician and insist that he immediately see the child. They call the teacher and raise questions as to why the teacher has been so demanding and lacking in understanding of their child, who is now sick. They walk with him to and from school or drive him in the warm car.

The onset of the school-phobic reaction is often triggered by specific happenings associated with school. The child may receive a low score on a test, be severely ridiculed by classmates, be scolded for not having completed an assignment, or be the victim of a physical beating by other pupils. These events also play right into the hands of the domineering or oversolicitous parent who feels compelled to protect, to somehow make up and replace something essential. (At the deepest level, such parents may feel their competency as parents is at issue.) As relevant historical details are uncovered, however, it is clear that such a child has a deep and well-defined fear for his security and adequacy. Generally he has no friends. He seems to feel more safe if he remains inside the house. He refuses to walk to and from school with his classmates and waits to be escorted or chauffeured by his parent or older sibling. While waiting to be picked up at school, he may request to be near the teacher or principal.

With the onset of acute symptoms, the child becomes visibly more apprehensive. If questioned as to why he does not want to go to school, he may offer a story of a wild animal roaming near the school, his fear that the school might burn down, or his concern that there may be a terrible explosion at school. When reassured about these fears, others of equally doubtful plausibility rise; endless expressions of fear the food in the cafeteria will make him ill, the janitor doesn't like him, or a gang of pupils plan to waylay him can be recounted. The fear often begins with some localized aspect of the school, but quickly generalizes. In a short time, even bringing the child close to the school can be sufficient to bring on nausea, vomiting, blind running, loss of sphincter control, or active resistance in the form of crying, biting, kicking, holding breath, or fainting. Outbursts of crying and temper tantrums are common. The child actively resists being kept in school, especially if he has been away for a week or two. When the child is permitted to remain at home, these more acute symptoms subside, giving rise to a false sense that recovery has been effected. Of greater long-term consequence, however, is the subtle reinforcement of those same acute symptoms which a return to the home can accomplish. This factor makes the treatment of school phobia a matter demanding carefully coordinated management.

In some respects it is unfortunate that the label "school phobia" has come to be extensively applied to this condition since it is something of an incorrect depiction of the problem. The term implies a behavior disorder limited to a marked fear of school. On investigation, school is found to be only one of a number of fears which such children have. These children tend to fear many "familiar" and all new situations (attending a movie, watching a ballgame, going to the store, going to Sunday school). To be more exact, they are panicked by any situation in which they are alone and away from their parents. As Leton (1962) and White (1964) point out, it just happens that school is a major common demand for all children. Attendance at school is legally compulsory. When the child does not attend school, this fact is invariably called to his parents' attention. But no official is likely to check on whether or not the child attended a movie or ballgame.

Studies of the etiology of school phobia make it increasingly apparent that separation from the parent figures prominently in this behavior disorder. The child is struggling to cope with the problem of weaning himself from his parents. A certain amount of self-independence is a real developmental task which children in our society must attain in order to make the initial school adjustment satisfactorily. It may be that the rigors of coping with this developmental task contribute to the peak of incidence of neuroses, which is seen at about grade 4 or 5.

It has also been pointed out that the relationship with the mother seems to be more critical than that with the father. Studies by Leton (1962), Levison (1962), White (1964), and Coolidge and his associates (1964) have identified a conspicuous reciprocal relationship in which the child is very dependent upon the mother. The mother nurtures the child's dependency on her as gratification for the mother's own needs to be important and needed. Such mothers are very susceptible to the child's apparent upset condition, fears, and failures, which they tend to interpret as tangible evidence of their child's need for mothering. The parents' actions are more understandable as efforts to cover up their personal inadequacies rather than as realistic attempts to help the child. The parent may assume the role of an intervening bulwark, protecting the child from what the parent may claim are actions by school officials and clinicians to mistreat or be mean to the child.

TREATMENT

The treatment of school phobia has become a matter of increasing concern. Various treatment procedures have been advocated, including removal of the child from school, control by medication, some type of psychotherapy, or a form of behavior modification such as desensitization. There is a growing recognition that prolonged treatments, such as psychoanalysis or psychotherapy, generally are not necessary. Most cases of school phobia can be treated effectively by a variety of short-term techniques. The general treatment strategy should follow these steps:

1. The child should have immediate attention. The longer the problem exists without intervention, the more chronic and resistant to treatment it becomes.

2. The child should be given a thorough physical examination by the family physician. This step is necessary to settle once and for all any questions of physical health which are an integral aspect of the symptoms.

3. Persons carrying out the treatment must be assured that the child is tough and won't "fall apart" as they impose treatment demands on him.

4. The parents must be involved in the treatment program and given specific roles or functions to carry out. The parent should not be made to feel guilty. The parent must be reassured as to the toughness and resiliency of the child.

5. Medications, as prescribed by a physician, can be a significant source of support for alleviating many of the acute symptoms and thus helping to keep the child in school.

6. The child should be kept in school and any relevant modifications of his school program should be considered. The child must have potent support for his attending school.

What seems critical to the effective treatment of school phobia is placing the child back in the school with a minimum of delay. For each day, for each hour, that the child is permitted to remain outside of school, there seems to be a proportional increase in the severity of symptoms and the level of panic regarding return to school. Such a course of events is a characteristic feature common to psychoneurotic reactions. If the child maintains that he is afraid of school to the point that he cannot go to school, he is likely to behave in a way that justifies his complaint. If his simple complaint that he is afraid of school does not work, then he may do other thing to "prove" that he is really sick. Thus nausea, vomiting, diarrhea, stomachaches, or headaches can be anticipated as the child is kept in school. It is recommended, however, that the child attend school, even though there may be an increase in the severity of symptoms for a few days. The increase in intensity of symptoms can be planned for in the knowledge that the child is resilient and will not be traumatized or bear permanent injury by reason of having to be in school. Everyone must firmly believe that the child can adjust to school and that the problem is to find out what modifications and changes are needed to enable the adjustment to be made.

It is important to include the parents in the treatment regimen from the beginning. Ideally, the parent should be given specific assignments which are obviously part of the treatment procedures. One of the first such contributions that the parent might make is to secure a complete physical examination for the child. There are always questions about physical-health factors, and these must be answered as a part of the treatment program. Hopefully, the pediatrician will see fit to prescribe medications which render the child less anxious and more tractable. Care should be exercised to prevent the parents from feeling they are at fault, for parents of school-phobic children often have problems of guilt or question their adequacy as parents. The school social worker, nurse, or other person working with the parent must convey reassurances that the child is not really going to come apart at the seams and can, with assistance, make a satisfactory adjustment to school. Showing the parent real samples of the child's satisfactory work at school can be especially meaningful support for the parent.

Most of all, the child himself needs to have reassurance and support for the times that he is at school. It must be repeatedly communicated to the child that he can and will overcome his fear, and that everything being done is to accomplish that purpose. In some instances, a slight reduction of the child's school day might be considered. Such giving-in to the child should be avoided as a routine measure, however, since this can obviously play into the child's symptoms. An approach more recommended entails adjustment to the pupil's school program. Beneficial results can come from school tasks which hold guaranteed success experiences. Carefully planned assignments should enable the pupil to receive support and encouragement from his teacher and classmates. Praise for real successes and recognition for efforts in attending school will soon act to alleviate the condition.

The behavior-modification approach is illustrated in Garvey and

Hegrenes' study (1966) which used desensitization (or counterconditioning) to eliminate a boy's fear of school. The child, Jimmy, had been treated for six months in a traditional psychotherapeutic situation. Treatment was stopped when school was closed for the summer. After the summer the child was still unable to attend school. A desensitization procedure was then started. Having obtained the cooperation of the school, the therapist worked with the child for 20 to 40 minutes every day. The therapist used the following steps:

1. Sitting in the car in front of the school
2. Getting out of the car and approaching the curb
3. Going to the sidewalk
4. Going to the bottom of the steps of the school
5. Going to the top of the steps
6. Going to the door
7. Entering the school
8. Approaching the classroom
9. Entering the classroom
10. Being present in the classroom with the teacher
11. Being present in the classroom with the teacher and one or two classmates
12. Being present in the classroom with a full class.

These steps were carried out over a period of 20 consecutive days. At the end of that time, the child resumed his normal school routine with no return of the symptoms during a two-year followup period. The authors explain that

since Jimmy and the therapist had a good relationship, the presence of the therapist may be considered as a relatively strong stimulus evoking a positive affective response in the patient. As a consequence, because there was reduced anxiety in the presence of the fear stimulus, instead of an avoidance response, Jimmy was able to make an approach response which was reinforced by the therapist with strong praise.

It was felt that if the child had been forced into the classroom, the therapist might have acquired a negative stimulus value. Garvey and Hegrenes think that their method requires less time but that their results are just as effective as those of the methods of traditional psychoanalysis.

PROGNOSIS

In a followup study conducted by Coolidge, Brodie, and Feeney (1964), a group of 66 children were restudied in 1963 after having been diagnosed as "school phobic" during the period between 1953-1958. Of the 66, 10 could not be located, and 7 were eliminated because they were found to have more pervasive disorders such as epilepsy. The remaining 49 subjects had a median age of 16 years (median age was 7 years at the time of the original diagnosis). For 2 of the 49 subjects, there was insufficient information to assess, but the other 47 were evaluated as to current emotional adjustment appropriate to their age. One group of 13 subjects (3 boys, 10 girls) were found to be making satisfactory adjustments and were rated as "normal" adolescents. A second group of 20 subjects (7 boys, 13 girls) showed definite limitations in their adjustments which could still be regarded as neurotic. The third group of 14 subjects (9 boys, 5 girls) were found to be having serious adjustment problems, ranging from severe character disorders to frank psychoses. This group had all but given up trying, had indefinable goals, and were struggling to simply "stay in the boat." Although errors in original diagnoses are apparent in these outcomes, a more important consideration for the welfare of children generally is the indication that the children in the group were experiencing critical adjustment problems and desperately needed assistance. The findings offer compelling support for the advisability of active intervention rather than waiting to see if the child will outgrow his adjustment problems.

Psychoneurotic reactions respond to a variety of treatment procedures, including medications, rest, formal psychotherapy, and behavior-modification techniques. The treatment regimen requires the collective contributions of clinicians, teachers, and parents. There will be crises and stormy points, but there is reason to expect that any one of several methods will work. Although data on recovery are sporadic and incomplete, the outcome for school phobia seems especially favorable. If "returned to school" is taken as the criterion, meaning that the child soon was able to resume usual school participation and to continue normal school attendance during the 5–10-year period of followup observations, then from 71 to 94 per cent of the school-phobia cases reviewed met this criterion. The improvement rate seems unrelated to the type of treatment, or, in fact, to whether any treatment was received.

Robins' (1966) findings suggest that a preponderance of antisocial symptoms (aggression, sexual deviancy) indicates a poor prognosis. Data from Coolidge, Brodie, and Feeney (1964) caution that boys are less likely to rise above their neurotic problems than are girls. Both studies indicate that low academic achievement and borderline sociocultural status are associated with a poor prognosis.

SUMMARY

This chapter has considered how maladaptive patterns of behavior developing from anxiety can lead to psychoneurotic disorders. Some psychopathologists have emphasized the importance of a particular traumatic event, but anxiety generated by a chronic conflict between opposing drives or wishes seems more often to have etiological significance. Persisting high levels of anxiety precipitate neurotic patterns of behavior. Susceptibility to stress as well as effectiveness of tension-discharge systems may be constitutionally influenced. Prevailing responses of parents and other significant persons are of foremost influence in producing anxiety.

A characteristic of neurotic behavior is its quasi-success in coping with the threat; denial renders the child unaware of a threat; phobias separate him physically from the threat; and obsessive-compulsive thoughts and acts create a protective shield which cannot be penetrated. Once established, the neurotic reaction pattern absorbs a disproportionate amount of the child's resources and inhibits the making of new and possibly more effective adjustments The fact that so many factors can act to perpetuate a neurotic disorder underscores the advisability of early intervention for correcting the condition.

A widespread interest in psychoneuroses has encouraged extensive study of the condition by clinicians and laboratory workers. Information gained in these investigations has contributed much illumination for understanding all behavioral phenomena. Clarification has been made of the subtle ways by which constitutional factors may influence adjustment processes. It has been demonstrated that imprecise trial-and-error efforts to reduce an uncomfortable tension level may ultimately develop into specific and durable behavioral patterns. The role of reinforcement in accounting for maladaptive outcomes is equivalent to that in fostering favorable adjustment outcomes. Whether the person is constitutionally predisposed or whether the neurotic patterns are a consequence of the particular pressures and release channels present in his life situation, psychoneurotic reactions seem to require several years to become manifest. Thus they are not ordinarily identifiable until the child is 8 or 9 years old. Initially more common in boys, by adolescence the psychoneuroses are more prevalent in girls.

A number of approaches have been found to be about equally effective in the treatment of neuroses. This conclusion is compatible with suggestions that a variety of conditions can give rise to a neurosis. Identification of psychoneuroses demands the making of difficult discriminations, with physical illnesses, temporary stress reactions, and personality disorders being the most frequently confused. The complexities encountered in the diagnosis and management of childhood psychoneuroses can most effectively be dealt with by the combined efforts of the teacher, social worker, physician, and psychologist. Since school attendance is legally compulsory for the child, the child's school environment assumes a position of central importance in coordinating treatment. Recognizing this fact by making maximum use of the school's total resources may hasten the satisfactory resolution of the neurotic disorder.

SUGGESTED READINGS

Berkowitz, P. H., & Rothman, E. R. *The disturbed child.* New York: New York Univer. Press, 1960.

Freud, A. *Normality and pathology in childhood.* New York: International Universities Press, 1965.

Jersild, A., Markey, F. V., & Jersild, C. L. Children's fears, dreams, wishes, daydreams, likes, dislikes, pleasant and unpleasant memories. *Child Develpm. Monogr.* No. 12 (Columbia Univer.), 1933.

Lippman, H. S. *Treatment of the child in emotional conflict.* (2nd ed.) New York: McGraw-Hill, 1962.

Shaw, C. R. *The psychiatric disorders of childhood.* New York: Meredith, 1966.

REFERENCES

Bronfenbrenner, U. The split-level American family. *Sat. Rev.,* 1967, **50,** 60-66.

Coolidge, J. L., Brodie, R. D., & Feeney, B. A ten-year follow-up study of sixty-six school-phobic children. *Amer. J. Orthopsychiat.,* 1964, **34,** 675-684.

Davis, S. W. Stress in combat. *Sci. Amer.,* 1956, **194,** 31-35.

Dollard, J., & Miller, N. E. *Personality and psychotherapy.* New York: McGraw-Hill, 1950.

Eysenck, H. J., & Prell, D. B. The inheritance of neuroticism: an experience study. *J. ment. Sci.,* 1951, **97,** 441-465.

Frank, G. H. The role of the family in the development of psychopathology. *Psychol. Bull.,* 1965, **64,** 191-205.

Freud, S. *An outline of psychoanalysis.* New York: Norton, 1949.

Fries, M., & Woolf, P. Some hypotheses on the role of the congenital activity type in personality development. In R. S. Eissler, A. Freud, H. Hartmann, & M. Kris (Eds.), *The psychoanalytic study of the child.* Vol. 8. New York: International Universities Press, 1953. Pp. 48-62.

Funkenstein, D. H., King, S. H., & Drolette, M. E. *Mastery of stress.* Cambridge: Harvard Univer. Press, 1957.

Garvey, W., & Hegrenes, J. Desensitization techniques in the treatment of school phobia. *Amer. J. Orthopsychiat.,* 1966, **36**, 147-152.

Gottesman, I. I. Heritability of personality: a demonstration. *Psychol. Monogr.,* 1963, **77** (9).

Horney, K. *The neurotic personality of our time.* New York: Norton, 1937.

Kurlander, L. F., & Colodny, D. "Pseudoneurosis" in the neurologically handicapped child. *Amer. J. Orthopsychiat.,* 1965, **35**, 733-738.

Leton, D. A. Assessment of school phobia. *Ment. Hyg.,* 1962, **46**, 256-264.

Levison, B. Understanding the child with school phobia. *Except. Child.,* 1962, **28**, 393-398.

Lewin, K. A. *Dynamic theory of personality.* New York: McGraw-Hill, 1935.

Maher, B. A. *Principles of psychopathology.* New York: McGraw-Hill, 1966.

Morse, W. C., Cutler, R. L., & Fink, A. H. *Public school classes for the emotionally handicapped: a research analysis.* Washington, D.C.: Council for Exceptional Children, 1964.

Mowrer, O. H. *Learning theory and personality dynamics.* New York: Ronald Press, 1950.

Parsons, T. Age and sex in the social structure of the United States. *Amer. sociol. Rev.,* 1942, **7**, 604-616.

Proctor, J. T. Hysteria in childhood. *Amer. J. Orthopsychiat.,* 1958, **28**, 394-406.

Robins, L. N. *Deviant children grown up.* Baltimore: Williams & Wilkins, 1966.

Rosen, B. M., Bahn, A. K., & Kramer, M. Demographic and diagnostic characteristics of psychiatric clinic outpatients in the U.S.A., 1961. *Amer. J. Orthopsychiat.,* 1964, **34**, 455-468.

Sears, R. R. A theoretical framework for personality and social behavior. *Amer. Psychologist,* 1951, **6**, 476-483.

Shields, J., & Slater, E. Heredity and psychological abnormality. In H. J. Eysenck (Ed.), *Handbook of abnormal psychology.* New York: Basic Books, 1961. Pp. 298-343.

Sullivan, H. S. *The interpersonal theory of psychiatry.* New York: Norton, 1953.

White, R. W. *The abnormal personality.* (3rd ed.) New York: Ronald Press, 1964.

4

Learning
Disabilities

This chapter will look at several types of particular disabilities
whose importance stems from the fact that they impair the capacity
to profit from new experiences. Identifiable as discrete deficits, attitudes,
or ways for processing stimulation, these disabilities are distinguished
as precise conditions in contrast to the more general impairments
observed in cultural deprivation or mental retardation, for example.
These specific deficits are of importance in that they present barriers
to the acquisition of new knowledge or skills and in that they may

become the focal point for compounded adjustment difficulties, often with a prominent emotional overlay.

The treatment of learning disabilities is a matter which rightly demands the interested concern of many specialist persons because of the associated complexities in performance and because of the large number of children who are involved. Specific learning disabilities frequently are manifested as degrees of academic nonachievement and undoubtedly contribute significantly to the large number of children (estimated by Kessler [1966] to be three-fourths of pupils of elementary-school age) referred for individual study and treatment because of poor school achievement.

Specific learning disabilities are usually uncovered by means of a case study which entails the detailed assessment of a child's intellectual ability, emotional development, social maturity, and experiential background. When the information from such diagnostic studies is evaluated in depth, there has frequently been an inability to ascribe the disability in functioning to any one specific cause.

Let us review a case study of a child who was entirely competent in all abilities, including motor functions, so that he accomplished the early developmental tasks of locomotion and manipulation within the normal range of time. The parents initially had no fixed pattern of responding to the child's developmental accomplishments. As he became older, however, they grew to be concerned about the possibility of injuries and began to anticipate the probability that the child might hurt himself. Acting in accordance with social expectancies that they be good parents, they began to restrict their child's participation in those activities which they regarded as holding chances for injury.

The parents' anxious concern about the child's ability to cope successfully with new situations was recognized by the child, who then began to doubt himself. The child became more sensitive to his inadequacies and sought to avoid any new demands because he was not sure whether or not he could be successful. Since he was reluctant to try, he gave only casual attention to new situations and new objects. He could see nothing to be gained from looking carefully or listening intently. In fact, he much preferred to shut out such information because it only seemed to be another situation in which he might fail. The indifference and unconcern resulted in his not developing his ability to remember, organize, and relate visual and auditory stimuli. When he entered first grade, he learned the letters of the alphabet but he could not recognize words made of combinations of these same letters. He could not consistently associate the correct sound with a letter.

His anxious concern grew as he failed while his classmates were successful. Specific auditory and visual memory deficits placed him at a distinct disadvantage in learning to read. He failed more frequently. His failures gave his parents more reason to think that the child was basically inadequate. Finding substantiation for believing that the child was inadequate, the parents then began to react to him in terms of expected failure. The child responded to his parents' expectations of failure by more confusion, anxiety, and inability to remember. In this way a mutually reinforcing pattern of anxious inability to remember, failure, and resulting heightened level of anxiety with associated impairment of memory became established and influenced the child's effectiveness in dealing with other tasks.

A clearer picture of the mutual interrelationships among factors which contribute to success in meeting any demand has been gained from work with children who have specific learning disabilities. At first glance the prospects for intervention into such an apparently self-reinforcing and cyclical pattern of behavior seem formidable. These same qualities of mutual reciprocity and interrelatedness, however, have served as the basis for highly successful treatment programs directed toward the correction of specific learning disabilities, as will be seen elsewhere in this chapter.

DEFINITIONS

Even though there is currently a widespread interest in the child with specific learning disabilities, this type of disordered functioning is not a new concept. Persons concerned with adjustment failures in the past have recognized these same problems, as is all too evident from a review of the work describing past attempts to correct disabilities encountered in children. Some of the terms to be found include aphasic (impaired use or understanding of speech), brain-injured, dyslexia (difficulty in reading), interjacent educationally retarded, emotional blocking, word-blind, underachiever, and idiot savant.

An analysis of the variety of terms reflects an interest in these problems on the part of persons trained in such fields as general medicine, neurology, psychiatry, education, and psychology. In the general field of clinical work, there has usually been an abundance of diagnostic labels, but frequently a paucity of appropriate treatment procedures. A certain amount of classification, description, and labeling, nevertheless, is an initial requisite to the identification of problems and disabilities preliminary to formulating adequate steps for the amelioration of these difficulties.

Definitions proposed by authoritative persons in the field suggest that a specific deficit is being considered but that the disability manifests itself as a specific inability to learn or progress at the expected rate in a particular area of competence or in a specific training situation. What is meant by this type of disorder may be clarified by the consideration of some examples of learning disabilities.

EXAMPLES

1. *Visual Disabilities.* Frequent mention is made of *visual* (spatial) difficulties in which there is an inability to differentiate figure from background, to recognize reversal or inversion of letters and forms, and/or to perceive forms with usual consistency in the face of measured "normal" visual acuity.

2. *Motor Disabilities.* Another commonly encountered area of deficit entails *motor* disabilities, such as the inability to write or reproduce figures accurately, awkward and gross motor coordination, and/or clumsiness and ineptness in performing fine motor skills.

3. *Language Disabilities.* Certain *language* disorders are also cited as examples of specific learning disabilities. These include conditions ranging from mutism, omission or substitution of sounds and words, to confusion of tenses and acceptable syntax arrangements. Possibly closely related to these language disorders is another group of specific disabilities which are classed as *communication* deficits and include such problems as the inability to acquire usual competency in reading, to achieve in arithmetic, and/or to spell correctly.

4. *Auditory Disabilities.* Included in the group of *auditory* disabilities is the inability to discriminate sounds when these are presented as isolated elements, such as the sounds of syllables which make up a word. Audiological examination with the audiometer shows that hearing as thus assessed is "normal." More frequently, auditory deficits are seen as the inability to repeat more than five or six words in a sentence, a group of "nonsense" words, or a series of digits.

5. *Emotional Disabilities.* A large number of specific learning disabilities may be recognized on the basis of an *emotional* condition

which impairs effective functioning. In this category are disruptions associated with such characteristics as impulsivity, inattentiveness, daydreaming, aggressiveness, restlessness, negativism, and uncooperativeness. It is of interest to note that this group of disabilities encompasses a range of traits extending from active assertion to the opposite extreme of passive withdrawal.

6. *Social Disabilities.* A little understood and probably frequently unrecognized group of learning impairments may be classed together because they seem to represent deficits in organizing or relating to *social* surroundings. It is possible that misperceptions of social relationships figure prominently in this group of disabilities which is also comprised of more easily identified disabilities as erratic judgment, irresponsibility, nonparticipation, and irritability.

7. *Combinations of Disabilities.* Not infrequently, deficits are observed which involve several of these areas of functioning, with the result that the learning disability is referred to as *visual-motor, social-emotional,* or *language-communicative.* There are several possibilities for such combinations based on discrepancies revealed by the evaluation of various kinds of responses or behaviors varying as to level of complexity. Sometimes the functional interrelatedness of two or more major systems contributing to particular performance is reflected in the use of the term *association disability* (visual-motor association, auditory-language association, auditory-visual association). Other workers recognize the basic interaction of several systems in producing behavior but believe that deficiencies in one area may be of *primary* importance, whereas deficits in another related area are of *secondary* importance (primary motor incoordination with secondary irresponsibility and secondary social-learning disability, for example).

DIFFERENTIAL DIAGNOSTIC CONSIDERATIONS

OVERVIEW OF ASSESSMENT PROCEDURES

The assessment of learning disabilities follows the same plan and relies on the same procedures as are invoked in seeking to identify the sources of any difficulty which is limiting a child's functioning effectiveness. The diagnostic process is a judgmental one, based on the critical scrutiny of four major areas: physical health, developmental history, comparisons of capacity and achievement, and family and home situation. The diagnostician explores these areas until he feels that he has sufficient information for making a decision.

In collecting information, some specialists make use of laboratory tests, X-ray pictures, and electrical measures of performance. Other specialists rely more on the question-and-answer probing of the interview. Possibly the most important source of data is observation as the child functions in varied situations. Observation is frequently made in the controlled condition for administration of a standardized measuring scale, or by asking the child to remember a series of words or digits. Although gained in less formal conditions, taking note of the child's participation in play groups, his manner of fitting in with his classmates, even the way he walks, sits, and waits in the examiner's office supplies valuable information.

Ideally, a diagnostic study should answer all questions posed by the adjustment difficulty, ranging from the cause and nature of the disability to suggested treatment and prognosis. In practice, it is seldom that any specialist covers all the major areas of investigation in detail. His evaluation will rely heavily upon the findings elicited by the particular set of techniques in which the specialist has been trained. For example, the physician (pediatrician, neurologist) will depend predominantly on findings concerning physical health and developmental history. The educator will be advised by information obtained from comparisons of capacity and achievement and from the family and home situation. The social worker is primarily interested in surveying the developmental history and the family and home situation. The psychologist will count mostly on data supplied by comparisons of capacity and achievement and from developmental-history materials. Experience in dealing with behavior disorders, which tend to be more vague and uncertain than most somatic disabilities, has shown that effectiveness in treatment demands the collaboration of all these specialists. A complete picture of the disorder is formed only on having available information elicited from each of the four major areas outlined below (with sample coverage):

1. *Physical Health*
   a. General physical health (stamina, fatigue, regularity of functions, complaints of pain or discomfort).
   b. Review of systems (survey of functioning of sensory, digestive, skeletal, motor, and endocrine systems).

c. Neurological examination (balance, coordination, reflexes, responsiveness to pain and pressure stimuli).

d. Prior illnesses (age of onset, severity, type, incapacitation).

e. Accidents and injuries (age, nature, associated deficits, treatment).

f. Possible significant hereditary influences.

2. *Developmental History*

a. Accomplishment of developmental tasks (age of sitting, standing, walking, talking, completion of toilet training).

b. Language acquisition (making speech sounds, vocabulary, ease of speaking and understanding).

c. Growth of interests (activities enjoyed, activities disliked, passive versus active participation).

d. Emotional controls (intensity of emotions, appropriateness, stability).

e. Adjustment to school (favored subjects, disliked subjects, educational goals).

3. *Comparisons of Capacity and Achievement* (focus is on school adjustment for school-age child)

a. Indices of general capacity (intelligence, aptitudes, language).

b. Measures of general achievement (attainment in reading, writing, arithmetic).

c. Measures of specific abilities (memory, dexterity, listening, eye-hand coordination).

d. Speech fluency (enunciation, inflection, articulation, smoothness of expression).

e. Personality organization (goals, motivation, reality orientation, self-evaluation).

f. Capacity for independent work (distractibility, remembering instructions, understanding directions).

g. Progression in school (age of entrance, failures, achievements).

4. *Family and Home Situation*

a. Parent-child relationships (acceptance-rejection, permissiveness-restrictiveness, consistency, mutuality).

b. Socialization (place in family group, friends, relations to neighborhood and community, conformity).

c. Adequacy of home and neighborhood (intactness, recreational facilities, sources of stimulation, ease of getting about).

d. Prevailing models and value standards (personal responsibility, type of gratification encouraged, release outlets available, social standards).

ASSESSMENT OF SPECIFIC DISABILITIES

In practice, a specific learning disability is identified on the basis of findings gained in a series of assessments which contrast potential with performance. The first phase consists of establishing whether or not there is a real discrepancy between capacity and attainment, thus establishing a deviation which might be the manifestation of a specific learning disability. Indices of general capacity, usually expressed as mental age, chronological age, achievement age, learning age, vocabulary age, or motor age, are obtained. General level of functioning is ascertained according to performance on measures of educational achievement, motor coordination, language comprehension and usage. The actual level of performance is compared with the expected level of performance as suggested by the MA (mental age), CA (chronological age), or other appropriate normative scores. A learning disability is said to exist when there is a significant discrepancy between the measures of capacity and performance.

The second phase of the assessment is directed toward the more detailed investigation or description of the learning disability. Preliminary study (first phase) may show that a child has, for example, a test age of 8 years on a scale measuring general intellectual capacity, but scores only at the level of the average child of 6 years on a measure of language comprehension and usage. Subsequent study would attempt to account for the discrepancy by evaluating abilities which contribute to language acquisition and use.

Standardized as well as informal analytic measuring techniques may be utilized in this second phase of the diagnostic study. The child may prove to have normal auditory acuity, but have an inability to remember or fuse sounds into the patterns which make up words. Another line of investigation would center about assessment of the speech and vocal processes as indicated by an articulation measure, or by a test such as the Illinois Test of Psycholinguistic Abilities. This second phase would be pursued until the deficits associated with the impaired performance are sufficiently identified to suggest an appropriate approach to the correction of the disability.

The tendency to have expanded diagnostic categories for classifying specific learning disabilities reflects the fact that a deficit may influence more than one type of functioning. The child with a visual perceptual disability may encounter difficulty in reading and in walking and become irritable because of these failures. The problem of identifying a learning disability is rendered difficult, however, by the awareness that the blind learn to read and to walk. It is advisable to keep in mind that there is a hierarchy of relationships between abilities and performance.

The child who has difficulty in remembering letters in a fixed sequence, such as would provide a consistent clue for the visual recognition of words, can be expected to have low performance in reading. This expectation would be especially justified if his training in reading emphasizes an approach which places a high demand on visualization abilities. The same child may find that his visual memory-sequencing deficit results in his having some difficulty in playing baseball. The difficulty in baseball will probably not be as marked as it is in reading since baseball-playing requires mainly motor-ability responses which are indirectly based on visual clues. A careful evaluation of the child's capacity to respond orally to problems which are presented to him verbally may show that he has no difficulty with these types of tasks since the performance required of him does not even indirectly involve visual memory-sequencing ability.

DIFFERENTIATION FROM OTHER DISORDERS

Efforts to delineate learning disabilities as separate from another type of impaired functioning are evident in descriptive-type diagnostic classifications such as "academic retardation without mental retardation." The problems observed in the child with a specific learning disability should not be attributable to such global conditions as ataxia, blindness, deafness, mental retardation, or social-emotional disorder. It is necessary to differentiate a specific learning disability from such conditions which sometimes manifest a closely similar set of characteristics, including achievement discrepancies.

Social and Emotional Maladjustment. A study carried out by Schroeder (1965) investigated the reading and arithmetic achievement of elementary-school pupils who had been diagnosed as falling into one of these five categories: psychosomatic, aggressive, having school difficulties, school-phobic, and neurotic-psychotic. Schroeder concluded that the wide ranges and variations in achievement observed did not support the classification of all the pupils into one large category such as "emotionally disturbed." A similar study of emotionally disturbed children of elementary-school age referred to the Child Psychiatry Service of the State University of Iowa was conducted by Stone and Rowley (1964). They found that only 52 per cent of their sample (N = 116) had lower than expected deviations, where 29 per cent had higher than expected deviations when achievement in reading and arithmetic was compared to mental age. In addition to these differences in academic achievement, the degree of emotional disturbance and disorganization observed in the socially or emotionally maladjusted pupil is much greater than that observed in the child with specific learning disabilities.

Organic Dysfunction. It has also been found that not all children with brain damage have specific learning difficulties even when the condition is so obvious as to lead to a classification of epilepsy (Maher, 1966). The mentally retarded present a rather uniform and general retardation in achievement which is, however, consistent with indices of their general capacity, such as mental age. Although the child with a specific learning disability presents characteristics which allow for a differential diagnosis from brain-damaged, emotionally disturbed, or mentally retarded, some children within these same groups are found to have specific learning disabilities which may or may not be associated with their other disorders.

INCIDENCE AND DISTRIBUTION

Reports of the incidence of learning disabilities must be interpreted in the light of several problems which are encountered in any attempt to quantify these difficulties. Perhaps the most prevalent problem rests in the lack of agreement among the various professions as to just what constitutes a specific learning disability. Earlier in this chapter, we provided a list of terms encountered in the literature pertaining to learning disabilities. Each of these terms can be seen to have slightly different implications as to the manifestation of the disability, its origins, and its possible treatment. The persistence of these varied labels reflects the many points of differences about learning disabilities. Sometimes the differences are slight and technical, but in other instances they are considerable.

As might be expected, these differences in what constitutes a learning disability must be considered in reports of the frequency of learning disabilities since incidence depends on definition. It follows that those persons who accept the more general categories (as, for example, "underachiever") in classifying learning disabilities will report a higher number of cases identified than will be reported by those persons who favor a more restrictive and narrow definition of the problem ("dyschronometria"—difficulty in telling time).

Bateman (1964), in her review of developments in the field of learning disabilities, suggests that from 5 to 10 per cent of the general school population may have learning disabilities which are identifiable as reading problems and that deficits in other academic areas also occur but with less frequency. Myklebust and Johnson (1962), who provide for a large number of disabilities grouped under the general category of dyslexia, state that "at least five percent of school children have some type of psychoneurological learning disorder." Bakwin (1949) notes that from 2 to 3 per cent is frequently cited for the incidence of cerebral damage, and Bender (1956) has suggested a frequency of about 1 per cent for the number of children who would be classified as brain-injured.

The differences which seem to account for the variation in reports of number of children with specific learning disabilities are not easily reconciled, but they can be understood as reflecting differences in the definition of a learning disability. There is a paucity of reports in which entire populations have been exhaustively studied by any of the existing diagnostic criteria, and most of the information used for making estimates of the incidence of learning disabilities has been gained from such restricted population groups as children referred to child-study clinics, remedial-reading clinics, psychiatric hospitals, or school psychologists. Incidence figures vary with the orientation of the reporting agency.

Detailed investigations of carefully selected samples would do much to clarify the exact incidence of learning disabilities, which probably falls somewhere in the range suggested by Bateman (1964), a frequency of from 5 to 10 per cent of school children. One such attempt was reported by Burks (1960), who evaluated all pupils (524) in a public elementary school (kindergarten through eighth grade) with a rating scale designed to identify the hyperkinetic child. It was found that 8 per cent (42) of the children showed a large number of the diagnostic criteria from a moderate to a severe degree.

FACTORS INFLUENCING REPORTED INCIDENCE *in learning disabilities*

1. *Sex.* Although estimates of the incidence of learning disabilities vary considerably, there is rather general agreement among all investigators that the condition is more commonly observed in males than in females. Myklebust and Johnson (1962) report that dyslexia "occurs at least five times more frequently in males than in females." This proportion seems to be remarkably consistent with, and even overshadows, some of the differences which are found in the definitions of what characterizes a learning disability. The finding has sometimes been used to support the claim for some sex-linked genetic factor influencing the disabilities, but it can be interpreted with equal plausibility as supporting the impact of socialization upon development and functioning. Sociologists and child-development specialists, like Talcott Parsons and David P. Ausubel, have pointed to the greater cultural demands for achievement which confront the boy and render him more susceptible to the consequences of all failure experiences.

2. *Socioeconomic Status.* The incidence of learning disabilities appears to follow a pattern which is associated with socioeconomic levels. The interpretation of data which support this contention is, however, complicated by several factors. Eisenberg (1962) has described a "deprivation syndrome" affecting persons in lower socioeconomic groups who, as a result, tend to have less advantage of adequate medical care, less educationally appropriate stimulation, less opportunity to gain usual social rewards, and who may acquire a different set of motivational values in comparison to persons at higher socioeconomic levels. All of these conditions may adversely influence the functioning effectiveness of members of lower socioeconomic groups. The diagnosis of learning disability is generally made on the basis of lower than average performance in several areas of functioning, but diagnostic procedures may not always be sufficiently refined to take into account influences associated with lower socioeconomic status. No small part of the problem in making this differentiation is the fact that members of the lower socioeconomic class are less likely to be able to afford the costly diagnostic and treatment services which may be required to identify a learning disability. There is then limited opportunity to study a large number of such cases.

3. *Age.* The obvious influence which specific learning disabilities can have on school adjustment has resulted in more information being known about school children than is known about any other age group.

Regardless of the explanations which must be considered, not the least pervasive of which centers about the contribution of maturation to learning disabilities, the picture indicates clearly that there is a peaking of the incidence of learning disabilities at about the second or third grade. There is then a progressive decline in the incidence with each successively higher grade level. The frequency may approximate as much as 20 per cent at the peak point and then diminish to approximately 2 or 3 per cent in the advanced high-school grades (Burks, 1960; McCarthy & Kirk, 1963). A portion of the reduced incidence in the higher grade levels is undoubtedly accounted for by the dropping-out of pupils who have become discouraged with the school failures they experience because of their specific learning disabilities.

4. *Assessment Techniques.* Previous mention was made of the difficulties in diagnosing learning disabilities because of different persons' viewpoints as to what constitutes a learning disorder. Closely related to this factor is the nature of the instruments and techniques used to assess human performance. The evaluation of children is an arduous task which is rendered more laborious by the limited language facility of the young child. Emphasis upon verbal responses and communicative ability is inherent in most psychoeducational measuring devices. Often there is no suitable standardized measuring instrument for eliciting a specific type of functioning in detail (such as auditory blending and sequencing, or visual memory), and the examiner must invent his own techniques. At best this individualistic procedure may yield qualitative information which is difficult to communicate precisely to other interested professionals.

5. *The Diagnostic Team.* Much confusion also rests in the prevailing system of diagnosis on the basis of evaluation by a "team" of specialists. Each such specialist tends to consider the child only from the vantage of his particular training, and in fact may exercise great care to avoid impinging upon the "area" covered by another member of the team. In practical situations the theoretical advantages of the "diagnostic team" are often unable to rise above the built-in walls which delimit the various disciplines. There is a lack of necessary interdisciplinary communication and misunderstanding as to who is to bear the primary diagnostic and treatment responsibility.

6. *Lack of Followup Reports.* The uncertainty as to who is the responsible person contributes to another problem, namely, the lack of adequate followup study for many children who have been seen for

diagnostic evaluation. Such followup observation is essential to the perfection of appropriate treatment procedures. Followup could, for example, give some indication as to which children have specific deficits as distinct from those children who are only evidencing delayed developmental or maturational patterns.

THE MAJOR THEORETICAL APPROACHES

When the teacher observes that a pupil is consistently unable to keep up with classroom assignments, he may refer the child for study by other specialists in the school staff. The referral request includes a brief account of the difficulty, such as "unable to progress in arithmetic even though his work in all other areas is average" or "does average work in reading and other subjects but consistently fails in spelling where he cannot differentiate words as *lake* and *like*." The problem often centers about a marked lack of attainment in a particular area in the face of average achievement in other areas and indications of at least average intellectual ability. Frequently, the difficulty is a lack of progress in acquiring reading skills.

The several child specialists on the school staff (often, psychologist, social worker, nurse) will carry out an evaluation of the pupil's capacity for doing school work. They will assess and consider his personality, learning abilities, social development, and physical health. In addition to the measures of his present performance, the staff will compile a historical account of his past adjustment and development. Inabilities to be successful with particular tasks and previous failures in the developmental sequence will be carefully noted. In a case conference, information obtained by these several specialists will be shared and added to by the teacher's impressions. From the case-conference discussion will evolve a picture of the pupil's capacity for learning, his strengths and his deficits. The complete description will indicate the pupil's potential for achieving and will identify the factors limiting his ability to perform. The proceedings of a case conference in one school are paraphrased here:

The school nurse, in reporting the pupil's physical health and development, indicated frequent illnesses of the upper respiratory system, ear infections, and associated high temperatures. The pupil had received prompt medical attention for these illnesses and was even hospitalized twice. He is regarded as having good health. The social worker's account of the home and family relationships described a family group in which there was a limited amount of verbal interchange to the point that the pupil's pattern of delayed speech acquisition was not a matter for concern on the part of the parents. The psychologist pointed out that the pupil was of better than average intellectual ability; however, the many doubts about his ability made it difficult for the pupil to make full use of his intellectual ability. The psychologist raised the question of whether the pupil was deliberately performing at a level much below his real capacity for attainment.

In expanding upon the pupil's difficulty in spelling, the teacher brought out that the pupil has previously attended school in another city, where there was more emphasis upon training visual skills and less attention given to drills or other practice in auditory abilities. The teacher stated that the pupil was one of the worst readers in her class and seemed to be having increasing difficulty in this area. She wondered if his poor reading skills had not led the other children in the class to think of him as being inadequate in other activities. He was usually among the last chosen for team games.

In later phases of the case-conference discussion, it was recognized that performance (spelling) emerges from the integration of various abilities (attending, hearing, writing), which in turn originate from the action of several organ systems (skeletal muscle, auditory, central nervous system). An injury or defect in any one of these organic components can be expected to result in impaired performance.

Performance is also influenced by the nature of the pupil's personality organization which must take into account any deficits as well as assets and then formulate defenses or compensations to maintain his individual psychological integrity. At still another level, functioning is modified by factors within the situation itself. The task of spelling words correctly and the approval of the teacher and classmates constitute a particular set of expectations and consequences which require specific abilities and reactions. Organic injury, psychological makeup, and environmental demands may thus be involved in this pupil's inability to spell.

The concepts of interaction and interrelatedness are central to understanding the problems of specific learning disabilities. They also make it necessary to consider several approaches in establishing the type of learning disability, its etiology, and its treatment. In the following sections, we will discuss the three major ways in which specific learning disabilities may be regarded: the psychoneurological approach, the psychodynamic, and the psychoeducational. Discussion will include prominent characteristics, rationale, assessment, suggested treatment, and a critical appraisal of each approach. It will be noted that the three approaches contrasted have certain commonalities and areas of overlap (see Table 10, pp. 152-153).

THE PSYCHONEUROLOGICAL APPROACH in L D

Characteristics

From the psychoneurological approach, recognition of the child with specific learning disabilities is made on the basis of the presence of general behavioral characteristics and specific functional deficits. A list of these characteristics as suggested by Strother (1963) includes:

1. *General Personality Characteristics*
   a. Hyperactivity (restlessness, aimless activity, random movements).
   b. Distractibility (uncontrollably drawn to all new stimuli).
   c. Impulsiveness (spontaneous and compelling inclination to respond).
   d. Emotional instability (sudden mood changes, exaggerated and inappropriate emotional responses).

2. *Specific Disabilities*
   a. Perceptual disorders (errors in form discrimination, form constancy, spatial orientation).
   b. Motor disorders (incoordination, awkwardness, clumsiness).
   c. Language disorders (errors in processing auditory components of speech, inability to associate words with objects, confusion as to time and sequential patterns).
   d. Concept-formation and reasoning disorders (inability to grasp concepts, inability to make associations between ideas, faulty judgment of relevance of associations made).

It must be pointed out that the list presented by Strother is very comprehensive and seeks to incorporate a variety of conditions into a more comprehensible categorization. Groupings such as dyslexia (difficulty in reading), aphasia (inability to use or understand speech), hyperkinesthesis (increased muscular movement), and agraphia (inability to write) often proved to have limited value in the practical problem of treating these same conditions. It is generally recognized that no one child will likely exhibit *all* of the characteristics, although a child showing several of these characteristics would be considered as falling into the classification. The absence of a fixed pattern of behaviors and deficits which would be manifested by all children with specific learning disabilities has been the source of no small amount of the confusion in dealing with this type of disorder. Not only does the combination of these characteristics observed in any child vary, but

TABLE 10. A SUMMARY OF THE PSYCHONEUROLOGICAL, PSYCHODYNAMIC, AND PSYCHOEDUCATIONAL APPROACHES TO LEARNING DISABILITIES

Theoretical Approach	Etiological Factors	Diagnostic Procedures	Some Major Proponents	Treatment Methods	Diagnostic Terminologies
Psycho-neurological	Trauma, injury, or damage to central nervous system.	Neurological examination, EEG findings, case history.	Bakwin Bender Birch Burks Doman Myklebust Reitan Strauss	Depressant drugs, stimulant drugs, surgical intervention, physical therapy, corrective devices, developmental training.	Alexia, aphasia, dyslexia, agraphia, strephosymbolia, dyscalculia, brain-injury, autistic, minimal brain dysfunction, hyperkinetic, word-blindness, dyspraxia, agnosia, dysjunctive, achronometria.
Psycho-dynamic	Impaired parent-child relationships, conflicting social values, excessive early stimulation, inadequate failure, deficits in ability, inadequate self-concept, maladaptive habits and attitudes.	Projective techniques, measures of general and specific abilities, interview, case history, observation, measures of achievement, interpretation of physical-health data.	Bettelheim D'Evelyn I. Harris Pearson Sperry Weisskopf	Psychotherapy with parent and/or child, environmental intervention, educational remediation.	Passive-aggressive personality, oral character, anxious personality, emotional block, insecurity, immaturity, delayed developmental sequence, reading disability, motor incoordination, mild social and emotional maladjustment, inattentiveness, poor self-concept, inadequate control of emotional impulses, inadequate experiential background.

| Psycho-educational | Etiology of minimal consideration; some mention of the correlates or factors which appear to be associated with the disability. | Case history, observation, measures of achievement, performance in specific situations requiring particular skills, consideration of measures of general abilities, review of physical-health data. | Barsch Bateman Bond Frierson Frostig Hewett Kephart Kirk McCarthy | Compensatory training, corrective remediation. | Perceptual handicap, educational disabilities of auditory or visual perception, perceptual speed and tracking, visual or auditory discrimination, selective capacity to attend, skill in auditory and visual fusion, auditory-visual association, visual and auditory memory, kinesthetic sensitivity, laterality, language temporal sequencing, eye-hand coordination, spatial orientation, educationally retarded. |

153

there is a wide range for the same characteristic when observed in different children.

Perhaps the most obvious of these characteristics, and certainly the one most distressing to parents and teachers, centers about the continual and intense motor activity exhibited by such children. The combination of hyperactivity, distractibility, and impulsivity is so pronounced that these children have been referred to as "motor-driven." The inappropriate emotional control and resulting lability are also prominently observed characteristics. Although the personality characteristics are gross and rather easily recognized, the specific disabilities are considerably more difficult to detect. These specific disabilities, which may be slighted or overlooked in a usual evaluation such as a neurological examination, may, nevertheless, exert a profound influence on the child's development and performance.

Etiological Considerations

Although adherents of the psychoneurological approach to specific learning disabilities accept a variety of characteristics as constituting the syndrome, these impairments are taken as evidence of injury or damage to the central nervous system. Initially the treatment of learning disabilities was relegated to physicians, who naturally attempted to understand these problems from the framework of their particular training. The central nervous system was regarded as the center for regulating and coordinating all functioning. It was believed that, in the course of development, the central nervous system becomes organized into many specialized areas, directive centers for particular activities and responses. Information on the location of these specialized areas led to the preparation of "maps," with coded numbers referring to designated centers. One such brain map, prepared by Brodmann, is shown in Figure 2.

Any effort to review the extensive research findings pertaining to brain functioning would lead to discussions beyond the scope of this chapter. Although a controversial issue, some evidence, largely obtained from studies carried out on adults, can be interpreted as lending general support to a localization-of-function theory. Thus the frontal-lobe area (9-10-11 in Fig. 2) appears to coordinate intense emotional experiences and to carry out general inhibitory functions. The temporal lobe seems to hold a center regulating verbal activity (44-43). In the parietal lobe, areas 4-1-3-2 mediate motor and

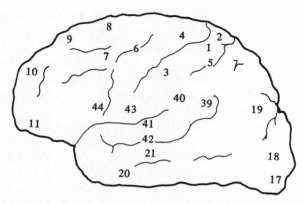

FIGURE 2. *Some localized cerebral centers, after the Brodmann system.*

sensorimotor functions. The occipital lobe holds visualization centers (17-18). The integration of all incoming stimuli from the major sense modalities appears to be vested in areas (5-7-19-39-40) of the parietal-occipital-temporal lobe. Especially in adults, injury or damage to these areas of the brain frequently results in impaired functioning in the particular type of performance regulated by the center.

The psychoneurological approach has given much importance to etiologies, possibly reflecting the influence of the training undergone by physicians. The field of medicine has had great success in dealing with the identified causes of disorders. The emphasis on anatomical-physiological factors has led to a consideration of such factors as heredity, diseases, and accidents as these may result in injury or damage to the central nervous system. In discussing factors resulting in brain damage, Bakwin (1949) listed diseases and infections, tumors, anoxia, metabolic disturbances, toxins, pyrexia, and injuries as being of primary etiological significance. He felt that damage from anoxia is probably the most frequently encountered.

Assessment Procedures

Despite the acceptance of brain injury as being responsible for impaired functioning, assessment procedures used in the psychoneurological approach are not pointed to the direct examination of the brain. The present development of assessment techniques does not make it possible to conduct a detailed scrutiny of the intactness of the human brain. Instead, the diagnosis is arrived at on the basis of interpretations drawn from observed functioning, with inferences as to the mediating role of the central nervous system.

Indications of the intactness of the central nervous system are suggested by walking a line with the eyes closed (balance), inserting marbles on a board with cutouts (dexterity), touching finger to nose (accuracy), reactions to heat, cold, pain, light, strong odors, sounds, and touch (sensitivity). The electroencephalograph (EEG) provides a record of the electrical activity of the brain as tasks of varying degrees of complexity are performed (rest, reading, solving abstract problems). X-ray pictures of the brain, placed in sharper detail by injections of air into cerebral passageways, may provide evidence of blocked passages or tumors.

The findings may be supplemented by other measures. Motor-visual coordination is revealed in writing and copying figures. Visualization effectiveness is evident in the discrimination of forms or by reading. Auditory abilities are ascertained by audiometric examination or by repetition of words and sentences. A careful appraisal of speech facility may be revealing of specific deficits. In some instances, the influence of drugs or medication on these functions may be of importance in establishing an impairment. It is interesting in practice that the psychologist is more inclined to pay heed to neurological findings than the neurologist to consider psychological assessment findings.

The making of a diagnosis of specific learning disability, now frequently referred to as "minimal brain dysfunction" following the deliberations of a task force on terminology and identification (Clements, 1966), also entails differentiation from other conditions of neurological impairment. The distinction is usually made on the basis of the rather generalized impairment associated with mental retardation, cerebral palsy, encephalitis, psychosis, cultural deprivation, and such, in contrast to the more limited impairment observed in specific learning disabilities. The ultimate diagnostic choice may depend upon information provided by a detailed developmental and clinical history.

Treatment Approaches

In the past, treatment of specific learning disabilities was largely delegated to the physician. The specific disabilities encountered were mostly seen in adult clients, as consequences of some injury. Initially, the medical concern was for describing, classifying, and seeking neuroanatomical correlates for the specific deficits observed (Bateman, 1964). There was little attempt at correction, especially in the presently accepted techniques of retraining, prior to the work of Orton (1925), a physician. Orton's interest in education may have inadvertently contributed to some of the confusion which prevails concerning who is responsible for the treatment of specific learning disabilities. Attempts to dodge a charge by other professionals has added to physicians being caught in a kind of "buck-passing" situation regarding treatment of these disorders, which are puzzling to everyone.

Certain corrective procedures for remedying defects of the visual, auditory, motor, and central nervous systems can be performed only by a physician. These include surgery, the administration of medications, and in some instances the fitting of hearing aids and corrective lenses. Advances in medical treatment have been extensive. Drugs are available for selectively increasing a child's attentiveness by reducing his reaction to stimuli (tranquilizers) or by making him more responsive to stimuli (stimulants). Making a diagnosis has been facilitated by more refined electrical apparatus such as the electroencephalograph. Progress in refining and standardizing the neurological examination is being carried out by Reitan (1958), who has usually been successful in pinpointing cerebral focal points of malfunctioning.

Even so, there are instances in which surgical or medical procedures cannot be used in treatment. For example, careful neurological examination may reveal that a child has a deep and centrally located cerebral lesion. Surgical correction may be contraindicated, and there may be no medication which will act selectively on the lesion. The child must learn to live with and in spite of his defect. Treatment in such cases becomes largely a matter of education and training. Physicians are presently apt to be concerned with the possibility of correcting the disability by some training program. They generally do not become so directly involved in the amelioration by education as did Orton, but may cooperate with teachers or other educators in developing a total corrective program. The pediatrician is likely to consider a referral to a psychologist or to a psychoeducational clinic known to have developed extensive developmental training programs for correcting specific disabilities.

THE PSYCHODYNAMIC APPROACH *in* ᒪᗪ

Characteristics

A second major approach to understanding specific learning disabilities places emphasis on psychological as opposed to organic dysfunction. The psychodynamic framework focuses on the individual arrangement of energies, skills, and abilities as these become organized by experience. Of particular importance is the capacity for handling emotions and for achieving new learning. From the psychodynamic view, specific learning disabilities are seen as any impairment which might prevent learning. Consideration is directed to the processes for coping with demands and to pressures associated with the demands. Characteristics of concern in the psychodynamic approach to the identification of specific learning disabilities can be grouped under six major categories:

1. Emotional (negativism, inattentiveness, anxiety, self-depreciating passive aggressiveness, depression, dependency).
2. Social-impulsive (immature, poor peer acceptance, antisocial-compensating, hostile).
3. Sensory (hyperresponsive, visually incompetent, tone-deaf, insensitive).
4. Physical (uncoordinated, clumsy, awkward, malaise, disoriented).
5. Communication (stammering, inarticulate, sparse vocabulary, uncomprehending).
6. Performance discrepancy (underachieving, poorly motivated, nonreader).

Actually, the characteristics acknowledged by proponents of the psychodynamic approach do not differ greatly from those recognized in the psychoneurological approach, as Mesinger (1965) pointed out. There is an expansion to encompass environmental demands and attitudinal factors in the categories of "academic" and "social." In this way, the child's reaction or "adjustment" to his deficit is given weight equal to that of the particular deficit itself. This may have important implications in formulating a treatment program. One of the most profound features of emotional influences upon behavior is the possibility of a self-perpetuating circular reaction such as failure-aggression-failure or anxiety-failure-anxiety.

As was true for the psychoneurological approach, there is no specific set of characteristics which form a "specific learning disability syndrome" within the psychodynamic framework. Possibly because of the broader framework in which the child's functioning is evaluated from the psychodynamic approach, the child with specific learning disabilities is more likely to show multiple deficits involving three or more of the major groups of characteristics from all six areas because of the interrelatedness of performance made by the same person.

Teachers are more likely to be aware of characteristics within the "academic" and "emotional" categories whereas parents may be more concerned about those of the "emotional" and "communication" categories. Characteristics in the "sensory" and "physical" categories are perhaps the most frequently overlooked by teachers and parents, especially since the detection of these impairments may require special equipment and training.

Etiological Considerations

The psychodynamic approach places primary concern on the modification and development of the individual as a result of his individual experiences. It holds that emotions, as the motivational sources for maintaining and sustaining performance, play a crucial role in learning (Berlyne, 1964). Unchanneled energy results in an uncontrollable overflow which disrupts performance. Too little energy leads to insufficient involvement and failure to learn. In other instances, energy expended may find no satisfaction and attach itself to inappropriate objects or tasks, with consequent perseveration or fixation.

Emotions evolve out of experiences, especially those of success and failure. The most important experiences for humans are social learnings incurred in contacts with other persons. Social learning, a major field of study in its own right, places emphasis on the social possibilities for rewards and the channeling of emotions (frustration, aggression, anxiety) into socially acceptable outlets. A personal directional-integration center (self-concept) develops from individual experiences of success and failure. Concurrently, concern must be given to the acquisition of consensually agreed cues and meanings (attitudes) which serve as the basis for interpreting all situations and events.

Just as it is not possible to be exact in pinpointing brain damage, so are emotions and experiences impossible to present in tangible forms. In the light of this difficulty, the assumed influence of emotions is implied by stating that the impaired performance, which is demonstrable, is associated with one or another emotional feeling. These somewhat abstract relationships may be made more comprehensible by a synopsis of examples of psychodynamic factors which Weisskopf (1951) found to be associated with specific learning disabilities in children referred to school psychologists for study. These factors are briefly described below:

1. *Conscious Refusal to Learn.* A boy feels real hostility toward his parents and other adults. He readily expresses his dislike for all adult persons, including teachers, who he claims try to "use" him. His rejection of adults has generalized to a point that he refuses to do anything he associates with being adult, such as reading. A girl has strong loyalties to her parents, who have only limited educational attainment. They do not value educational achievement, and she feels that applying herself at school would be inconsistent with the wishes of her parents and might even alienate her from them.

2. *Overt Hostility.* A girl has intense feelings of resentment. She is hypercritical and has a continual chip on her shoulder. Her anger spills over at the slightest provocation. She sees only the possibilities for battle in any situation, and it is impossible for her to enter into and profit from the usual classroom learning relationships.

3. *Negative Conditioning.* A negative emotional response (fear, anger, dislike, failure) to a particular task (reading) may be acquired out of previous associations. Reading, having been presented with someone or something already feared or disliked, becomes capable by itself of producing these negative emotional reactions. A child's first-grade teacher would walk around the room rapping knuckles with a ruler. The teacher placed great stress on reading. The child's panic-like reactions to this teacher continued in response to reading lessons from other teachers in later years.

4. *Displacement of Feelings.* This process involves the transfer of feelings originally aroused by some object or person to a similar object or situation. A child is extremely jealous of a favored brother who excels in reading. The resentment is transferred to the act of reading which is the sibling's strong point. A variation of this impairment is seen in the case of the child whose parent is an avid reader. The child is unable to express his hostility toward the parent in an open or direct fashion, but feels free to dislike the reading which is so impor-

tant to the parent. Displaced hostility is seldom recognized by either the parent or the child.

5. *Resistance to Pressures.* Our culture has been repeatedly cited for its undue emphasis on achievement. Rendered overanxious by his sparse food intake, a child's mother begins forcibly to cram food into the child, and is surprised that the child capitalizes on the possibility for asserting his rights by even stronger refusal of foods. Similarly, the overambitious parent pushing for intellectual attainment runs the risk of resistance that may take the form of lack of interest in reading.

6. *Clinging to Dependency Status.* The overprotected and babied child may, consciously or unconsciously, choose to preserve his infantile status and secure attention through being helpless. Such children may reject everything associated with growing up, including the self-reliance evidenced by being able to talk well or being successful in school. The arrival of younger siblings may accentuate this pattern on the part of an older child, who can interpret being sent to school as an attempt to get him out of the house so that his mother can give all her attention to the new baby.

7. *Limited Persistence.* This factor is operative in the child who launches into a task but meets with some initial difficulty. He quickly becomes discouraged and stops trying. As a rule, such children come to school with marked feelings of inferiority and uncertainty. Their homelife has not provided them with security and self-confidence. The parents may have been hypercritical, rejecting, or plagued with self-doubts. These children seem predisposed to failure and are easily convinced that they are stupid, readily accepting an inferior status.

8. *Fear of Success.* For some children, almost any successful form of self-expression may stir up feelings of intense anxiety and distress related to unacceptable fears of destruction or damage. Success in reading may symbolize entering into an adult activity and therefore competing with a parent. Such competition, in turn, may imply the possibility of dreadful forms of retaliation. The child may seek safety in self-destruction and passivity. This type of reaction, involving deep-seated unconscious conflicts, tends to be highly resistant to all remedial help.

9. *Extreme Distractibility or Restlessness.* When tension builds up

to a level exceeding the usual capacity for control, the child may seek relief in the form of an outlet. Release in motor activity is often chosen. The child is unable to sit still, does not remember directions given him, and falls behind in learning. The realization that he has failed leads to discouragement and heightens the level of tension. The child becomes unable to direct his attention selectively and is helplessly impelled to react to all objects, persons, and situations. The ensuing disruption and disorganization make it impossible for him to persist at a task except under the most controlled conditions.

10. *Absorption in a Private World.* A child may become so absorbed in his own thoughts that he can give only intermittent attention to his real surroundings. Memorizing the complicated rules and logical formats of mathematics requires much more effort and gives much less satisfaction than does the preoccupation with daydreams. The reverie may entail the excitement of hitting a homerun, scoring a winning touchdown, finding romantic adventure; or it may be concerned with morbid fantasies of burning cities and destroying whole races of people. In either instance, the child's abilities are diverted from opportunities for real praise and recognition gained from being successful with a task.

11. *Exaggerated Emotional Responses to Instructional Materials.* Instructional materials are selected to have meaning for the learner. Stories are about people, families, and friends. They tell of incidents, happenings, and situations. The meanings given such content will vary according to the needs and experiences of the child. The sudden surge of emotional feelings experienced by a child from a broken home as he reads a story dealing with happy family life may obscure any new learning presented by the story.

12. *Suppression and Constriction.* Some children are faced with being unable to find outlets for unacceptable feelings of destruction, guilt, or hatred. They seek to handle these impulses by denial, compartmentalization, and noninvolvement. The rigid controls established over these emotional feelings and the effort required to constantly keep up a guard exacts a considerable reduction in the capacity for any new learning. The total inhibition manifests itself in such impairments as the unwillingness to express ideas, the inability to recite or answer questions, and the deliberate tuning-out of any new information.

Assessment Procedures

It should be apparent by now that a wide range of behaviors is encompassed in the classification "specific learning disability." It may well be that variability of behavior is the one incontestable characteristic consistently associated with this disorder. The psychodynamic conception of learning disabilities as impairments influenced by many different factors gives compelling support to the total evaluation of the child's potential for intellectual, emotional, and social performance. The detailed assessment will include an examination, observation, and study of the child. Generally this threefold task can be adequately carried out by a psychologist, but provision should also be made for psychiatric, neurological, audiological, speech, or social-worker consultation if indicated. Examinations by other specialists, such as an ophthalmologist or otologist, may be suggested by evidence of visual or auditory defects. A developmental history and account of the child's family life and home background can serve as an important source for the interpretation of identified deficits in performance.

Measures of potential for achievement are compared with measures of actual attainment. Mental age or test age from the Stanford-Binet Intelligence Scale or the Wechsler Intelligence Scales may be used as the basis for predicting a certain level of attainment on an achievement test. If some of the achievement scores (reading, arithmetic, vocabulary) do not fall within the expected range, a specific learning disability is suspected. The low-performance area is investigated in greater detail. Frequently, the discrepancy is between expected and actual attainment in reading.

From the psychodynamic point of view, it is also necessary to differentiate consistent nonachievement in limited and particular areas from the more general lack of achievement seen with mental retardation or with speech and hearing disabilities and from the inconsistent achievement typical of the severely emotionally disturbed. To make such a differential diagnosis, information obtained from the psychological examination must be carefully interpreted in the light of findings presented in a case history of physical health and family relationships and in reports of examinations carried out by other specialists.

Suggestions of factors contributing to the learning disability are sought in the nature of the child's social and emotional adjustment. The assessment of social and emotional development via personality scales comprises the unique contribution of the psychologist. In carrying out the personality evaluation, the psychologist makes extensive use of specific measures and observations. Favored measuring devices include projective and paper-and-pencil self-report tests of personality. On the basis of responses to a series of inkblot pictures, the Rorschach test supplies information regarding such important personality characteristics as aggression, fantasy, introversion, emotional controls, intellectual efficiency, and general approach to a task. From stories elicited by ambiguous pictures, the Michigan Picture Test or Thematic Apperception Test (TAT) provide clues as to the person's needs, sources of satisfaction, reactions to success or failure, currently perceived pressure of demands, and individual attitudes and value systems.

More specific information regarding particular attitudes, values, and demands is suggested by paper-and-pencil measures, such as sentence-completion tests, Sixteeen Factor Personality Inventory, or an adjustment inventory. The general social acceptability of the individual's personality makeup is indicated by other paper-and-pencil scales and inventories such as the Minnesota Multiphasic Personality Inventory (MMPI). There are many other personality measures and assessment techniques. It must be cautioned that giving meaning to data gained from these measures is a highly skilled matter and demands extensive training and practice.

The interpretation of material from personality tests in fact frequently requires the consideration of other impressions. Thus the psychologist finds it necessary to observe the child's reactions in a variety of situations: the unstructured setting of the playroom and the more formal organization of the classroom. The importance of precisely identifying attitudes and feelings which may contribute to specific learning disabilities often makes it appropriate for the psychologist to supplement his entire battery of objective measures by carrying out a detailed interview with the child.

Ideally, the psychologist should be able to complete his evaluation of specific learning disabilities by a detailed assessment of basic motor, visual, and auditory skills. Such information, generally provided by a diagnostic reading test or one of several special scales (Bender Visual Motor Designs Test, Wepman Auditory Discrimination Scale, Frostig

Developmental Test of Visual Perception), would be of great value in planning a remedial program for correcting the disability. Some psychologists working in the school are competent to do this type of assessment, but unfortunately the majority of psychologists have not had such training.

Treatment Approaches

The treatment of specific learning disabilities by psychotherapy is only a particular application of techniques which are extensively discussed in Chapter 9 of this text. Common sources of psychopathology and resulting impaired functioning associated with specific learning disabilities are inadequate parent-child relationships and consequent heightened aggression or dependency, self-perceptions of inadequacy and inferiority, excessive levels of anxiety and concern about failure, and confusion resulting from unsuccessful experiences in coping with tasks encountered in the past.

Psychologists, psychiatrists, social workers, and counselors have attempted to correct these conditions and the associated impaired performance by a variety of methods. The techniques applied have tended to be of the more conventional types, such as regularly scheduled counseling interviews, play therapy, psychoanalysis, and group-therapy sessions. Some therapists prefer to see only the parent; others see only the child. In another arrangement, both the parent and the child are worked with but in separate sessions. A recent development entails the entire family participating in a therapy session as a unit.

Innovations in the psychodynamic approach are being explored. One such change finds the trained psychotherapist serving as a consultant and directing a nonformally trained therapist (such as the classroom teacher), who actually carries out the therapy. Another approach centers about the use of intensive retraining in the classroom with behavior-therapy techniques. Psychologists, especially those working in the schools, have been particularly inclined to recommend the treatment of learning disabilities by remedial educational methods.

Wider application of the less conventional forms of psychotherapy has been urged by Cohn (1964) and by Bower (1966). They point out that since specific causes of learning disabilities are generally not known, treatment must necessarily be nonspecific. An approach which emphasizes support and assistance for the child to grow and develop in ways consistent with his intact abilities is more promising than one which insists on the child giving up self-respect and security to correct his disabilities by conventional psychotherapy procedures.

THE PSYCHOEDUCATIONAL APPROACH In L.D.

Characteristics

Relatively new but growing in acceptance is the psychoeducational approach to specific learning disabilities. Perhaps the most comprehensive list of deficits indicative of a specific learning disability from this point of view is that presented by Bateman (1964). The list organizes the skills and abilities which are maximally called upon in ordinary classroom learning into four main groups:

1. *Sensory Skills*
   a. Auditory and visual perception.
   b. Visual and auditory discrimination.
   c. Auditory and visual fusion.
   d. Visual and auditory memory.
   e. Kinesthetic sensitivity.

2. *Motor Skills*
   a. Eye-hand coordination.
   b. Laterality.
   c. Perceptual speed and tracking.

3. *Language Skills*
   a. Temporal sequencing.
   b. Verbal facility.
   c. Language comprehension.

4. *Association Skills*
   a. Selective capacity for attending.
   b. Auditory-visual association.
   c. Spatial orientation.

It is of interest that these characteristics have evolved primarily from the observation and comment of educators, those professional persons most involved in dealing with specific learning disabilities. There is less emphasis on "personality" traits such as hyperactivity, negativism, distractibility, or impulsiveness, which are apparently of greater significance to adherents of the psychoneurological and psycho-dynamic approaches. The differences in emphasis may be a reflection of the teacher's interest in identifying what skills the child does have for learning rather than what he does not have.

Another difference is the specificity with which the learning disability is described. This feature contrasts especially with the rather general classifications, such as "emotional instability" or "motor inco-ordination," which have a major position in other lists of learning-disability characteristics. These disabilities are so explicit as to make it unlikely that they would be recognized by parents or other profes-sional persons (physicians, psychologists) without a considerable familiarity of classroom learning activities.

Etiological Considerations

There is a common belief that "diagnosis" consists of a search for the *cause* of a disability. Diagnosis, in such a limited sense, reflects the medical model and its concern for specific etiologies. The psycho-educational differs most from other approaches in that there is a minimal interest in the cause of a disability. From the psychoeduca-tional viewpoint, diagnosis is to be understood as a detailed *description* of a disability. Reliance is placed on being able to identify and describe behavioral deficits sufficiently to then prescribe appropriate correction by direct training or by compensatingly drawing upon other skills and abilities. A psychoeducational diagnostic statement such as "read-ing disability associated with auditory memory deficit" implies that there is a correlational rather than a causal relationship between the reading problem and the auditory defect. As Bateman (1964) has stated, "The very fact that we cannot exchange parents or repair damaged brains has led to the present day concern of many with behav-ioral and symptomatic rather than pathological or etiological factors."

The most substantial support for the ahistorical position of the psychoeducational approach comes from studies of learning. It has been repeatedly demonstrated that performance can be shaped or altered, a task can be successfully completed, without detailed knowledge of the learner's nervous system or his remote prior experiences. Although from a practical point of view there is little attention given to original causes, suggestions as to the causes may be implied in correlates included in the description of the disability. It may be noted, for example, that the child who has an inability to maintain correct verb tenses has limited language stimulation in his home, or poor auditory discrimination, or temporal confusion.

Pragmatically, the deemphasis on usual etiological considerations has been reinforced by the observation that successful educational treatment of a disability seems to be unrelated to its supposed cause. The remedial teacher has about equal success with those children who have hostile uncooperative attitudes toward reading, who have minimal brain dysfunction, or who have visual sequencing deficits. Even the most exhaustive diagnostic study frequently produces only implicit etiological factors, which can seldom be verified. The teacher is still faced with the problem of having to provide learning experiences with which the child can be successful. Etiological correlates are deemed useful only insofar as they contribute to the planning of appropriate educational experiences.

Assessment Procedures

The identification of a specific learning disability with the psycho-educational approach entails obtaining evidence of specific lack of attainment in view of other indications of normal general ability in intelligence, vision, audition, and locomotion. Even though the focus is on the current functioning capacity rather than on an extensive history of the nature of the previous adjustment, mental retardation, severe emotional disorders, and physical handicaps (orthopedic, hearing loss) must be ruled out. This is not to deny that some children in some of these categories (mentally retarded, emotionally disturbed, poor vision) may have specific learning disabilities. Rather the concern is for making the most effective educational placement.

Specific learning disabilities are identified on the basis of interpretations made of the child's functioning as observed in a variety of performance situations. The diagnostic study is directed to providing an educationally useful description of the disability. It is often carried out by a psychologist or a remedial educational specialist. The assessment must frequently make use of nonstandardized or informal techniques and procedures.

Standardized measuring scales developed for normal groups are seldom suitable for the evaluation of children with specific learning disabilities. For example, a child with a suspected learning disability may be shown, one at a time, a series of words of varying complexity. He is allowed to look at each word for a fixed time and then asked to write the word from memory. He may be asked to tell what was said as the examiner sounds out the phonic elements of words (m-e, t-o-p). The interpretation of performance elicited by such techniques places considerable demand upon the ingenuity and experience of the diagnostician. Fortunately, the number of standardized psychoeducational measuring scales suitable for this detailed assessment is increasing, although they tend to be limited to the evaluation of skills required for reading. Those currently available include the Illinois Test of Psycholinguistic Abilities, Frostig Developmental Test of Visual Perception, Kephart Perceptual Rating Scale, Parson's Language Scale, and Wepman Auditory Discrimination Scale.

When assessed from the psychoeducational point of view, the child with a specific learning disability is likely to be described in educationally relevant terms. The disability is described in terms of impairments to achievement in basic areas of academic attainment such as writing, arithmetic, reading, remembering, listening, and communicating. This tendency represents a significant step in recognizing the potential which the school holds with respect to the correction of specific learning disabilities.

Treatment Approaches

Although not a new approach to the correction of learning disabilities, the psychoeducational method of treatment has gained increased acceptance. Recognition of the validity of educational training has been underscored by studies indicating the positive role of experience in the development of abilities. Advances and improvements in other aspects of society are analogously to be observed in the educational system. More reliable psychoeducational measuring devices, the addition of other professional specialists in support of the classroom teacher, and the development of many ingenious methods and materials for instruction have made the school more effective in dealing with all problems. A greater understanding of the fortuitous possibilities for strengthening weaknesses or compensating for deficits has encouraged the school to correct specific learning disabilities.

The psychoeducational approach includes diagnostic study, treatment, and followup evaluation of the pupil. Specialists trained in fields other than education, such as nurses, speech therapists, social workers, counselors, psychologists, and physicians, may assume significant roles in the diagnosis and evaluation. The actual treatment is provided in the main by such educational specialists as special remedial teachers and regular classroom teachers. Speech therapists, social workers, and psychologists may participate in lesser degrees.

The special teacher is likely to work with a pupil on a one-to-one basis, or with very small groups homogeneously placed on the basis of common educational disabilities, presenting a sequence of experiences which have been individually planned for the pupils. Some major areas of concentration advocated by specialists in the field are:

1. Motor Development (Bender, 1956; Schilder, 1937; Kephart, 1960).

2. Perceptual Training (Frostig, Lefever, & Whittlesey, 1961; Wepman, 1960; Kephart, 1964).

3. Language Training (Myklebust, 1964).

4. Concept Formation by Motor-Perceptual-Language Integration (Strauss & Lehtinen, 1947; Gellner, 1959; Epps, McCannon, & Simmons, 1958).

5. Reading Skill (Bond & Tinker, 1967; Harris, 1964; Monroe, 1932; Durrell, 1956).

6. Stimulus Control (Bender, 1956; Strauss & Lehtinen, 1947).

Some workers attempt to correct a disability by direct training of the deficit; others prefer to present a task in a way that is consistent with the identified strengths of the pupil. Yet another technique entails strengthening deficits by associating them with stronger abilities. The actual training experiences presented to any one pupil are geared to the pupil's particular learning disabilities and assets and are therefore individual and unique. There is no research evidence at this time to indicate the superiority of any one method. Several sets of general guidelines are available for planning an educational treatment program. Those suggested by remedial-reading specialists (Bond & Tinker, 1967; Monroe, 1932; Fernald, 1943; Harris, 1964) are perhaps the most detailed. Others warranting considerations, although in some instances less specific, have been proposed by Frostig, Lefever, and Whittlesey (1961), Hewett (1964), Kephart (1960), and Whelan and Haring (1966).

CRITICAL EVALUATION OF APPROACHES

The major approaches to the treatment of specific learning disabilities have been outlined according to the etiology emphasized. Since all three are widely used, a critical appraisal of each approach can serve to clarify the inherent limitations and applicability. They will be contrasted from the standpoint of evidence supporting the rationale, principal inadequacies, and general effectiveness for correcting learning disabilities.

THE PSYCHONEUROLOGICAL APPROACH

Rationale and Supporting Evidence

When the problem of brain damage and resulting behavioral deficits is examined, the key question is the relationship between performance and neuroanatomical structure. The psychoneurological approach assumes that behavioral functions are carried out under the direction of localized cerebral centers. It is generally accepted that the brain does indeed carry out coordinating and directive activities. Unfortunately, even when a deficit is identified, it is not possible to verify actual brain injury. The data from which localization of function is assumed are sparse and mostly obtained from adults. Inferences following injuries, post-mortem investigations, observation of electrical stimulation, the effects of drugs, and examination of infrahuman animals are the principal sources of information about the brain.

Although the available data may be interpreted as suggesting a general localization of cerebral function, the picture is by no means consistent. The assessment procedures are as yet gross and relatively little specific information regarding brain functions has been discovered. The amount of damage may be more important than the locus of the injury (Hebb, 1949). Complex types of performance may be more impaired by any injury than are simple automatic types of performance (Teuber, Battersby, & Bender, 1951). Maher (1966) observed that a cerebral injury might result in temporary losses which disappear after a time, or that disabilities might suddenly appear long after an injury was incurred. The situation is well summarized by Eisenberg's comment, "thus, knowledge of the relation between nervous structure and function, however useful it may be, cannot suffice for an understanding of the problems of the brain-damaged child" (Eisenberg, 1957, p. 74).

Major Inadequacies

The concern with making a diagnosis and the interest in ascertaining the cause of a disability, typifying the psychoneurological approach, have produced a large number of diagnostic terms. Diagnoses expressed in such technical terms as dyslexia, aphasia, or agraphia have limited utility, even in communication with other medical specialists. In discussing the recent tendency to explain learning disabilities as "minimal brain damage," Cohn (1964) cited three reasons which contraindicate such a position:

1. The signs and symptoms are only qualitative indicators.
2. Minimal clinical signs have not been neuropathologically demonstrated to be related to minimal brain pathology.
3. The type of clinical signs elicited has been found to depend on the basic philosophy of the examining neurologist.

Cohn, who has had extensive experience and followup observation of school children with neurological damage, believes that, to be useful, neurological evaluation should identify those sensory and motor channels which can be used in learning.

General Effectiveness

The psychoneurological approach has only limited efficacy. The mere labeling of a condition is, in itself, of no real therapeutic value. To be useful, the diagnosis must suggest treatment procedures. Frequently, no medications, surgical interventions, or corrective prostheses are implied by diagnoses of learning disabilities made by the neurologist. As a group, physicians have generally been slow to appreciate the possible corrective benefit of special training to correct a disability. Even when special training is considered, there may be no way to coordinate this treatment. The cost of treatment suggested by neurological evaluation varies from moderate to so expensive as to be prohibitive for most families.

Even otherwise highly competent and well-trained neurologists may consider only gross performance in making an evaluation. It is a rare neurologist, for example, who is trained to assess in detail the child's capacity for learning to read. When effective, treatment prescribed in the psychoneurological approach can result in dramatic improvement which tends to be permanent. When ineffectual, it is likely to be lengthy, expensive, and entail certain discomfort and risk for the patient.

THE PSYCHODYNAMIC APPROACH

Rationale and Supporting Evidence

The psychodynamic approach to specific learning disabilities holds that any impairment in functioning mirrors impairments in the individual's experiences. Although deficiencies in the number and quality of objects and situations to which an individual is exposed are recognized, particular significance is given to deficits in relationships with other people. Experiences which are so intense as to be overwhelming experiences which have inadequate or inappropriate consequences, or no experience may all lead to deficits. These deficiencies in experience are difficult to identify, and their influence on behavior is not easy to demonstrate. Existing psychological measuring devices have a marked inability to differentiate low achievement associated with brain injury from low achievement due to social and emotional maladjustment or to mental retardation (Yates, 1954; Klebanoff, Singer, & Wilensky, 1954). Factors identified as contributing to a disability are thus vague and not readily verifiable. The same experience may facilitate or impair performance. A child deprived of the rewards associated with a comfortable, happy home may either work harder or give up.

Major Inadequacies

Adherents of the psychodynamic approach are likely to waste many hours in an exacting diagnostic study which only identifies possible causes. When identified, these are, moreover, historical and cannot be directly changed. McWilliams (1965) has described the psychodynamic approach to diagnosis as more a matter of ruling out rather than of finding etiological factors. Lack of an adequate personality theory and the interrelatedness of performance and ability contribute to superficial and circular explanations of disabilities.

Deficits are frequently pictured as resulting from multiple causes. Although Bond and Tinker (1957) believe that emotional maladjustments tend to be consequences of deficit-induced failures, they admit also that failures in performance may result from emotional maladjustment. It is puzzling to find that treating either the disability or the emotional problem leads to improvement in performance. Treatment of the emotional aspects of a disability seems to take longer to show improvement in performance than does direct treatment of the disability.

General Effectiveness

The psychodynamic approach is regarded as being moderately successful in correcting specific learning disabilities. Despite comprehensive diagnostic study and extensive use of measuring devices, evaluations of the efficacy of treatment give somewhat confusing results. The outcome is about equally effective when the child is seen alone, when only the parent is seen, or when both parent and child are seen. The same is true whether play therapy, psychoanalysis, or counseling is used. Followup evaluation of therapeutic outcomes is complicated by the lack of precise statements of causal factors and because the influence of the causal factors is difficult to prove or disprove.

The detailed psychodynamic evaluation is time-consuming and can be relatively expensive. It tends to provide a picture which emphasizes the individual's deficits and may thus be threatening and undermining to the child. The psychodynamic approach can contribute to the fragmentation approach, cautioned against by Bower (1966). The child can be confused by treatment given by a team of specialists who communicate minimally among themselves and when no one assumes responsibility for coordinating the treatment program. On the other hand, psychodynamic evaluations are couched in behavior traits, such as negativistic, inattentive, or hyperactive. These are moderately useful educationally and serve to communicate meaningfully even though they do not suggest much in the way of specific corrective training.

THE PSYCHOEDUCATIONAL APPROACH

Rationale and Supporting Evidence

The psychoeducational approach is highly pragmatic. If it has a rationale, it is the belief that each child must be provided with opportunities which will promote the maximum development of his abilities. The realities of life are such that each person must acquire ways of meeting demands and expectations which society makes. Success with one type of task is likely to be followed by success in dealing with another type of task. That capacity for learning and performing can be improved with training is well substantiated by studies investigating effects of early stimulation and deprivation on future performance.

Training is the chief concern of the school. There have been an implicit acceptance of the infeasibility of redoing the child's past experiences and a commitment to working with the pupil as he is. This view has led to the recognition that each pupil brings assets and deficits for new learning experiences. Although much of the educational training is provided in a group organization, there has been an increasing awareness of the necessity for matching individuality of capacity with individuality of instruction. This trend has made it more important to carry out an educational diagnosis which identifies in detail the pupil's potential for education.

Major Inadequacies

Most of the inadequacies associated with the psychoeducational approach to specific learning disabilities can be attributed to past reluctance to become more actively involved in providing training. The potential of education has been more acknowledged than made use of. Educational offerings, presented in the curriculum, have been very general and geared to the majority two-thirds of pupils. Necessary diversification from formal academic instruction to include motor development, perceptual training, concept formation, and stimulus control has created organizational problems. Sometimes there is no administrative supervisor who can pull these varied activities into a coordinated sequence. Followup of pupils who are provided with these services is often lacking.

Related to the organizational difficulties associated with providing educational programs for specific learning disabilities are problems related to personnel for staffing such programs. Effective educational treatment requires specially trained teachers who must have support and assistance from psychologists, physicians, nurses, social workers, and guidance counselors. Of practical importance is the availability of assessment and remedial materials which are sufficiently specific for identifying and correcting particular disabilities. The lack of organized coordination, properly trained staff, and adequate assessment and instructional materials may contribute to the overlooking of critical factors of a medical or home and family nature. Although probably infrequent, when they exist such factors should have appropriate correction in order to facilitate the educational treatment.

General Effectiveness

Although not free of all problems, the psychoeducational approach seems to offer a highly favorable way for correcting specific learning disabilities. It has the advantage of being only a particular extension of educational activities already established. Thus it can minimize a pupil's impression of being singled out or embarrassingly put on the spot. The pupil is better able to see the direct benefit of his treatment, and improvement in his performance can bring immediate rewards from many sources—classmates, teachers, and parents.

Increasing assuredness on the part of the school as to its effectiveness in correcting learning disabilities can only enhance the psychoeducational approach. The cost of remedial programs is much less expensive than psychoneurological or psychodynamic treatment programs. The educational diagnoses of specific learning disabilities, expressed as visual-memory deficit, auditory-discrimination disability, and such, are readily translated into educational programs. Better administrative organization, refinement of diagnostic techniques, a greater number of specially trained teachers, and earlier intervention will make the psychoeducational approach even more telling.

FUTURE TRENDS

It seems obvious that interest in the alleviation of specific learning disabilities will increase. The coming-together of various specialists dealing with these problems will improve communication and promote an exchange of ideas. New understanding of relationships, more acceptance of responsibility by schools, and successes with existing methods will encourage the continuation of these same procedures. Advances will be made in all areas for dealing with specific learning disabilities. New medications, surgical methods, and therapeutic techniques will be developed, but the greatest progress is anticipated in education. Educational programs, supported by psychoneurological and psychodynamic advances, bid to become the major treatment procedures.

As operated by the schools, educational programs will provide for systematic identification by group screening of pupils. Treatment results will be regularly evaluated by routine followup of pupils served. Teachers especially trained for correcting specific learning disabilities will draw on particular techniques and measuring scales. Applications of procedures adapted from behavior-modification findings and measurement devices, such as the Illinois Test of Psycholinguistic Abilities and the Frostig Developmental Test of Visual Perception, already show considerable promise. Diagnosis and treatment will be closely integrated, with treatment being initiated at a much earlier time, perhaps eventually on a preventative basis in the form of intensive preschool readiness training. The key to making these developments possible rests in the formulation of an acceptable organizational plan which will supply necessary administrative control for the educational management of specific learning disabilities.

There are indications that some of these trends are becoming actualities. A real step in the school's accepting responsibility for treatment of learning disabilities is seen in the agreements reached by the joint committee from the United States Office of Education and the Council for Exceptional Children. The committee dealt with the educational treatment of "major learning disorders."

SUMMARY

Specific learning disabilities are manifested as particular impairments in performance. Examples are inabilities to remember, make visual or auditory differentiations, follow usual patterns for sequential arrangement of words in a sentence, keep the orientation of geometric figures, carry out a particular arithmetic operation, or copy letters in the spatially correct form. Generally limited to a single area (motor, visual, auditory, emotional), they may take the form of deficits in integrating two major areas, such as motor-visual association or auditory-emotional association. The disability persists in the presence of indications of average or better general ability.

Learning disabilities must be differentiated from mental retardation, social and emotional maladjustment, and language, hearing, or visual defects. The distinction is not always easily made. A specific learning disability is a limited deficit. Some persons who are mentally retarded, language-disabled, or emotionally maladjusted are found to have specific learning disabilities, but others do not. It seems more likely that specific learning disabilities can contribute to or speed up the development of a more severe and general behavior disorder.

Typically seen as a reading problem in school-age children, the impairment in performance has accompanying feelings of failure and frustration. Besides fostering a discouraging tendency to give up trying, the lack of success in attempts to master a task can have unfortunate emotional consequences. Bond and Tinker (1957) have described the pattern as seen in disabled readers thus: "The frustration brings feelings of inferiority accompanied by personality and behavior deviations. The emotional maladjustments developed in this way are then a handicap to further learning. In this way a vicious circle is formed."

Learning disabilities reach a peak incidence of about 8 per cent of children in the primary grades and are five times more prevalent in boys than in girls. Although constitutional defects, emotional blockings, and faulty training experiences are frequently cited as having etiological significance, the actual causes of specific learning disabilities are not well understood. Because of the uncertain origins, the evaluation of learning disabilities requires extensive diagnostic exploration and the compilation of findings made by physicians, audiologists, social workers, nurses, teachers, and psychologists.

The correction of specific learning disabilities has important consequences for rendering the individual more adequate and effectively able to profit from new learning opportunities. Medical procedures, parental support, and individual counseling are often a part of treatment approaches. Remedial education is being increasingly recognized as an effective corrective procedure. This recognition puts pressure on the schools to do a better job of educating all pupils. It is frightening to consider that a pupil may learn how *not* to learn as well as how to learn. The possibility for correction by educational training has also served to focus attention on the early identification of specific learning disabilities and on the development of efficient group corrective methods.

SUGGESTED READINGS

Bakwin, H. (Ed.) *The pediatric clinics of North America: symposium on developmental disorders of motility and language.* Vol. 15, No. 3. Philadelphia: Saunders, 1969.

Frierson, E. C., & Barbe, W. B. (Eds.) *Educating children with learning disabilities.* New York: Appleton-Century-Crofts, 1967.

Johnson, D. J., & Myklebust, H. P. *Learning disabilities.* New York: Grune & Stratton, 1967.

Van Witsen, B. *Perceptual training activities handbook.* New York: Teachers College Press, 1967.

REFERENCES

Bakwin, H. Cerebral damage and behavior damage in children. *J. Pediat.,* 1949, **34,** 371.

Bateman, B. Learning disabilities—yesterday, today and tomorrow. *Except. Child.,* 1964, **31,** 167-178.

Bender, L. *Psychopathology of children with organic brain disorders.* Springfield, Ill.: Thomas, 1956.

Berlyne, D. Emotional aspects of learning. *Annu. Rev. Psychol.,* 1964, **15,** 115-142.

Bond, G. F., & Tinker, M. A. *Reading difficulties: their diagnosis and correction.* New York: Appleton-Century-Crofts, 1957.

Bower, E. C. The psychologist in the schools. Paper read at meeting of Illinois Psychological Association, Chicago, October, 1966.

Burks, H. F. The hyperkinetic child. *Except. Child.,* 1960, **27,** 18-26.

Clements, S. D. *Minimal brain dysfunction in children.* Washington, D.C.: National Institute of Neurological Diseases and Blindness, 1966.

Cohn, R. The neurological study of children with learning disabilities. *Except. Child.,* 1964, **31,** 179-186.

Durrell, D. D. *Improving reading instruction.* Yonkers, N.Y.: World Book, 1956.

Eisenberg, L. Psychiatric implications of brain damage in children. *Psychiat. Quart.,* 1957, **31,** 72-92.

Eisenberg, L. The sins of the fathers: urban decay and social pathology. *Amer. J. Orthopsychiat.,* 1962, **32,** 5-17.

Epps, H. O., McCannon, G., & Simmons, Q. D. *Teaching devices for children with impaired learning: a study of the brain-injured child from research project fifty at the Columbus State School.* Columbus: Ohio School for Retarded Children, 1958.

Fernald, G. M. *Remedial techniques in basic school subjects.* New York: McGraw-Hill, 1943.

Frostig, M., Lefever, D. W., & Whittlesey, J. R. B. A developmental test of visual perception for evaluating normal and neurologically handicapped children. *Percept. mot. Skills,* 1961, **12,** 383-394.

Gellner, L. *A neurophysiological concept of mental retardation and its educational implications.* Chicago: J. Lewinson Research Foundation, 1959.

Harris, A. J. Reading in educational psychology. *Annu. Rev. Psychol.,* 1964, **15,** 258-260.

Hebb, D. O. *The organization of behavior: a neurophysiological approach.* New York: Wiley, 1949.

Hewett, F. M. A hierarchy of educational tasks for children with learning disorders. *Except. Child.,* 1964, **31,** 207-214.

Kephart, N. C. *The brain-injured child in the classroom.* Columbus, Ohio: Merrill, 1960.

Kephart, N. C. Perceptual-motor aspects of learning disabilities. *Except. Child.,* 1964, **31,** 201-206.

Kessler, J. W. *Psychopathology of childhood*. Englewood Cliffs, N.J.: Prentice-Hall, 1966.

Klebanoff, S. G., Singer, J. L., & Wilensky, H. Psychological sequences of brain lesions and ablations. *Psychol. Bull.*, 1954, **51**, 1-41.

McCarthy, J., & Kirk, S. *Illinois test of psycholinguistic abilities*. Institute for Research on Exceptional Children, University of Illinois, 1963.

McWilliams, B. J. The language-handicapped child and education. *Except. Child.*, 1965, **32**, 221-228.

Maher, B. A. *Principles of psychopathology*. New York: McGraw-Hill, 1966.

Mesinger, J. F. Emotionally disturbed and brain-injured children—should we mix them? *Except. Child.*, 1965, **32**, 237-238.

Monroe, M. C. *Children who cannot read*. Chicago: Univer. of Chicago Press, 1932.

Myklebust, H. R. *The psychology of deafness, sensory deprivation, learning, and adjustment*. New York: Grune & Stratton, 1964.

Myklebust, H. R., & Johnson, D. Dyslexia in children. *Except. Child.*, 1962, **29**, 14-25.

Orton, S. T. "Word blindness" in school children. *Arch. Neurol. Psychiat.*, 1925, **14**, 581-615.

Reitan, R. Validity of the trail making test as an indicator of organic brain damage. *Percept. mot. Skills*, 1958, **8**, 271-276.

Schilder, P. The psychological implications of motor development in children. *Proc. Child Res. Clin.*, 1937, **4**, 38-59.

Schroeder, L. B. A study of the relationships between five categories of emotional disturbance and reading and arithmetic achievement. *Except. Child.*, 1965, **32**, 111-112.

Stone, B. F., & Rowley, V. N. Educational disability in emotionally disturbed children. *Except. Child.*, 1964, **30**, 423-426.

Strauss, A. A., & Lehtinen, L. E. *Psychopathology and education of the brain-injured child*. Vol. I. New York: Grune & Stratton, 1947.

Strother, C. R. *Discovering, evaluating, programming for the neurologically handicapped child with special attention to the child with minimal brain damage*. Chicago: National Society for Crippled Children and Adults, 1963.

Teuber, H. L., Battersby, W. S., & Bender, M. B. The performance of complex visual tasks after cerebral lesions. *J. nerv. ment. Dis.*, 1951, **114**, 413-429.

Weisskopf, E. Intellectual malfunctioning and personality. *J. abnorm. soc. Psychol.*, 1951, **46**, 410-423.

Wepman, J. M. Auditory discrimination, speech, and reading. *Elem. Sch. J.*, 1960, **9**, 325-333.

Whelan, R. J., & Haring, N. E. Modification and maintenance of behavior through systematic application of consequences. *Except. Child.*, 1966, **32**, 281-290.

Yates, A. J. The validity of some psychological tests of brain damage. *Psychol. Bull.*, 1954, **51**, 359-379.

5

Mental Subnormality

Retarded

The reader may wonder why a chapter on the mentally subnormal, more commonly referred to as the "mentally retarded," is included in a textbook dealing with behavior disorders. It is true that mental subnormality is not usually regarded as a behavior disorder in the same sense that a psychoneurosis or a personality disorder is a behavior disorder. Yet there are certain similarities to be found between the performance of the mentally handicapped and that of the behaviorally disordered. Commonalities in the procedures invoked for the management of mental subnormality and functional disorders are also apparent. In some instances, mental subnormality and behavior disorders can be traced as consequences of remarkably similar antecedent

181

conditions. It follows that opinions of behavioral scientists about mental subnormality are not uniform.

In this chapter, conceptions of mental subnormality will be reviewed primarily in order to illustrate the relationship with other behavior disorders. Work with the mentally handicapped has contributed significantly to the understanding of all behavior deviations. The clinical treatment of children has been greatly advanced by refined diagnostic techniques and more effective treatment procedures, many of which were originally tried out with the mentally subnormal.

OVERVIEW

The condition of mental subnormality is one of the oldest concerns to those who deal with behavior deviations. The simpleton or village idiot is to be found in all cultural groups and all ages. In years past, the mentally subnormal were often victimized and sometimes dealt with inhumanely by more able members of society. Benefactors who sought to intercede and assist these unfortunate individuals initiated trends which have provided answers to many puzzling questions about behavior. Attempts to intervene by approaches which offered nothing more than humane treatment were ultimately sufficiently successful to contradict former explanations of deviant behavior as the work of demons and evil spirits.

The relatively modest gains obtained by mere humane treatment were adequate for spurring other approaches and investigations. It became apparent that some disorders were apparently acquired (formerly designated as "dementia"), whereas others appeared to be constitutional in origin ("amentia"). Subnormal mentality was found conjointly with organic defects in some instances, but not in others. These observations contributed to the coining of the concept of "functional impairment," a condition of disability in performance with no identifiable related organic defect.

Overshadowing the question of organic or functional etiology was a rather consistent subpar performance in meeting many everyday life demands. This observation provided an avenue for developing techniques of identifying mental subnormality on the basis of quality of performance in selected situations. The fledgling movement of psychoeducational measurement, which had floundered for many years, was given powerful support by the success of Alfred Binet's measuring scale. Scores from the Binet scale could be used successfully to identify those children whose less-than-average intellectual potential rendered them unable to profit from the usual classroom curriculum. Assessment of intellectual ability, whether by newly developed scales or by newly refined older scales, continues to be a significant step in identifying mental subnormality.

Physicians were frequently in charge of treating the mentally subnormal. As might be expected, their concerns focused on the role of constitutional factors. Organic defects identified as having etiological significance in some mentally subnormal persons, such as the blocked circulation associated with hydrocephaly, were sometimes correctable by surgery. Impaired organic functions, such as the hypothyroid deficiency condition of cretinism, could sometimes be restored by medication. These findings served to stimulate a continual quest for medical intervention procedures which could be applied to behavior deviations.

In addition to the medical intervention approaches, interest centered about efforts to control mental subnormality by manipulating the environment. The assumption that mental subnormality is the consequence of inadequate acquisition of necessary experiences suggested two main lines of correction. One approach, illustrated by the classic work of Itard and Sequin, was based on the possibility that there had been a total lack of exposure to most ordinary experiences. A program of intense stimulation was then provided for the individual. The essential role of stimulation in developing capacity for coping is today well accepted and has been extended to form the base of programs for the culturally disadvantaged, as will be seen in the next chapter.

A second line of environmental intervention rests on the possibility that the mentally subnormal person encounters adjustment difficulties because of specific experiential deficits. Support for this contention is gained from observations that the mentally subnormal do not do well in certain situations but may be successful in other situations. They may, for example, fail in the face of highly academic demands in the usual school situation but perform satisfactorily in some occupational settings. This approach to correcting adjustment problems capitalizes on identifying the "success-possible situation" and then providing necessary specific training which will be demanded of the individual. Well illustrated in the work carried out by Goddard at the Vineland Training School, this approach has been widely extended to the correction of many behavior problems.

CONCEPTIONS

CURRENT DEFINITIONS

The varied background of professional workers, the necessity for evaluation in different social situations, and the fact that several factors contribute to mental subnormality have posed many problems in defining the condition. As a way of overcoming some of these differences, representative groups have gotten together from time to time and agreed upon a common definition. These conferences have generally been sanctioned by the American Association for Mental Deficiency. The most recent definition, agreed upon in May 1960, states: "Mental retardation refers to sub-average general intellectual functioning which originated during the developmental period and is associated with impairment in adaptive behavior" (Heber, 1961). Heber, who has been the spokesman for the AAMD, has offered explanations for the intention of the definition. Intellectual functioning is to be ascertained by performance on a standardized intelligence test. Subaverage intellectual functioning is indicated by scores below minus one standard deviation (IQ below 84 on the Stanford-Binet Intelligence Scale, as an example). Impairment in adaptive behavior, a crucial criterion, is to be evaluated from the standpoint of maturation, learning, and social adjustment. Maturation is understood as rate of development as evidenced by attainment in such sensory-motor skills as sitting, walking, and talking. Learning is interpreted as the capacity for achievement in the acquisition of academic skills. Social adjustment refers to essential aspects of adult living such as personal self-reliance and independence, gainful employment, and the ability to conform to social demands and standards of the community.

The definition is commendable in that it seeks to make classification contingent upon several factors, rather than relying on a single characteristic (as, for example, IQ). Requirements of irreversibility and specific etiology, prominent in previous definitions, have been dropped from the new criteria. Possibly the most important aspect of the definition is the fact that a group with diverse training and backgrounds can come to agreement about a condition which is recognized as being complex.

TYPICAL TRAITS

Work with the mentally subnormal has generated a number of traits which are deemed typical of the condition. Some of the more frequently mentioned traits will be discussed as falling into three major areas.

1. *Intellectual.* The feature most commonly ascribed to the mentally subnormal is that of having less than average intellectual ability. Individuals with less than average intelligence are regarded as being conceptually impaired. There is a diminished capacity for dealing with such intangibles as abstract concepts and symbolizations. Such persons are limited in the degree to which they can make associations and generalizations. Stated succinctly, the mentally subnormal person is looked upon as being mentally "dull."

2. *Personality.* As a consequence of a basic conceptual limitation, the mentally subnormal person finds it easier to deal with tangible materials and specific tasks. Since this preference is not always available, the mentally subnormal person sometimes functions with a prevailing air of uncertainty as to what is expected of him. When not sure of how to approach a task, the mentally subnormal person may be slow in responding or even take a wait-and-see position. The hesitation and slowness could be interpreted as perseveration or dependency. Difficulty in comprehending exactly what is expected of him may predispose the mentally subnormal person to fail frequently. The fact that the mentally subnormal are subject to demands which are developmentally inappropriate for them could foster a low degree of persistence, diminished aspirations, and a feeling of helplessness. Even though these possibilities exist, it must be acknowledged that they are only tendencies. Such traits may or may not be found in any given mentally subnormal person. A number of studies investigating the personality of the mentally subnormal have been carried out. The findings gleaned from these explorations have provided almost overwhelming evidence that the complete range of behaviors and personality configurations can be found among those of less than average intellectual ability.

3. *Social.* As is often the case for any impairing condition, there has been a proneness to ascribe a number of unfavorable social characteristics to the mentally subnormal. Included are allegations of being dirty, dishonest, lazy, dumb, irresponsible, uncontrollable, weak, crude, criminal, and physically unattractive. The mentally subnormal person may have difficulty in identifying social standards and values and so learns them at a slow rate. A majority of mentally subnormal children may live in environments which do not present favorable models for approved social learning. Thus, the situation with respect to social traits found in the mentally subnormal is the same as for personality traits. A large number of mentally subnormal persons may have unfavorable social traits, but not all persons of less than average intellectual ability are socially maladjusted. A complete range of desirable and undesirable social traits are to be found in all degrees and in all combinations when any one mentally subnormal individual is considered. The situation was aptly described by Gardner (1966), who reviewed studies investigating the social and emotional adjustment of retarded children. He concluded that although the mentally retarded person is usually depicted as socially unacceptable and having greater adjustment problems, unequivocable data in support of these contentions are difficult to come by, if for no other reason than that the mentally subnormal have a low mental age, find academic work difficult, cannot read at a level comparable to the average child, can fail frequently, and may have other than a middle-class value orientation.

CLASSIFICATIONS

SINGLE-GROUP CLASSIFICATIONS

The high frequency of associated adjustment difficulties contributed to grouping mentally subnormal persons since they typically required assistance from physicians, social workers, educators, psychologists, and vocational counselors. Individuals were usually not referred for help until they had become enmeshed in rather severe adjustment difficulties. Too frequently, "treatment" consisted mainly of diagnostic appraisal. At first, diagnostic techniques were gross and unrefined. Measures from scales assessing intellectual ability were in the form of a single global score (IQ). Diagnosticians had little opportunity for continued contacts with persons classed as mentally subnormal and could not detect what types of adjustments the mentally subnormal might make. It was assumed that the mentally subnormal person experienced chronic adjustment difficulties. There were only limited recommendations that might be offered, such as institutional or special-school placement. The diagnostic appraisal suggested a common predicament for the adjustment problems of the mentally subnormal because the individual had less intellectual ability than a situation demanded. It was sufficient to establish that the person had a diminished capacity for meeting demands.

This state of affairs encouraged professional workers to deal with mental subnormality as a general condition. The orientation of the clinician was a manifestation of his particular training. Physicians, accustomed to identifying dysfunctions having physiological or anatomical origins, viewed the problem as a defect of the nervous system and used the term "mental deficiency." Psychologists, trained to evaluate the effectiveness of performance, saw the mentally subnormal as having limited intellectual capacity for meeting many life demands and used the term "mentally handicapped." For the educator, who saw the mentally subnormal child as being slower than average in school progress, the term "mentally retarded" was preferred. Even though all clinicians were aware that the condition existed in varying degrees, not much attention was given to the degree of impairment since the limited choices available for treatment made a qualitative evaluation adequate. The classification terminologies and levels of impairment used in the United States are contrasted in Table 11.

The initial terms used to designate degrees of incompetency (idiot, imbecile, moron) have been replaced with severe, moderate, mild, or custodial, trainable, educable. Diagnostic study is carried out by a physician, psychologist, or educator, frequently in collaboration. The diagnostic assessment culminates in the mentally subnormal person being classified according to the terminology used by the diagnostician's professional discipline.

Proposed Two-Group Classification

From time to time, clinicians have become specialized in the problems of the mentally subnormal. As a consequence of years of working with and observing the mentally subnormal, these workers have advocated a more specific approach to mental subnormality. Sarason and Gladwin (1959) have been especially inclined to see the differences

TABLE 11. CLASSIFICATION TERMS AND LEVELS OF IMPAIRMENT FOR MENTAL SUBNORMALITY USED BY THE MEDICAL, PSYCHOLOGICAL, AND EDUCATIONAL DISCIPLINES

	Medical	Psychological	Educational	Associated IQ Range (Approx.)
Generic term	Mentally deficient	Mentally handicapped	Mentally retarded	
Degree of incapacitation	Mild Moderate Severe	Mild Moderate Dependent	Educable Trainable Custodial	55–80 35–55 Below 35

between what they designate as the endogenous (familial) type and the exogenous (organic defect) type of mental subnormality. Accumulating evidence supports the practice of recognizing two types of mental subnormality which have a small cluster of overlapping characteristics but a larger number of differentiating characteristics.

The necessity for differentiating between the two kinds of mental subnormality has currently found a strong advocate in Zigler (1966, 1967). He has presented an impressive case for recognizing one type of mental subnormality as the outcome of a predominantly organic defect. Another type is the consequence of the interaction of familial with psychosocial factors. Even though there are as yet no reliable or convenient diagnostic methods for classifying a mentally subnormal person as being of one or the other type, the differentiation is a useful and promising one. The identification of specific organic deficits and pathology is largely an unresolved barrier. Even where identifiable, there are few specific medications or surgical procedures for correcting many such deficits, and treatment is still an educational matter.

Although in practice the terms "mentally deficient" and "mentally retarded," depending upon the practitioner's orientation, are used to refer to all mentally subaverage persons, it is possible in discussion to speak separately of the two types of subnormality. There is, moreover, a certain benefit in maintaining the distinction which adds to the understanding of the condition of mental subnormality. Accordingly, this presentation will follow closely the differentiation as outlined by Zigler (1967). The terms "mentally handicapped" and "mental subnormality" will be used in the more general sense, as suggested by Sarason, to include both types or all cases.

Characteristics of the Mentally Deficient (Defective)

There are relatively few traits common to all individuals of less than average intelligence. Other than a small cluster centering about comparable scores on measures of intelligence, the picture is confusing. Zigler has suggested that a part of the disagreement can be attributed to the failure to recognize the two types of mental handicap and what he believes to be rather distinctly associated characteristics.

Pointing out that the term "mentally deficient" itself stresses the salient characteristic of this group, that of a physiological or anatomical defect, Zigler has listed several other distinctive traits. These include a tendency to have a lower degree of measurable intellectual ability (IQ of less than 50) and a high frequency of other physical disabilities including sensory and motor defects. The mentally deficient are inclined to have poorer general health, markedly less stamina, and to appear disjunctive. They have very limited intellectual potential which appears to become even more reduced when observed over a long period of time. Poor motor coordination, speech problems, and general frailty predispose the majority of them to a dependent status.

Characteristics of the Mentally Retarded (Familial)

Zigler (1966) points out that the chief characteristic of this group is also aptly conveyed by the term "retardation." By way of illustration, he draws upon the analogy of a person who has tuberculosis but may in many situations not be incapacitated. Contending that the mentally retarded may well constitute the lower end of a normal continuum of intellectual ability as represented by a distribution of IQ scores, Zigler holds that the mentally retarded is the larger of the two groups of mentally handicapped. Generally speaking, the mentally retarded include those persons with an IQ from about 50 to 75, although there is some overlap in IQ of the two groups, as is demonstrated in Figure 3.

Persons in the mentally retarded group, approximately 75 per cent of all mentally subnormal persons, are very comparable to the average person from whom they differ mostly in degree. Their impairment shows itself most clearly in specific situations demanding a high degree of ability to deal with the abstract. They tend to have good physical health, fair motor coordination, and in general attain an adequate degree of personality integration even though they take longer to realize their potential. Athough less persistent, less self-confident, and more dependent, the expectation of eventual self-sufficiency and inde-

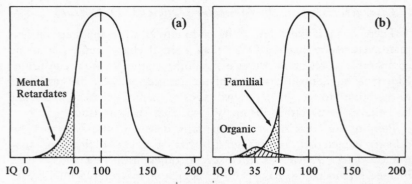

FIGURE 3. (a) *Conventional representation of the distribution of intelligence.*
(b) *Distribution of intelligence as represented in the two-group approach.*
(*Source:* E. Zigler. Familial mental retardation: a continuing dilemma.
Science, 1967, **155**, 292-298. Copyright 1967 by the American Association
for the Advancement of Science.)

pendent adjustment is justified for these "late bloomers." The mentally
retarded, also referred to as the "familial" retarded, and by Sarason
as the "garden variety" retarded, as a group make the most promising
responses to rehabilitation programs.

IDENTIFICATION

Each of the several major approaches used in identifying the mentally subnormal person has advantages as well as limitations. None
is free from error. The orientation of the clinician, the purposes of
the classification, and the stage of refinement of diagnostic techniques
are only a few of the factors influencing identification. In practice,
specialists working with the mentally subnormal typically emphasize
one or another approach, but most of them consult information
collected from several sources before making a final diagnosis. A
developmental history, scores from intelligence scales, and school-
achievement results are suggested as minimally essential data. Under-
standably, most specialists defer making a final diagnosis of mental
retardation in other than the most severe cases until the child has
been observed for several years.

FAMILIAL AND DEVELOPMENTAL HISTORY

A carefully compiled account of the individual's origins and development is one of the major aids used in diagnosis. Physicians are

particularly likely to rely on this method, which begins by reviewing the adequacy of the adjustment made by parents, siblings, and other near relatives. A majority of the mentally subnormal have close relatives who also are subaverage, and this evidence of familial tendencies can only be revealed in a carefully obtained history. The exploration next considers possible sources of trauma from illnesses and injuries the child may have incurred. Rounding out the history-taking is a detailed review of the developmental attainments of the individual.

The mentally subnormal consistently lag in age of sitting up, feeding self, walking, dressing self, talking, and toilet training. They are slower in all anatomical, physiological, motor, and social functions, so that the pattern indicated by the history may clearly justify a diagnosis of mental subnormality. The "defect" type of mental handicap is probably most readily identified by a history. Making a diagnosis from a history of developmental slowness can become difficult because other conditions, such as motor, sensory, or emotional disabilities, can also lead to lags in accomplishment. This makes it necessary to give importance to the consistency of the retardation and to agreement with other findings.

MEASURES OF INTELLECTUAL ABILITY

Scores from scales assessing intellectual ability are the single most frequently used criterion for rendering a diagnosis of mental subnormality. The field of psychoeducational measurement was given great impetus by Alfred Binet's success in identifying young children who could not be expected to do well in school because they had less than average learning ability. Assessing intelligence continues to be a favored method for diagnosis by psychologists and educators, who may be inclined to rely too heavily on the IQ. A number of scales measuring intellectual ability have been developed. Even though scales with high verbal content have proved to be the most dependable predictors of school achievement, most measuring scales offer a balance of verbal and nonverbal tasks.

It may well be that the usefulness of scores from intelligence measures as indicators of mental handicap is explainable by the fact that this measure taps what many regard as the most outstanding and immutable characteristic of mental subnormality: the capacity for learning. Explanations of the wide appeal of intelligence scores must also consider the ease and convenience with which IQ scores can be obtained from "objective" and "standardized" measuring devices. Reliance on measures of intelligence is so universal that intelligence tests have a clearly marked point designating which scores are indicative of mental subnormality. This point commonly includes scores which are lower than one standard deviation below the average.

The IQ score is an indicator of capacity, but it is the application of that capacity which is at issue. Applying learning ability to making a suitable vocational or social adjustment is influenced by motivational and other psychological variables which are not necessarily given specific consideration in computing an IQ. Intelligence scores are, and doubtless will continue to be, given wide acceptance in diagnosing mental subnormality. This condition persists in spite of the well-known unreliability of such scores in predicting specific adjustment outcomes in adults. The practitioner with years of experience in working with the mentally handicapped is well aware of the pitfalls inherent in too much reliance on the IQ and withholds making a definitive diagnosis until other relevant data are available.

SOCIAL COMPETENCE

Historically, the mentally subnormal have been identified on the basis of being unable to finish school, keep a job, stay out of jail, or provide for a family. No one would deny that there are many persons among the unemployed, school dropouts, convicted law violators, and similar groups of socially incompetent who prove to be mentally subnormal. Such data have been generated by frequent psychosocial investigations and are easy to come by. It is strange that the suggestion of equating social incompetence and mental subnormality as implied by such studies persists in the face of refutation of the contention which is inherent in the very same investigations. No study has found that all jobless, all law violators, or all persons of any socially incompetent group are mentally subnormal. Most persons included in such socially deviant groups are in fact of average or above-average intellectual ability. The condition known as "sociopathic personality disturbance" is a particularly relevant example illustrating this point.

There is some justification for expecting a greater percentage of mentally subnormal persons to encounter failure in meeting social demands. Skill in meeting social expectations is apparently largely the outcome of acquisitions gained in being acculturated. Social learning frequently entails dealing with values and attitudes, intangibles which may be elusive for the mentally subnormal. Society holds a number of possibilities for acceptable adjustment, and it is unlikely that any one person is in fact equally competent in all areas. The mentally subnormal person can be expected to be less proficient in academic skills because of the high degree of abstraction involved. But the pioneering work of Goddard offers ample evidence for showing that most mentally subnormal persons have sufficient abilities for making an adequate adjustment. Rosen (1967) is currently actively engaged in this same objective by correcting deficiencies in the existing educational and institutional programs. Too often, sheltered institutional life has promoted tendencies for dependency and denied realistic opportunities for the mentally subnormal.

The criterion of social competency must then be carefully weighed in arriving at a classification of mental handicap. Zigler (1966) has pointed out that a greater frequency of mentally subnormal persons are in lower socioeconomic groups and acquire values and behavior patterns typical of these groups. It is these values and standards which may be the critical factor in meeting demands of a predominantly middle-class society. Social competency is, unquestionably, a relevant criterion for identifying the mentally subnormal. In practice, this ability is difficult to evaluate. What constitutes a good parent, a steady worker, a respectable citizen, and so on cannot be easily measured. Social maturity is attained at different rates and in different degrees. It should be considered in classifying a person as mentally subnormal, but its significance must be decided only in the light of other information.

PERSONALITY FACTORS

The survival of efforts to identify the mentally subnormal on the basis of distinctive personality traits is possibly best explained as another indication of a wish to reduce behavior to simple units which could be easily quantified. The major personality traits proposed for inclusion in the mentally subnormal configuration have been referred to in the discussion of characteristics of the mentally handicapped. Those most frequently cited include perseveration, dependency, a preference for dealing with the concrete and tangible, slowness and limited ability to deal with the abstract. Slight variations in the phrasing of these qualities are to be encountered in literature dealing with mental subnormality, but the emphasis is about the same.

In part, the search for a typical personality associated with mental subnormality has been given some impetus by refinements in procedures for assessing personality. Advancements in the field of projective techniques have particularly contributed to this line of interest. However great the convenience and interest, to date no personality pattern has been discovered which is exclusively associated with mental subnormality. Continued investigation of the problem has in fact produced an increasing amount of evidence which contraindicates such a contention. A study carried out by Zigler and Butterfield (1968) suggests that the trait of dependency is a consequence of the docile adjustment demanded by institutionalization. After investigating the social adjustment of mentally subnormal children in public schools, Lapp (1957) concluded that the low social acceptance common for such children was not related to any identifiable personality trait. The low acceptance was simply a realistic reflection of the fact that the mentally subnormal had very little to contribute to an academically oriented group. In short, identification of mental subnormality on the basis of a purported characteristic personality is at once the most hazardous and the least substantiated procedure.

PERFORMANCE IN LEARNING

A difference in the ability to learn a task is the most consistently observed quality of the mentally subnormal. An excellent summary of studies contrasting the learning ability of persons with less than average intelligence and those of average intelligence is presented by Lipman (1963). As a group, the mentally subnormal take longer to learn a task, reach a peak performance at a lower attainment level, and seem to retain less. There are considerable individual differences, so that explanations of these differences must take into account the degree of mental subnormality and individual variations in relevant personality traits. In his detailed analysis of performance in various situations and with varied tasks, Maher (1966) emphasizes the influence of previous experiences, the nature of the task, and the procedures used to measure learning as contributing to the generally poor performance of the mentally handicapped.

Irrespective of what factors may be influencing the outcomes, the mentally subnormal are identifiable on the basis of performance in learning. The distinction becomes more obvious when the task is a complex one and involves the making of abstractions. Although the mentally subnormal are identifiable on the basis of characteristics revealed in learning a task, the special situations in which this feature becomes apparent are not generally available to or used by the clinical diagnostician. Diagnosis from such performance is more cumbersome and requires more time than most practitioners are willing to invest. Differences in learning ability have had more application in designing experimental treatment programs than in routine diagnosis and treatment.

DIFFERENTIAL DIAGNOSTIC PROBLEMS

Emotional Maladjustment. Perhaps the most common problem in diagnosis is encountered in evaluating low performance which is the result of impairment associated with an emotional disorder. Unless skillfully managed, most preschool children will be inhibited and upset by the diagnostic process. The examiner is a stranger who makes specific demands to be carried out in fixed time limits. These temporary emotional reactions are generally easily managed, but chronic emotional disorders present greater difficulties. Emotional disorders are frequent in children and are often sufficiently severe to markedly limit the child's efficiency in coping with a task. The differentiation can be facilitated by keeping in mind that erratically uneven performance, disturbances of affect, and bizarre behaviors typically accompany emotional disturbance. In contrast, the performance of the mentally subnormal is uniformly below average, affect remains congruous, and behaviors are appropriate. The performance of the mentally subnormal is consistent and suitable but quantitatively less than average.

Language Disorders. Another major diagnostic problem centers about the differentiation of language disorders from mental subnormality. The magnitude of this problem can be appreciated when it is considered that auditory impairments and associated language difficulties make up one of the three most frequently encountered areas of impairment found in children. Psychoeducational measuring scales routinely used in the diagnostic study of children tend to have high verbal content. The child with a language disability is thus penalized in this situation and may perform much below average, suggesting mental subnormality. The question of a hearing loss can only be resolved by competent audiometric evaluation, which should be routinely included in all diagnostic evaluations of children. Where a hearing loss is identified, the classification as mental subnormality should be deferred. The developmental history will often show that the language-disabled child has a rate of attainment in other areas (sensory-motor, social) which falls in the normal range. The developmental accomplishment of the mentally subnormal child falls below that of the average. The performance of the language-impaired child, although below average in situations demanding language facility, rises to the average range in situations where minimal language facility is required. The functioning of the mentally subnormal child is consistently low in verbal and nonverbal situations.

In general, the differential diagnostic questions can be resolved on the basis of the consistently below-average performance which typifies the mentally handicapped child. Total evaluation of all aspects of the child is the only safeguard for bringing to light deficits which may impair performance in specific situations. In some instances, mental subnormality may be found in combination with other disabilities. Making a diagnostic choice in such cases may be dictated by what is most likely to facilitate the child's getting the necessary treatment. In other instances, there may be "reasonable doubts" which make it inadvisable to make a specific diagnostic choice. In such situations, it is best to mention the possible classifications suggested and to defer choosing a final category until supplementary information is obtained from longer close observation of the child.

INCIDENCE

At this point it may be apparent to the reader that the number of mentally subnormal persons will vary according to the diagnostic characteristics being followed and the method of identification. An accounting of the mentally subnormal is made difficult by the lack of agreement among clinicians as to what constitutes mental subnormality.

Illustrative of the difficulties encountered in a search to identify the mentally subnormal is the following incident shared by the authors. While engaged in a research project studying the incorporation of on-the-job training experiences into a high-school program for mentally handicapped pupils, it became apparent that classroom teachers were not referring for individual psychological evaluation all potentially eligible pupils. A preliminary group screening had given some indication of the number of pupils with below-average intellectual ability. This situation was announced to the teachers in a group meeting, and teachers were scheduled for individual conferences in which the referral criteria were reviewed. In the individual conferences, each teacher acknowledged that there were pupils meeting the criteria who had not been referred. Several of the teachers even admitted that the nonreferred pupils (who were, not altogether incidentally, almost entirely girls) were "probably" mentally handicapped. The teachers justified not referring these pupils on the basis of the pupils being "good" girls, that is, compliant and "clean." Boys not referred were described as cooperative and "willing to try as best they can." In this rather typical public-school system our rather comprehensive survey indicated that about 6 per cent of the approximately 10,000 pupils were mentally handicapped. Allowance should be made for the concern for educational classification. Only about two-thirds of the total mentally handicapped group in this school system were in special classes.

An incidence rate of 3 per cent of the general population is frequently cited as designating the portion of mentally subnormal. This figure evolved from surveys made many years ago and was probably based on estimates gained from experiences with the more severe cases and extreme degrees of social maladjustment. Nevertheless, various explanations, including genetic ones, have been offered to substantiate this figure, which was cited as recently as 1965, by the President's Panel on Mental Retardation.

Although a few specialists believe that 3 per cent is too high an incidence figure, the majority believe the figure is too low. It is interesting to note that the criteria cited by the American Association for Mental Deficiency, often referred to as the Heber (1961) definition, establish a basis for regarding all who score below minus one standard deviation from the average on measures of intelligence as being mentally subnormal. If literally interpreted, this could be equivalent to an incidence rate of about 16 per cent, or a staggering 32 million persons from a population totaling 200 million. It must be pointed out that this is the result of taking only one of three criteria (intellectual capacity, developmental rate, social adjustment) in the Heber definition, and most properly it only establishes a group of persons who may potentially prove to be mentally subnormal after additional study. Very few behavioral specialists are willing to concede that the incidence of mental subnormality is even close to 16 per cent. The more conservative rate of 5 or 6 per cent is regarded as reflecting the workable incidence of mental subnormality.

The actual incidence of mental subnormality is and may well remain an unknown since it is unlikely that the entire population of the United States will ever be assessed. Even if such a massive undertaking were carried out, it might only serve to illustrate what is already apparent, which is that the frequency of mentally subnormal persons varies according to many sets of factors. When the preschool-age group is considered, the incidence is lowest. There is a sharp and sudden rise in incidence with the start of school, another peak at about the age persons ordinarily graduate from high school and take a job, and another peak occurring with aging. In general, more males than females are identified at all levels as being mentally subnormal.

Whatever the actual frequency of mentally subnormal persons may be, these variations in incidence are of interest in themselves. They suggest very clearly that mental subnormality is a complex condition which is not identifiable by any one single criterion. It is apparent that social inadequacy is an important criterion for identifying mental subnormality. This raises a question as to just what is implied by mental subnormality—a lower than average intellectual potential or a demonstrated social incompetency? Clarification of this question might help to explain why mental subnormality is more prevalent in the lower socioeconomic groups, where the bulk of the Negro population fall. Greater understanding of the nature of mental subnormality is essential to the development of effective countermeasures for correction of the condition.

ETIOLOGICAL CONSIDERATIONS

The distinction between mental deficiency and mental retardation is a useful one in a discussion of factors which have been found to contribute to mental subnormality. Agents and conditions resulting in specific organic damage are frequently found associated with mental deficiency. Many of these have been specifically identified. Mental retardation seems to be the outcome of factors which are less specific and not easily identifiable. In some instances the processes seem to be reversible, but in other cases they override any efforts for control. In some cases the origins of mental subnormality appear to involve complex interrelationships between the individual and his surroundings. It is almost axiomatic that traumas incurred early in development have widespread and general consequences, whereas those traumas incurred at later stages tend to have specific and limited effects.

MENTAL DEFICIENCY

Internal factors seem to predominate in the etiology of most mental deficiency, a situation reflected in the term "endogenous" sometimes used to designate this variety of mental handicap. Factors which can lead to mental deficiency can be arranged in four groups:

1. *Hereditary.* This group includes genetic factors and aberrations such as amaurotic idiocy, trisomy 21, phenylketonuria, and glactosemia.

2. *Prenatal.* Of significance in this group are traumas, nutritional deficiency, anoxia, infections (virus, rubella), blood incompatibilities (Rh reactions), irradiation, and toxins.

3. *Natal.* Prematurity, asphyxia, and traumas are important factors in this group.

4. *Postnatal.* Toxins, neurotropic infections (virus, encephalitis, meningitis, chicken pox, mumps, scarlet fever), pyrexias, and, rarely, traumas are included in this group. Dietary deficiencies should also be considered.

Because many of the consequences of these internal or organic etiological factors occur before birth, it is not possible to give reliable estimates of the relative contribution attributable to each factor. Collectively, they account for about 25 per cent of the total group of mentally subnormal.

MENTAL RETARDATION

The picture with respect to the factors giving rise to mental retardation is considered more complicated. Although hereditary factors appear to be involved in part, it seems that environmental situations and conditions which act on the individual are the more prevalent. This emphasis is reflected in the term "exogenous" which is sometimes used to designate this variety of mental subnormality. Exogenous factors tend to be less specific and to have consequences which vary widely in degree for any individual.

1. *Familial.* Genetic factors included in this group are of a multiple type. In contrast to the more specific and direct-acting genetic factors associated with mental deficiency, these multiple factors probably have a cumulative action.

2. *Environmental.* In this group are the minimal conditions associated with what is designated as limited opportunity. Inadequate diet,

little contact with other persons, marginal educational opportunities, insufficient medical care, and general lack of attention and stimulation are most frequently cited.

Despite acknowledgment that the environment influences mental retardation, there is no general agreement as to which conditions can be conclusively counted upon to give rise to mental retardation. As Zigler (1966) has stated, what constitutes a "good" as opposed to a "poor" environment is difficult to define. Illustrative of the puzzling information is the finding that a higher than expected incidence of mental retardation is associated with inadequate dietary intake; yet no diet has been found which produces a mentally superior child. Severely retarded children are also to be found in homes which offer an abundance of all the cultural advantages.

MANAGEMENT CONSIDERATIONS

The diversity of conditions which contribute to mental subnormality makes it mandatory to think in terms of an equivalent number of treatment measures. Mental handicap is a prevalent and persistent condition, second only to emotional disorders in terms of human resources lost to society. Advances in technology, particularly in the field of medical science, and the growing cultural gap between the advantaged and disadvantaged groups of our society could add materially to what is already a sizable social problem.

MEDICAL PERSPECTIVES

The field of medical science has made many significant contributions for dealing with problems of mental subnormality. At present, medical treatment is probably most indicated for the defect group. Surgical techniques have been perfected for correcting hydrocephaly. Mysteries of the developmental arrests induced by metabolic dysfunctions of cretinism, glactosemia, and phenylketonuria have been unraveled. Recently a serum has been developed which counteracts the devastating effects of the Rh-negative blood-incompatibility reaction. The marauding consequences of measles, scarlet fever, chicken pox, and polio have been practically eliminated by the development of specific vaccines.

Less heralded, but possibly of far greater long-term benefit, are the reductions in the incidence of mental handicap which will derive from continual improvement in general medical care. More mothers are given prenatal service, more children are born in hospitals, and pediatric services are routinely provided more children with each passing year. Although a part of the consequences from these same advances is an increase in the number of defective children who will survive, the benefits will far outweigh the disadvantages. A comprehensive program for the management of mental subnormality will always require medications, surgical intervention, and ongoing research investigations from medical specialists.

INSTITUTIONAL PROGRAMS

Formerly regarded as centers for the protective isolation of the mentally handicapped, institutions specializing in the care of these individuals have recently been undergoing many changes. New objectives have been incorporated into intensive treatment programs. As an initial step, residents are put through a detailed diagnostic evaluation, in which physical-health status, sensory-motor systems, personality traits, and social skills are reviewed in addition to the customary attention to intellectual ability. Interestingly, such detailed scrutiny frequently turns up a picture of an individual with low but adequate intellectual ability. His adjustment potential is reduced by one or more areas of impairment, with emotional and sensory-motor difficulties being prominent.

Backup programs for rendering the individual more suitable for independent adjustment outside the institution concentrate on correction of these secondary deficits by means of a coordinated educational program. In addition to training in basic academics, the educational program must make provisions for the acquisition of competency in the selection of clothes, use of public transportation, management of money, finding a job, and related social skills and habits. Rosen (1967) has been instrumental in establishing a model program at the Elwyn Institute in Media, Pennsylvania.

Not all mentally subnormal persons can be made capable of independent life adjustment by such programs, and it must be recognized that there may always be a certain population of severe cases which will require permanent custodial care. At no time, however, have a majority of mentally subnormal persons been institutionalized. Institutionalization is more likely to be a consideration in the management of mentally defective individuals and for persons with multiple disabilities, one of which is less than average intellectual ability. Success in placing qualified residents in real-life situations may require initial supervision by specialists on the staff of the training institution, or an arrangement such as halfway houses.

PUBLIC-SCHOOL PROGRAMS

Management of subnormal mentality by an educational approach in placing qualified residents in real-life situations may require initial of maturation. The educational approach is then usually more appropriate for the mentally retarded, the uncompounded "garden variety" child where difficulties appear to be consequences of a slower than average rate of attainment. Such persons are suitable for education in the special classes of the public schools as indicated by educational designations of "educable mentally handicapped," "educable mentally retarded," and "slow learner." They have IQ scores ranging from about 50 to 75 and are usually identified on the basis of inability to do work assigned in regular classes. They are referred to qualified school staff members for individual psychoeducational evaluation. Recommendations made on the basis of the psychoeducational findings may suggest special-class placement.

Public-school special classes for the educable mentally retarded are usually about half the size of regular classes and have a teacher trained in the educational problems of the retarded. Assignments are made on the basis of mental age so as to avoid excessive failures inherent in demands which are too high. Basic skill in reading, arithmetic, and writing is mastered to about the fourth-grade level by most pupils in these special classes by the time they are 14 or 15 years old. Subsequent school experiences then shift to emphasize social and vocational skills, with the pupil spending about half the day in selected job-training situations. "Graduation" can be at any time the pupil gives satisfactory evidence of being able to function independently on the job, usually around the chronological age of 19.

Although most pupils in public-school programs are of the "educable" category, a smaller number are classed as "trainable." They have less total potential and obtain IQ scores ranging from about 35 to 50. Trainable mentally handicapped persons are not generally regarded as being capable of self-sufficient social and vocational adjustment. They seldom acquire even minimal skill in the basic academic areas. Special classes for this group emphasize training in self-care, personal safety, and basic household tasks. It is conceded that many of this group will require the protection of institutional placement. Institutional placement is usually made around 14 or 15 years of age. Actual outcomes and final placement vary according to the demands of the surrounding community and the possibilities for continued protective supervision such as a community sheltered workshop.

The number of special classes for the educable mentally retarded is increasing rapidly. Such specific programs can claim considerable success in aiding the mentally retarded. The reader wishing a more thorough review of investigations of adult adjustments of graduates from special classes for the mentally retarded should consult Carriker (1957), Porter and Milazzo (1958), Goldstein (1964), and Reynolds and Stunkard (1960). Generally favorable adjustment outcomes as evidenced by findings summarized from these investigations are:

1. Approximately 80 per cent of graduates become economically self-supporting.
2. Commonly held jobs are of a service nature but some are semiskilled.
3. About 80 per cent marry and maintain a family.
4. There is a higher crime rate compared to persons of normal intelligence, but the violations are of a minor nature (misdemeanors).

The picture is not entirely favorable, however, and many crucial issues as to the place of special classes must be regarded as not definitively answered. Some important studies which question the effectiveness of special-class placement are those carried out by Cassidy and Stanton (1959), Mullen and Itkin (1961), and Goldstein, Jordon, and Moss (1962). The investigations compared mentally retarded pupils in special classes with those in regular classes and came up with these interesting findings:

1. Pupils in regular classes did as well or better academically than those in special classes.
2. Pupils in regular classes had a higher self-esteem.
3. Pupils in special classes had a more favorable sociometric standing.

There are factors associated with special-class placement which may offer some explanation for these outcomes. As Dunn (1968) has pointed out, special classes are too often dumping-grounds for a ragtag of social misfits. The labeling of the child and the special class creates a basis for social stigma and isolation. Even when the child is truly mentally retarded, he is not identified for placement until his troubles in the regular classroom become so pronounced as to bring attention to his plight. The curricular offerings in many special classes may be only more of the same unappealing academic emphasis, albeit presented at a slower rate. In view of possible biasing influences from these limitations, it seems advisable to defer making a final evaluation of the efficacy of special classes. The mentally retarded are unquestionably of an educable potential, and when properly arranged, special classes can hold real possibilities for countering maladjustment tendencies of the mentally retarded.

REHABILITATION PROVISIONS

A plan which leads to placement of the mentally subnormal in a desirable situation is the most successful management of the condition. One way this objective can be accomplished is to create a situation which will accommodate the person. This approach takes little cognizance of the possibility for altering the mentally subnormal who is assumed to have known characteristics of a relatively immutable nature. Care must be exercised in designing such situations to guard against their becoming too artificial and removed from prevailing social trends; otherwise such contrivances encounter severe restrictions.

In one sense, custodial institutions may be thought of as a situation created for those of severely limited intellectual ability. A more common example, however, is the sheltered workshop. In many ways, the sheltered workshop is only an extension of conditions prevailing in ordinary institutions. In neither situation is the person entirely self-sufficient and on his own. Cost of care may be reduced by the sheltered-workshop arrangement, but the personal benefit is often slight for the mentally subnormal person. Adverse consequences are frequently aroused by such public-supported industries competing with private enterprise. All factors considered, sheltered workshops and institutions can probably make the most substantial contribution as temporary placements. As an example, essential training for later real-life demands may be most effectively carried out in a sheltered workshop where job conditions are simulated.

The more promising approach and the really strong point of all rehabilitation planning entails the shaping of the individual to fit existing situations. Situations of particular relevance in this effort are jobs where the person can earn an adequate living. The Office of the Division of Vocational Rehabilitation at the national and state levels has enjoyed huge successes in placing all types of handicapped persons, including the mentally subnormal, in jobs where they can be self-supporting. It is difficult to find another federal program which has such an outstanding record of accomplishment.

In making a placement, vocational-rehabilitation counselors can and do marshal all facilities and services which can improve the employability of the person. Included are medical, surgical, psychological, educative, and training services.

The individual is carefully assessed to identify his strengths and skills. Placement is made from the counselor's current knowledge of the job market and personality characteristics of the prospective employer. Success in placing the mentally subnormal has undoubtedly been enhanced by the emphasis on training for relevant social skills and personality traits. A tendency to be slow and a little dull is easily overlooked if the individual is clean, neat, polite, and dependable.

Again, no one approach holds the entire answer to the management of the mentally handicapped. The mentally retarded are more likely to be regarded as essentially suitable for eventual job placement than are the mentally defective. Vocationally oriented rehabilitation services are working in close cooperation with education programs in public schools and institutions. Cooperation can be expected to increase in the future since this avenue provides what may be the ideal treatment program.

PREVENTION

To some extent, prevention can be an aspect of the management and treatment of mental subnormality. From this perspective, applications from the fields of medicine and education assume importance. Although improvements in the field of medicine may lead to a slight rise in the mentally deficient group, there are promising advances which are available for controlling many subtypes of mental deficiency. These include genetic counseling, therapeutic abortions, continued elimination of defect-producing illnesses, compulsory tests for phenylketonuria, glactosemia, and Rh compatibility, and increased knowledge of the body's use of nutritional materials.

Many exciting possibilities are to be expected for extensions of educative procedures. Although the complex interactions which ensue developmentally between individual capacity and the environment are far from being adequately understood, the earlier belief that mental retardation is essentially an unchangeable condition is no longer tenable. An impressive array of hard data leaves no doubt that measured intellectual ability can be increased by controlled experiences systematically presented at critical periods of development. Studies carried out in orphanages and institutions for children have come to be referred to as "deprivation" studies. They show very clearly the importance of adequate stimulation in maximizing the development of intellectual potential.

A frequently cited deprivation study was carried out by Kirk (1958). At the start of the study, children 3 to 6 years old with IQ scores ranging from 45 to 80 were put into four groups. Two groups lived with their families in the community. Two groups were studied in an institution for the mentally subnormal. The 28 children in one community group and the 15 children in one institutional group attended a special preschool program for three years, while no special treatment was given the control groups. Assessment of intellectual ability at the end of the three-year period indicated that the 43 subjects provided with school experiences had significantly higher IQ scores, with individual gains of from 10 to 30 points. Of the 15 children in the institutional group, 6 now had IQ scores high enough to qualify them for adoption outside the institution.

The Kirk (1958) study has evoked considerable disagreement as to how the gains in IQ might be explained. Some reviewers have been impressed with the fact that 13 of the 43 subjects showed no gain in IQ after three years of schooling. Others have questioned the reliability of IQ scores obtained on 3-, 4-, and 5-year-old children and raised queries as to the adequacy of the family and home backgrounds of the subjects. Some knowledgeable persons feel that the efficacy of education for dealing with mental subnormality is still an unknown quantity. Dunn (1968) has openly urged a hard look at the present practices of placing mentally retarded children in special classes. He claims that socially and emotionally maladjusted problem children are hidden away in special classes intended for the mentally handicapped.

Studies reporting gains in IQ as a result of increased stimulation or intensive experiences have been criticized from many quarters.

Some have questioned the real importance of gains of 10 or 15 IQ points when the person is still markedly below average in intellectual ability. These critics may have a point since an IQ in itself offers very little from which to make a prediction. Other critics, impressed with the fact that there appear to be limits in the extent to which IQ gains can be attained, have suggested that intellectual ability itself is not changed by the early training. They explain the apparent gain as accruing from the child's acquisition of other habits and skills (attending, remembering, wanting to please) which enable him to make maxiumum effective use of his potential.

Let us hope that the critics have correctly analyzed the problem and that the chief influence of early education is made by instilling more efficient personality traits and social skills. If so, this opens a potent possibility for dealing with mental retardation since the adjustment failures of the mentally retarded appear to be more related to deficits in personality and social skills rather than in intellectual potential.

Aside from these practical applications of medical and educational techniques, the prevention of mental subnormality touches on obscure sociocultural variables. It is apparent that programs of population control must eventually include population selection. Rigorously followed, population selection could all but eliminate mental subnormality except for a few cases of mental deficiency. Living will become an increasingly demanding matter for all individuals, for they will have to cope with technological conditions of growing complexity. In order to accommodate persons of limited ability, artificial situations may have to be created which will hold demands commensurate with their limitations. This would be especially likely if subsequent study over the next few years indicates that intelligence level cannot be raised beyond a certain point by any educational program.

As Telford and Sawrey (1967) have so cogently pointed out, the more we succeed in efforts to render all persons uniform in ability, the more otherwise small differences become significant. At the present state of progress, capacity seems to be the outcome of many inherent abilities. Some of these abilities are favored by one procedure; others are enhanced by yet another set of conditions. We must conclude that there is at present no one approach, no one program, which is sufficient for dealing with the problem of mental subnormality. Continued investigation of the many inconsistencies is necessary to resolve the problems found in connection with mental subnormality.

SUMMARY

This chapter has dealt with one of the most ancient concerns: persons who encounter adjustment difficulties because they have less than average intellectual and other abilities. Although the authors have taken a position that the occurrence of less than average intellectual ability may not constitute a behavior disorder in one sense, the condition is of interest to the behavioral specialist for several reasons. The impairment of mental subnormality is most obvious in the mastery of a new situation, especially where the learning involves dealing with abstractions or symbolic materials. Mentally subnormal persons tend to be predisposed to a greater amount of failure and may thus be more susceptible to social and emotional problems. Knowledge gained in the treatment of the mentally subnormal has greatly increased the effectiveness with which all behavior disorders can be alleviated.

Mental subnormality exists in various degrees of severity and seems to be the outcome of an interaction between organic and environmental factors. It has been suggested that familial and environmental factors may be of greater etiological importance in accounting for as many as three-fourths of the mentally subnormal. The remaining cases, which include a preponderance of the more severely incapacitated, tend to have a higher frequency of anatomical and physiological defects. In practice, the impairment of mental subnormality can be difficult to differentiate from impairment associated with language or emotional disorders. A diagnosis of mental subnormality is made on the basis of considerations which include intellectual ability, social competence, and possible influences from significant etiological factors. Estimates of the incidence of mental subnormality range from 3 to as high as 16 per cent of the general population. The variations of incidence are a reflection of different sets of criteria for identifying the condition, which in any event seems to be about twice as frequently identified in males as in females. The incidence also shows interesting prevalence peaks which are clearly related to developmental demands for school, work, marriage, and aging.

Conditions of below-average intellectual ability respond favorably to a wide range of treatment approaches, but no one procedure can be counted on to correct all cases. Attention for the problems of the mentally subnormal requires the coordination of many approaches and specialists, but an intensive educative-vocational training program appears to be the most promising. The success of such a program is enhanced by adequate medical and casework services. Work with mentally subnormal persons has stimulated active research investigations seeking answers to puzzling questions about the development and correction of impairments. Findings gained in these studies have had widespread applicability for improving total human welfare.

SUGGESTED READINGS

Clarke, A. M., & Clarke, A. D. B. *Mental deficiency: the changing outlook.* New York: Free Press, 1965.
Grossman, H. J. (Ed.) *The pediatric clinics of North America: mental retardation.* Vol. 15, No. 4. Philadelphia: Saunders, 1969.
Robinson, H. B., & Robinson, N. M. *The mentally retarded child: a psychological approach.* New York: McGraw-Hill, 1965.
Sarason, S. B., & Gladwin, T. *Psychological problems in mental deficiency.* (3rd ed.) New York: Harper, 1959.

REFERENCES

Carriker, W. R. A. *A comparison of postschool adjustments of regular and special class retarded individuals served in Lincoln and Omaha.* Nebraska Public Schools Project No. 146. Washington, D.C., U.S. Office of Education, 1957.
Cassidy, V. N., & Stanton, J. E. *An investigation of factors involved in the educational placement of mentally retarded children: a study of differences between children in special and regular classes in Ohio.* Columbus: Ohio State Univer. Press, 1959.
Dunn, L. M. Special education for the mildly mentally retarded—is much of it justifiable? *Except. Child.,* 1968, **35**, 5-22.
Gardner, W. I. Social and emotional adjustment of mildly retarded children and adolescents: critical review. *Except. Child.,* 1966, **33**, 97-102.
Goldstein, H. Social and occupational adjustment. In H. A. Stevens & R. Heber (Eds.), *Mental retardation: a review of research.* Chicago: Univer. of Chicago Press, 1964. Pp. 214-258.
Goldstein, H., Jordan, L., & Moss, J. W. *Early school development of low IQ children: study of special class placement.* Urbana, Ill.: Research Institute for Exceptional Children, 1962.
Heber, R. F. Modification in the manual on terminology and classification in mental retardation. *Amer. J. ment. Defic.,* 1961, **65**, 499-500.
Kirk, S. A. *Early education of the mentally retarded.* Urbana: Univer. of Illinois Press, 1958.

Lapp, E. A. A study of the social adjustment of slow-learning children who were assigned part-time to regular classes. *Amer. J. ment. Defic.,* 1957, **62**, 254-262.

Lipman, R. S. Learning: verbal, perceptual-motor, and classical conditioning. In N. R. Ellis (Ed.), *Handbook of mental deficiency.* New York: McGraw-Hill, 1963. Pp. 391-423.

Maher, B. A. *Principles of psychopathology.* New York: McGraw-Hill, 1966.

Mullen, F. A., & Itkin, W. The value of special classes for the mentally handicapped. *Chicago Sch. J.,* 1961, **42**, 353-367.

Porter, R. B., & Milazzo, T. C. A comparison of mentally retarded adults. *Except. Child.,* 1958, **24**, 410-412.

President's Panel on Mental Retardation. *Report.* Washington, D.C.: Government Printing Office, 1965.

Reynolds, M. C., & Stunkard, C. L. A comparative study of day class vs. institutionalized educable retardates. Cooperative Research Project No. 192. Minneapolis: Univer. of Minnesota Press, 1960.

Rosen, M. Rehabilitation, research, and follow-up within the institutional setting. *Ment. Retard.,* 1967, **9**, 24-41.

Sarason, S. B., & Gladwin, T. *Psychological problems in mental deficiency.* (3rd ed.) New York: Harper, 1959.

Telford, C. W., & Sawrey, J. M. *The exceptional individual: psychological and educational aspects.* Englewood Cliffs, N.J.: Prentice-Hall, 1967.

Zigler, E. Mental retardation: current issues and approaches. In M. L. Hoffman & L. W. Hoffman (Eds.), *Review of child development research.* Vol. II. New York: Russell Sage Foundation, 1966. Pp. 107-168.

Zigler, E. Familial mental retardation: a continuing dilemma. *Science,* 1967, **155**, 292-298.

Zigler, E., & Butterfield, E. C. Motivational aspects of changes in IQ test performance of culturally deprived nursery school children. *Child Develpm.,* 1968, **39**, 1-49.

6

The Socially Disadvantaged

This chapter deals with what is unquestionably the most ambitious enterprise in the entire range of human behavior: the concern for persons who are regarded as having adjustment problems because their way of living runs counter to what may be arbitrarily designated as the main current of the stream of life. As with all the adjustment problems we have reviewed in this text on behavior disorders, those of the socially disadvantaged child are "new" only for those very recently come upon the scene. The problem has been around for as long as societies have advanced to a point where there are layers of organization, customarily referred to as "classes" or "subcultures."

Although our presentation will concern itself with the problem of the socially disadvantaged in the United States, the problem is a universal one.

The chief traits ascribed to the socially disadvantaged—poverty, matrifocality, legitimization of short-range hedonism, mistrust, reliance on magical phenomena—are found among groups of people in diverse parts of the world, including those where there are no distinct ethnic minorities, no unemployment, no history of slavery, and no police force (Lewis, 1966). Solutions proposed for dealing with the socially disadvantaged mirror the enormous complexity of correcting the problem. Some situations may warrant the revolutionary approach of creating basic changes in the structure of society by redistributing wealth, organizing the poor and giving them a sense of belonging, and changing leadership hierarchies. The major line of attack dictated by social planners in the United States has followed a more evolutionary plan of trying to incorporate the subculture of the lower class into the culture of the middle class.

In recent years much has been said about the socially disadvantaged and their problems. A bleak picture of otherwise able persons soaking up welfare benefits, persons uneducable and therefore unrehabilitatable, excessively large families whose children will contribute little more than to increase the number of criminals, dope addicts, and prostitutes, and the frank outbreaks of destructive waves of rioting— all makes dramatic reading. But how prevalent is such behavior? And is it, as often seems the case in news-media presentations, invariably associated with, or for that matter even attributable to, the socially disadvantaged? Even the brief mention of these happenings raises a host of issues which must be resolved in one manner or another since they center about a schism which if not integrated poses a sizable threat to our total society.

The problem of the socially disadvantaged, who are variously referred to as "culturally deprived," "educationally deprived," "culturally disadvantaged," as well as "disadvantaged" or "deprived," is one with many facets. Dealing with the adjustment problems encompassed may properly demand multiple approaches and solutions. Not the least of the difficulties encountered are ethical ones, such as the extent to which one segment of a social order is justified in imposing its will on another. It is impossible to discuss the situation meaningfully without considering the social and cultural framework in which the problem manifests itself. Our discussion will review this frequently neglected framework before proceeding to a description of the more salient characteristics of the difficulties and concluding with an evaluation of some of the more educationally oriented proposals for remediation.

IDENTIFICATION

Information relating to the culturally disadvantaged has poured forth in the past few years as this area has assumed its turn for consideration as a major social problem. Unfortunately, much of that which has found its way to the public has been of a shocking, extreme, and flamboyant nature. Such exaggerations may serve the purpose of capturing the attention of the audience, but they have fostered many misconceptions about the culturally disadvantaged. Let there be no doubt about it: the culturally disadvantaged are persons assimilated in and acculturated to a legitimate subculture. Members of this subculture are not necessarily intent upon breaking all the laws, burning the existing social order to the ground, spitefully destroying the educational system, furiously acting out a chronic hatred for all organizations, or chaotically consorted in the slums of major cities.

Anthropologists designate values, attitudes about life, customs, traditions, and patterns of living as the most important aspects of culture. Cultures evolve over long periods of time and are themselves enduring. Each culture provides its members with a design for living in the form of suggested solutions for common life problems. The members of the culture have available the distillate from previous efforts to cope with life problems. Regardless of the fact that these prescriptions for meeting life demands may seem inept or ineffectual, judged from the frame of reference of another culture, compelling testimonial as to their effectiveness, at least for the members of the culture concerned, is found in the durability of the culture over time. A culture which offers no rewards or benefits to its members simply does not long exist. Realization of this principle is essential to understanding the culturally disadvantaged and holds the only hope of an approach for changing the behavior of the group. Looked at from this perspective, as an effort to cope with one's surroundings, the allegations of ineffectiveness, failure, hostile counterreaction, or the product of scapegoating must be rejected as explanations of the problem. Attention can then be turned away from fruitless rationalizations of the negative factors to the less dramatic but potentially more constructive factors which govern the behavior.

CONTRAST WITH EMOTIONAL DISTURBANCE

In one sense, the culturally disadvantaged are socially maladjusted. This statement holds true if the condition of being out of step with the predominant social code is taken as a gross criterion. Most experts in the behavioral sciences, however, recognize the generality of such a criterion and its inadequacy for dealing with this problem. Social maladjustment is more properly a social deviancy, a reaction built upon frankly antisocial tendencies. Such patterns of adjustment—which range from mild lying, irresponsibility, disobedience, and shift-lessness through sexual deviancy and a disruptive disregard for others' property to the more severe acts of theft and fraud—are usually seen as single dominant traits of the personality organization. Social deviancy as nonconformity is to be found in varying degrees among the members of any culture, family, or social class.

The culturally disadvantaged must also be differentiated from the emotionally maladjusted. It may be true that some of the culturally disadvantaged are also emotionally maladjusted, but this is not a characteristic of all the culturally disadvantaged. Emotional maladjustment is a personal problem—the inability of the individual to effect a personally effective and satisfying organization, meshing his abilities with the demands of his particular culture. Emotionally maladjusted persons are generally chronically unhappy and are severely limited psychologically in the extent to which they can participate in their culture. In more extreme cases, the incapacitation reaches degrees of total breakdown. Emotional maladjustment is likely to respond to intervention by psychotherapy, medications, and rest. Acute episodes of emotional maladjustment often show a clear connection to specific events of an emotionally traumatic nature, such as the death of a loved person, the failure to gain a desired goal, or a harrowing experience.

The culturally disadvantaged person, in contrast, has problems only in the context of comparison with another culture. Evaluation in the setting of his own social group reveals no difficulties. The problems arise when he is weighed according to the standards of another and foreign culture. As Cloward and Ohlin (1960) summarized the problem, the so-called culturally deprived are, more correctly, caught up in a cultural conflict. A comparison of values and standards which prevail in "middle-class" and "lower-class" cultures points up the differences which are at the root of the conflict.

DIFFERENCES IN CLASS VALUES

In order to understand the problem clearly, it is constantly necessary to keep in mind that a culture is an organization of techniques, procedures, and ways for making an adaptation to conditions. The organization is, moreover, effective, in that it provides solutions to life problems and it rewards its members. If it is not effective, it does not long endure. This simple principle, well known to cultural anthropologists, is often obscured by the prevalent use of the terms "middle class" and "lower class." The comparison is, from the first, set up in such a way that "lower class" becomes equated with something that is negative, not good, and that really ought not to be permitted to go on. Other than perhaps Lewis' suggested phrase "culture of poverty," no less biased labels have been proposed. It is to be expected that behavioral scientists, who come predominantly from the middle class, are likely to defend and justify their origins. At this stage of the game, our concern is not to provide a new or more "objective" framework; the problem remains the same regardless of the terms in which it may be couched. Use of "middle class" and "lower class" is a choice made for convenience in communication.

The core of middle-class culture is achievement. All resources are organized for production. Participants in the system receive an abundance of material gains—houses, cars, refrigerators, clothing, dishwashers. The niceties of such affluence are comforting, but the actual cost of these gains is seldom objectively reckoned. There are in fact built into the system safeguards for preventing too careful an accounting, for the credit ledger is never closed. Things are always going to be better, greater gains are to be expected. All the person has to do is work and keep on working. If he is not getting the benefits, material rewards, it is because he is not working hard enough. A member of the middle class can easily persuade himself to participate in long-range programs and can be counted on to deliver his bit with reliance and punctuality. He skeptically rejects luck and fast success in favor of deliberation, control, and guaranteed small gain. The middle-class person, then, has his eye on the future. He is concerned with developing abstract intellectual skills for thinking and planning. He must live a carefully planned life pattern with calculated moves toward anticipated "improvement." Immediate rewards available today are inconsequential and are to be forestalled in exchange for a glorious tomorrow. The middle-class person is altruistic in a distant way, mostly by paying others to deal with those struggling at a lower level. To stay on his narrow, achievement-oriented path, he must know where he has been but especially where he is going. Priding himself on being responsible, he is intolerant of those who do not have a shoulder to the wheel of "progress."

By contrast, members of the lower-class culture are more likely to be "enjoyers" rather than "doers." Believing that no one person or group can really beat the system (So why fight it?), the lower-class person's orientation is current and directed to the here and now. It makes no difference how much or how hard you might work, events are largely prearranged. Some days he is lucky; other times he is unlucky. A dollar in his pocket will buy many pleasures. But in the bank—who knows if the bank will burn down or be robbed and the dollar lost for all time? Best to spend it while you can; tomorrow you may be dead. This transitory orientation accounts for many significant personality features of the lower-class person, who is spontaneous and impulsive in loving and in fighting. His belief in a kind of magic makes him adventuresome and ever ready to "travel on," where he may find new friends or greater fortunes. He is mistrustful of anyone who approaches him on the grounds of doing something today for a reward promised two weeks or a month from now. Makers of such offers are only scheming to take advantage of someone, trick him into doing a few days' work—for who can be sure what tomorrow will bring? He is aware of the plentiful supply of everything and sees nothing wrong with "borrowing" food or money from someone who has more than anyone really needs for a day. After all, doesn't he generously share his lucky fortune with everyone? Not only does he share freely his "wealth," but he also tolerantly extends to other persons his own low aspirations. He has no great ambitions, no accumulations of unnecessary objects, and sees no reason for others to have them either. Anyone who is ambitious and strives to acquire property is really creating a situation for bad luck. Such persons should be viewed with suspicion. The choice between having a television set or a bathroom is really no problem; one can find many places for toileting.

To sum up, the "culturally disadvantaged" child is going to encounter adjustment difficulties if he is expected to adapt to a set of values, beliefs, and mores different from what he has acquired. When evaluated according to the standards of his particular cultural group, he is very well adjusted. Teachers trained to work with the middle-class child may be puzzled by behaviors which only reflect differences between the values of the lower-class culture and those of the middle-class culture. Major differences in the values of lower-class and middle-class persons in the United States are listed in Table 12.

TABLE 12. A COMPARISON BETWEEN LOWER-CLASS AND MIDDLE-CLASS VALUES

Lower Class	Middle Class
Present time orientation	Future time orientation
Preference for concrete and tangible	Preference for abstract
Adventurousness and spontaneity	Responsibleness and control
Acceptance of "fate" without worry	Use of intellect to plan and think
Immediacy of gratification	Delay of gratification
Emphasis on physical activity and sensual, with tolerance for violence	Emphasis on beauty, altruism, and perfection
Indulgence and low aspiration	Criticalness and high aspiration

The incorporation of lower-class values into the personality organization of members of the lower class forms a basis for behaviors which differ with the values and standards of the majority middle class. Members of the lower class are said to be culturally disadvantaged to varying degrees as they are caught up in a cultural conflict.

INCIDENCE

Making a count of the precise number of persons who can be designated as culturally disadvantaged is a staggering task. As has been pointed out, the criteria for evaluation consist of values and ideals which are abstract and elusively resistant to quantification. There are no handy measuring scales which can be brought into service to carry out such a survey. It has been necessary to rely on extensive observations carried out in detailed field studies by cultural anthropologists and sociologists. These field studies have suggested certain indices which are rather sensitive indicators of class membership. Possibly because the lower class is a minority of the total population, it is often thought that the culturally disadvantaged can be identified as those members of minority groups. Thus, American Indians, Spanish-Americans, Chinese-Americans, and Negroes suggest themselves as the culturally disadvantaged. A large percentage of these groups may be culturally disadvantaged, but a sizable percentage of each group is not. The majority of the culturally disadvantaged are native-born whites. The culturally disadvantaged cannot be identified on the basis of residence in big-city slums, the Appalachian hill country, or the rural areas of the South, although many of the persons in these areas are culturally disadvantaged. Migrant workers, the unemployed, and the poor are groups which also contribute substantially, but not exclusively, to the number of culturally disadvantaged.

Number of years of school completed (less than 10 years), occupation (laborers, semiskilled, farm workers), and total annual income (less than $4,000) are generally accepted as providing a reliable composite index for designating the culturally disadvantaged. Depending upon the weight given the several indices, from one-fourth to one-third of the total population of the United States may be classed as culturally disadvantaged. Of interest to child-welfare specialists is the fact that culturally disadvantaged families tend to be large, with a result that from one-third to two-fifths of all children may be in the culturally disadvantaged group (Witmer, 1964).

CHARACTERISTICS

COMMON MISCONCEPTIONS

Descriptions of the culturally disadvantaged, although plentiful in number, are frequently found to be sparse in presenting a realistic picture. The tendency to relegate the culturally disadvantaged to an unfavorable condition is perhaps best understood as an example of the general tendency to defend and protect one's own reference group by minimizing all other groups. By way of accomplishing this goal, generous use is made of the defense mechanisms of social psychology. Stereotyping, exaggeration, overgeneralization, and repetition are relied upon to create an unfavorable impression. The defense mechanisms of social psychology often have a certain amount of half-truth which is exploited to give a basis for credence. More than merely "nasty habits," social defense mechanisms act to obscure the individuals who make up the group and to perpetuate themselves by increasing the gap between groups. If accepted, they provide a bleak, hopeless, and immutable picture. Therefore it is essential to examine some of the more grossly erroneous attributes leveled at the culturally disadvantaged.

1. *Social-Depravity Traits.* It is frequently alleged that the culturally disadvantaged are criminals, dope addicts, engaged in illicit enterprises (prostitution, stolen property), alcoholic, family deserters, and all on relief. The allegations are surprisingly persistent in the light of the extreme improbability associated with each of these contentions. A major theme in Lewis' accounts of the life activities of the culturally disadvantaged is a marked dislike and fear of jails. This attitude is rivaled only by their contempt for criminals and sexual deviates who take refuge in the rather disorganized living conditions of metropolitan areas where many culturally disadvantaged live. Family arrangements are loose, but may actually be closer to arrangements in other cultural groups where children are regarded as community property and all adults are "father" and "mother." It is surprising to find that many of the culturally disadvantaged spurn any form of welfare assistance, other than perhaps medical services, for simple reasons of not wanting to bother with the stack of papers to be filled out or because of a basic suspicion of all nosey outsiders. It takes only a minute to compute that the absolute number of criminals, dope addicts, and such is far less than the total number of culturally disadvantaged.

2. *Ethnic Traits.* Another group of demeaning qualities is based to a large extent on traits supposedly basic to particular racial groups. Negroes, Indians, Spanish-Americans, Chinese, and other members of distinctly recognizable racial groups are blanketed with charges of being unattractive, unclean, sensual, menial, and shiftless. This discrimination and prejudice has the added support of distortions associated with the fact that many members of such ethnic groups are culturally disadvantaged. They are belied by the fact that members of each of these ethnic groups can be found in all cultural classes.

3. *Personality Traits.* A cluster of unfavorable characteristics is often directed indiscriminately to the culturally disadvantaged by otherwise well-informed persons. The charges seem to be attempts to account for what is interpreted as inferiority, incompetency, and inadequacy. Possibly suggested by the poverty, dearth of material acquisitions, and generally lesser attainment of the culturally disadvantaged, these unfavorable traits include conceptions of being intellectually dull, having inferior physical and mental health, an inaptitude for schooling, irresponsibility, and dependency. Chief among these is intellectual and physical inferiority. Once again, the indiscriminate assignment of these traits of inferiority may find partial justification in a few trends and

tendencies. But when any one of these ascribed traits is objectively investigated, about as many negative as positive cases are discovered. For example, Barber (1957) found that all degrees of measured intellectual ability existed among the culturally disadvantaged.

CONTROVERSIAL CONCEPTIONS

The student who embarks on a review of reports on almost any subject will usually find that he doesn't have to look very far before he encounters differing opinions about what seems to be the same topic. These variations in observations of a problem are related to many factors, including personal biases and theoretical background of the research investigator and the complexity of forces which influence the phenomenon. When these factors are considered, it is not surprising that there are many conflicting traits ascribed to the culturally disadvantaged. Some of these are rather easy to explain (purported nonverbalness), but others defy any consistent explanation (patriarchal versus matriarchal orientation, attitude toward school). Knowing that these traits are controversial may keep the issues open so that needed followup investigations will be carried out and eventually indicate the way the pieces of the puzzle may be fitted together.

Intellectual Ability

The plethora of scales for measuring "intelligence" and academic achievement has probably made it all too convenient for such devices to be used in behavioral research. The findings are rather consistent in placing the culturally disadvantaged at a less favorable position on such scales. More specifically, groups of culturally disadvantaged are reported as having scores from 10 to 15 points below the IQ scores obtained by groups from the middle class. A typical example of these studies is that reported by Bloom (1964), who has drawn together a wide array of studies. There seems very little reason to question the picture of lower scores on measures of intelligence associated with lower-class status, even though there are consistent findings of occasional high IQ scores among such groups.

Our concern is for the interpretations which are given to such data. In the work by Bloom, data are given comparing culturally disadvantaged groups reared in rural Southern environments with culturally disadvantaged groups reared in metropolitan Northern cities. The "higher" IQ scores of pupils born and reared in Philadelphia (the actual mean difference by chronological age of 15 years was 7 points in the most divergent groups) were attributed to the greater stimulation and advantage of the urban environment. If this is so, how is it then that this same "favorable" environment is cited as the chaotic, disorganized, and deprived setting which is said to be at the root of the culturally disadvantaged person's problems? It may well be that measured intelligence of the type we usually obtain is not too relevant a factor. Riessman (1962) has one of the more comprehensive discussions of this entire matter of the significance of IQ and adjustment of the culturally disadvantaged. Many treatment programs for the culturally disadvantaged report in glowing terms increases of about 12 IQ points after two or three years of varied intervention and remedial efforts. Haggard (1954) was able to show similar gains in intelligence scores of culturally disadvantaged children after only three one-hour sessions in which the children were simply instructed in how to take tests.

In view of the uncertainty as to just what the widely used intelligence and achievement scales are really measuring, it is very surprising that the culturally disadvantaged do as well as they do. It has been suggested that existing intelligence and achievement tests are highly loaded in favor of middle-class cultural values. Accordingly, the scores obtained from such tests should predict success in coping with middle-class cultural demands and in the achievement of middle-class scholastic objectives. This the tests seem to do adequately. Whether this kind of success alone constitutes "intelligence" or is only one manifestation of intelligence is quite another matter. As was seen from the discussion of the mentally subnormal, variables included in the IQ are only a portion of factors involved in adjustment. Correlations between IQ and any given outcome (job success, effectiveness of adjustment, school success) seldom range as high as $r = +.70$. Such a correlation indicates that common factors account for less than one-half the performance in the two situations, with more than one-half the factors contributing unaccounted for. Depending on the sizes of the groups compared, smaller correlation coefficients and small IQ differences may be statistically significant. When it comes to predictions about individual outcomes, the IQ is seldom contraindicative for any plan. The range in IQ scores in any one group of individuals frequently exceeds the difference between two groups.

To say the culturally disadvantaged are less intelligent is one thing;

to say they are lacking in certain test-taking habits is another, and to say they are less "middle-class" is still another.

Verbal and Language Skills

A deficit in the areas of language and verbal proficiency is so frequently cited as to be automatically accepted by many persons dealing with the culturally disadvantaged. When the findings gathered by dozens of studies are considered, there is irrefutable evidence that the culturally disadvantaged as a group have a limited vocabulary and are less able to deal with the kinds of language items which make up the prevailing scales for assessing these functions. Our intention is not one of arguing these findings, which speak for themselves.

The crux of the matter is just what all these measures may mean. Language is an integral aspect of culture. The position has been taken that we are dealing with a conflict of cultures. It should not be surprising, then, that members of two different cultures are found to have differences in language. When the data reporting the difficulty which the culturally disadvantaged have with middle-class language are analyzed in a cultural context, some interesting patterns are discernible. Such analyses have been made by Bernstein (1960) and Riessman (1962). Bernstein carried out a comprehensive study of the total language patterns and contrasted "formal" and "public" language as used in communication. Formal language is characterized by following certain technical arrangements and prescribed structures; it is thus rigid and syntactical. These qualities of formal language are what the culturally disadvantaged person finds perplexing.

Riessman (1962) has made a compelling case for the culturally deprived having great language facility and fluency, but the language is that of his culture. This observation is readily verifiable in the behavior of the culturally disadvantaged. Their language is colorful, flexible, and richly descriptive. Riessman suggests that much innovation and creativeness in communication originates with the culturally disadvantaged. Greater use of nonverbal methods in communication is also made by the culturally disadvantaged, who may freely and spontaneously combine hand-clapping, body-swaying, and singing to express their feelings.

Family Structure

A consideration of the family arrangements of the culturally disadvantaged entails a look into one of the more jumbled aspects of this cultural group. Information on family relationships has suffered from efforts to squeeze the picture to fit the frame of recognized psychoanalytic explanations of pathology and from what appear to be ethnically related influences among some of the more numerous subgroups of the culturally disadvantaged.

One of the major points of controversy centers about a prevailing pattern of dominant influence by adult females (matriarchal) as opposed to adult males (patriarchal). Lewis (1966), who has collected extensive cross-cultural data, insists that the pattern is one of matriarchy. Riessman (1962), who has made extensive analyses of the lower-class culture in the United States, is equally convinced that a pattern of patriarchy is typical, except for the Negro group. Several investigators have attached considerable importance to the consequences of the absence of biological fathers from the home and subsequent devastating effects for the development of male children. An excellent review of these studies is presented by Herzog and Sudia (1968). They conclude that the importance of these findings has been exaggerated and overgeneralized and that the existing data do not permit a decisive answer on the consequences of father absence. They suggest that what may be needed to provide illumination of the problem is the direct study of children in fatherless homes, rather than the present inferential approach of attempting to isolate an elusive "single factor" from what are obviously multiple and interacting factors.

The family pattern of the culturally disadvantaged seems to be one technically designated as the "extended family." Such families are recognized by the presence of several parent figures. All adult females act as "mothers" and all adult males serve as "fathers." A person is either an adult or a child, and there is relatively little differentiation other than this simple dichotomy. Reports indicate that the amount of parent-child interaction seems to vary, but parents are frequently occupied with one or another crisis situation and have little time to spend with the children. Early independence in self-help is emphasized, with the children depending on one another much of the time. Parental attention is secured by creating crises which compete with those already confronting the parent. This may hold important consequences for the later school adjustment of the children. Regardless of the presence or absence of the real father or mother, the children grow up as recognizable males and females.

The pattern of compulsive masculinity (machismo) has been cited as a reaction to excessive female domination, but this may be erroneous labeling of behaviors which are of a physical, motoric, and tangible orientation. Even the females in the lower classes must daily carry out physical feats of lifting, carrying, and fighting which exceed the physical exertions of the most active middle-class male. When the matter of who is the figure of authority, the decision maker, is considered, there is growing question as to how much of this responsibility is assumed by the middle-class male, and many sociologists have long ago conceded that the females dominate the middle-class family.

There are as many positive claims as negative that can be made for the extended-family arrangement. Children in such families could be expected to profit from multiple identification models without having to be concerned with pleasing only one particular person by a specified pattern of behaviors. Attaining independence as an adult should be an easier transition, and sibling rivalry might be reduced, to mention a few possible benefits. In any event, the family ties of the culturally disadvantaged are strong, and the family constellation is visible and cognizant.

Physical and Motor Skills

The culturally disadvantaged are typically depicted as having a preference for the physical and the concrete, which finds expression in motor activities. For a long time it was considered more appropriate to assess the intellectual ability of the culturally disadvantaged with tasks which demanded skill in motor manipulation and visual-motor coordination. It was expected that the culturally disadvantaged would be more adequate in dealing with motor-manipulation items such as the assembly of cutout puzzles and the arrangement of blocks to copy geometric patterns. It was recommended that the culturally disadvantaged have chances to play in games and to work with tools as a way of fostering more appreciation for school. Another line of support for the contention of great motor skill has been that of citing the high percentage of Negro members of athletic teams. This feature has become so widespread that some Negro leaders have objected to the continued participation of black athletes on the grounds that it is a special case of Uncle Tomism.

The concern of this discussion is to explore the many facets of this reputed physical-motor attribute, for which we find some supporting and some dissenting opinions. In his monumental study of social-class patterns and practices, Davis (1948) noted a lower-class preference for physical activities as releases for emotional feelings of all kinds. Members of this group fought, used physical punishment, and engaged in all types of physical activities and contests more than did members of other cultural groups. More recently, Miller and Swanson (1960) have verified and expanded on what they term the "motoric orientation" of the culturally disadvantaged. This characteristic can be observed in a predilection for dealing with objects—handling them and juggling them. Such behaviors are sometimes referred to as a propensity for "thinking with one's hands." The motoric orientation is credited with accounting for the heavy use of gestures in communication, the physical rather than verbal expression of violence and affection, a marked interest in competitive sports, and an admiration for feats of strength and endurance.

Despite the claims for a high degree of agility and motor skill, there are puzzling gaps which call into question the generality of this assertion. Granted that many culturally disadvantaged persons have achieved success in boxing, football, baseball, and basketball, very few of their number have gained recognition as violinists, artists, or dancers. In the preschool programs there seems to be as much need for presenting experiences which will develop motor-coordination skills of the culturally disadvantaged as for language stimulation. Some social scientists have suggested that the concern for physical prowess is an expresion of compulsive masculinity to defend against total domination by females in a matrifocal culture. Yet other social scientists have emphasized the fact that the culturally disadvantaged live in a world where physical activities predominate. They often carry water, chop wood, have fewer labor-saving gadgets, and must typically use their hands in their work. Recently there have been discoveries of possible constitutional factors which suggest a greater potential for physical and motor skills, at least for those culturally disadvantaged who are Negro. This evidence consists of differences in the bones and musculature of the legs and in the observed accelerated motor development of Uganda infants in Africa (Gerber, 1958). These infants accomplish developmental motor tasks of controlling the head movements, sitting alone, grasping, and walking alone in less than half the time required by white Occidental infants. Regardless of what the causative factors may be, a true picture of motor-skill potential and development is essential for effective educational planning. Potential skills in the physical and motor areas can provide solid assets for acculturation.

Attitudes toward Education

The culturally disadvantaged are often credited with having attitudes of not wanting to do much to help themselves get ahead. The rejection of education particularly is said to be widespread. Excessive dropout rates and a disproportionate number of persons in the lower school-achievement range are taken as expressions of a dislike for education on the part of the lower class. The opportunity to add to their educational attainment by attendance in night-school programs, frequently made easily available to the culturally disadvantaged, has been received less than enthusiastically. The attitude is difficult to understand in view of the constant emphasis on "better education—better pay" and in the light of the actual opening up of better vocational opportunities as discrimination practices subside. Adding to the confusion is the well-known tendency for members of the lower class to give "lip service" to values and objectives of the middle class while acting according to the standards and values of the lower class.

Recent studies have produced findings which challenge the belief that the culturally disadvantaged dislike, or are even uninterested in, getting an education. Riessman (1962) collected responses from lower-class adults to an open-ended question, "What do you miss most in life that you would like your children to have?" More than half the respondents answered, "Education." Surprisingly, the answer was given more frequently by Negro than by white persons in the study group. This response takes on an added importance when it is remembered that open-ended questions do not provide any choices or selections for answers but require the respondent to furnish his own answer. Even more unexpected are data reported by Durkin (1961), who found that 55 per cent of a group of children identified on the basis of being able to read on entrance into school came from lower-socioeconomic families. Teaching a child to read demands consistent and concerted effort on the part of the older members of the family. In some areas, notably St. Louis, interest and follow-through have been generated among lower-class parents at least sufficient for getting children started in school and in preschool programs.

Yet the patterns of dropping out and low achievement continue and demand clarification. It seems likely that lower-class families are at least favorably disposed to getting their children started in school. Data gathered by Lewis (1966) suggest that what is from the start a tenuous venture may ultimately be undone by the cumulative effects of being unable to keep up with more academically oriented classmates. Not only are the culturally disadvantaged less proficient in dealing with the school's curricular offerings, which are increasingly of an abstract and intangible nature, but they are less likely to have suitable clothing, books, pencils, lunch money, and the like. They give up, often retaining a belief that they will return someday. No small part of the matter of dropouts may rest with the schools' curricular offerings themselves. School curricula have remained amazingly inflexible and unchanged. There is a distinct narrowing to more and more of an academic orientation with each higher grade level. Not only do such academic tasks have little that appeals to the culturally disadvantaged, but they demand a lot of effort. It would in many ways be more strange if all pupils remained in such a thwarting situation indefinitely.

When all is considered, the controversy as to attitudes and responses toward education may not be such a dilemma. Children from the lower classes like to learn, and they do learn. Riessman (1962) has provided a succinct resolution of the apparent inconsistency. He maintains that "education" must be differentiated from "what schools offer." The school program is only one kind of educational experience, requiring particular talents and offering specific rewards. If the schools really intend to provide universal education, they must greatly diversify the experiences and the rewards available so as to reach the members of all social classes. As matters presently stand, lower-class children may be at their greatest disadvantage in the school.

EDUCATIONALLY RELEVANT CHARACTERISTICS

Whatever the picture with regard to characteristics of the culturally disadvantaged, experiences and events which occur prior to entrance into school are of paramount interest to the educator. It is these early experiences that develop the skills, goals, and rewards which the child brings to school. The general process of development, in which learning occurs out of the interaction between the child and his surroundings, is the same for all children. The children themselves may be very similar at the start, but different surroundings, rewards, and coping skills foster comparably different personality organizations which must be approached in appropriate modes and channels if development is to continue.

Home Conditions

Lower-class families tend to be large, with children appearing in rapid succession. The parents have only marginal acquisitions of skills and attributes highly valued by the middle class. The situation is then one which does not facilitate the instilling of middle-class values. Under ordinary conditions, the parents are strapped in coping with the routine operation of the family. There are endless dishes to be washed, clothes to be washed and ironed, food to be prepared, beds to be made. Life for both parents has been described as a never-ending cycle of crises which begin anew with each day. Thus engaged, parents may have little time to give to any child. In many homes the potential parental time available for children is further reduced by parental absence from death, desertion, divorce, or diversion.

As a consequence, children in such situations have minimal chances for talk and discussion with their parents. They become independent at early ages and may learn more from and depend more on older siblings and peers than on adults. Punishment may never be administered in many instances, because time simply runs out. More commonly, punishment is delayed and/or given in a reverse form which is not easily related to the undesired behavior. Left to figure things out for himself, the child may decide that he should develop greater skills for avoiding detection or that he should try to change his "bad luck" to "good" in some magical way. Operating only with his own resources, his curiosity may not be directed into useful channels. He may take an object apart, destroying it by dismantling, with no regard for trying to figure out how it "works." Parents often have little time to deal with the children as individuals. The child has little choice for obtaining needed attention other than by generating a crisis situation greater than the one currently absorbing the parent's concern. The child may also learn very early that he must grab his share of everything quickly while he can because what is gone is gone.

It is difficult to calculate the consequences of not being read to because there are too many diapers to be changed as a part of getting everyone bedded down. The never-ceasing demands on the parent's energies must undoubtedly result in many similar situations where honest intentions go astray. The impact of countless broken promises of trips to the zoo, going to the movies, or getting a new toy can easily be a feeling of suspicion, mistrust, and a reaffirmation for the immediate and tangible. Learning to be "good" or to work hard for future reward has little chance under such conditions. Along with these diminished opportunities for listening, remembering, and persisting, there may be other deficits in chances to manipulate books, pictures, paper and pencil, and other materials that will be encountered in the classroom. The parent may have a minimum of these same skills to share with the child or to serve as a resource for assisting the child to gain proficiency in them.

Social Learning

Throughout this text, the importance of social learning as a contributor to the understanding of adjustment difficulties has been emphasized. The principle is a particularly useful one when applied to the problems of the culturally disadvantaged, for there are three major acquisitions which have important implications for education:

1. Home and family arrangements are such that lower-class children are early welded into a cohesive group. Needs for contacts of all sorts, approval, recognition, and support are satisfied by this group affiliation. Intrusive efforts by outsiders, including adults, are warded off as being not needed. In a similar way, any efforts which may cost group membership are to be avoided. The safest course of action is not to be too ambitious and to be careful not to achieve too much. A violation of either of these standards would jeopardize group status. Moreover, gains made by an individual would be attained at a cost of making others appear incompetent or bad, and no one intentionally wants to hurt his best friends.

2. A second feature of the learning of the culturally disadvantaged child grows out of his greater reliance on tangible units of experience. Specifics can be handled and are "for real." Possibly because he can be the victim of many broken promises of good things to come that never materialize, or possibly because of an inherent predisposition for specific rewards, the culturally disadvantaged child has a definite orientation for dealing with the concrete. He has little capacity for accepting criticism and making corrections just to get praise in the future. It is difficult for him to comprehend the difference between the "И" that he makes and the "N" the teacher holds out as the model.

He may see no important difference between a picture of a bear and that of a guinea pig. He finds it difficult to learn something by reading about it and is wary of those who seek to goad him with promises that he knows well may never materialize.

3. A third major tendency of significance is the culturally disadvantaged child's expectancy of concrete rewards. A pat on the head, a stick of gum, or a small stamp in the form of a rocketship is acceptable as a reward. Being told he is a good citizen, a good worker, or a good scholar elicits little other than confusion. He has had long experience with the withholding of rewards and is not bothered by the experience. In the same way, he is not concerned (guilty) that he has behaved badly because he cheated. Exhortations to be nice, to work hard, or to be a good sport are ineffective as techniques for increasing his output. His tendency to be self-reliant minimizes any inclination for accepting criticism of his work in a positive sense. Optimal performance is more likely to be in evidence when specific responses are provided in the form of definite and concrete rewards which are immediately given.

Educational Difficulties

By this time it should be clear that the culturally disadvantaged child has objectives, responses, and expectations which are different from those observed in the middle-class child. There are rewards, reinforcement patterns, and methods of approach which can be advantageously manipulated in controlling and influencing his learning. More correctly, the culturally disadvantaged child is confronted with a situation of cultures in conflict. Lindgren (1967) has provided an excellent picture of the ways in which the culturally disadvantaged child has difficulty at school:

1. The culturally disadvantaged child is unfamiliar with the roles which govern classroom organization. He appears impulsive, interruptive, and inattentive.

2. The culturally disadvantaged child is less able to learn from someone *telling* him how to do something or how things are. He prefers a demonstration and direct participation.

3. The culturally disadvantaged child is less likely to look to adults (teachers) as persons who will help him.

4. The culturally disadvantaged child prefers frequent changes in what he is doing and doesn't remember directions or instructions well.

5. The culturally disadvantaged child has trouble grasping the formality and correctness of syntax.

6. The culturally disadvantaged child finds it difficult to make abstract associations; shown a group of pictures and asked which one is good to eat, he may give a verbal response of something far removed from any of the objects pictured.

7. The culturally disadvantaged child is casual and finds it difficult to make specific differentiations necessary to identify the dirtiest, prettiest, and so on.

8. The culturally disadvantaged child has a low degree of constructive curiosity.

9. The culturally disadvantaged child may have a rather narrow range of experiences, so that he is uncertain as to whether an animal is a lion, cow, or buffalo or whether an eating place is a restaurant, cafeteria, or cafe.

ETIOLOGICAL CONSIDERATIONS

Offering explanations to account for the adjustment problems of the culturally disadvantaged may seem at first glance a redundant effort. This may be especially so since our presentation has emphasized the notion of a basic cultural conflict rather than a deficit in the strict sense. "Culture" is a system which, made up of many factors, serves as an organization of patterns by which individuals come to experience their surroundings. Cultural disadvantage might then be expected to originate from defect or impairment in the organization of patterns of living as these are experienced, in the individual's potentials for absorbing this experience, and in the unique personal organization which the individual acquires as a result of his cultural experiences.

CULTURAL-DEPRIVATION FACTORS

Many behavioral scientists have attempted to present the problems of the culturally disadvantaged in the frame of reference of deprivation. Impressed with the manifest lack of material objects, the minimal housing and dietary conditions, and the generally narrow experiences typical of the lower classes, the approach has been that of equating these shortages with a total lack of all experiences. To a large extent, these investigators have found additional support for the interpretation of experiential deficit in the large number of so-called sensory-deprivation studies. It has been conclusively established that the withholding of visual, motor, or other stimulation in infancy has devastating consequences for the adult animal. Such results are demonstrable only where there is complete denial of stimulation, whereas only small amounts of stimulation are adequate for the development of a normal capacity to deal with experiences. There is a suggestion that any depression in stimulation has a correlated reduction in the functioning capacity of the adult individual. Evidence for the latter contention comes from comparisons of persons in usual family situations with persons placed in foster homes and in institutions.

The data are open to other interpretations, however, since constitutional factors are usually not controlled and there is considerable doubt as to the permanency or irreversibility of the consequences of limited experiences on later development. In either case, it is difficult to make a convincing argument that the early years of the culturally disadvantaged are missing in any kind of experience. The differences, where identifiable, are more qualitative than quantitative. There is every reason to believe the culturally disadvantaged have as much visual, kinesthetic, auditory, and other stimulation as does the middle-class child. In fact, the noisy, active surroundings of the lower class can more readily be said to hold more stimulation than does the quiet and controlled atmosphere of the middle-class home.

What is different about the experiences is a basic one involving acculturation in two different cultures. The members of each of the two contrasting cultures successfully incorporate the language, customs, mores, values, objectives, and coping techniques of their own culture. Differences in the attributes of the two cultures form the root of conflict and adjustment problems when an individual attempts to live in a culture other than the one native to him. A core of values emphasizing responsible planning, attainment by continuous education, competitive acquisition of material possessions, and future time orientation can be expected to have associated behavior which differs markedly from that elicited by belief in luck, doubt about the future, taking immediate pleasures, and tolerant indulgence. If the two sets of values did not hold enough disparities, sufficient discrepancies to form the basis for a struggle would be found in membership and allegiance choices faced by any one individual in the larger society made up of several major subcultures. In many respects, a clash is built into such a society. The impossibility of saying which of the opposing sets of values is the better intensifies the expectation of contention.

CONSTITUTIONAL FACTORS

Even though the problems of the culturally disadvantaged center about conflicting value systems, explanations of the disagreement must be sought in a consideration of how a culture maintains itself. Culture is an abstraction, a kind of organization of organizations. Intangible as it may appear, it is highly durable and has a profound influence on the behavior of its members. When members of one culture make evaluations of the features of another culture, they often wonder how such a culture can exist. All cultures are maintained in the same way, that is, by giving solutions to life problems and rewards for solving them. This description is very simply stated, but in everyday operation the functions of culture have many implications. Cultures have a way of standing alone and being self-sufficient. As Lewis comments, the observed stability of behavior patterns manifested over four generations suggests a tenacious cultural pattern (1966, p. xxvii). It is unlikely that a culture as an abstraction can marshal strengths out of air. A culture's strengths must be drawn from the strengths of the members.

The integrity and durability of a culture boils down to success in supplying workable solutions and acceptable rewards for dealing with life's problems. In solving a problem, the individual must rely on patterns of skills, talents, and energies which are within his behavioral-response potential. These are potentials which are packaged in a genetic container. The capacity for experiencing rewards is also genetically stipulated. It is consistent with observations of behavior to conceptualize a pattern of a particular genetic potential finding a suitable environment, developing and maintaining itself, and thus perpetuating the entire relationship. Jensen (1968) has assembled impressive data indicating that hereditary factors may have a major role in determining social-class membership. Such a picture does not allow much leeway for educational intervention, but if true, cognizance of the relationships could ultimately lead to more effective educational procedures for modification of the arrangement.

There appear to be somewhat more subtle constitutional forces which can influence social-class membership. Relevant for this contention are findings discovered in research directed by Pasamanick. Reporting on data collected in association with events during pregnancy and child-health outcomes, Pasamanick and Knobloch (1961) were able to show connections between abnormalities during pregnancy or at birth and later impairments in the child. Mothers who have poor diets, are fatigued or harassed, have any type of illness, or received less than minimal prenatal medical care gave birth to children who showed a higher incidence of defects and deficiencies of all types. These significant events in pregnancy are commonly observed in lower-class mothers and could be one factor contributing to the kind of marginality of potential which sometimes seems to typify members of the lower class.

EGO-DEVELOPMENT FACTORS

It is possible that the process by which the individual becomes organized as a functioning person is the most significant source of problems encountered by the culturally disadvantaged. An excellent review of ego-development patterns for lower-class persons has been made by Ausubel and Ausubel (1963). The acquisition of an integrated set of values, attitudes, aspirations, and satisfactions centering about the self, designated as ego development, encompasses constitutional and cultural factors. This is sufficient to ascribe primary importance to this developmental process in and of itself. Turning to a more specific consideration of ego acquisition, there appear to be particular steps which have special reference to the subsequent adjustment of lower-class members. These have to do with the consequences of parent-child relationships, the opportunities for acquiring status, the types of approved behaviors, and the kinds of achievement motivation sanctioned.

Previous reference has been made of the small amount of interaction between parent and child in the lower-class family. Parents are busy coping with many crisis situations, are drawn to various diversions, hold limited resources for meeting any demand, or are simply exhausted. The net result is that the child has difficulty in effecting a necessary satellite relationship with the parent. He is denied an important source of positive self-esteem, and the fleeting encounters with parents are likely to be ones of harsh punishment. The multiplicity of parents he must obey and please can make for confusion in identification or deny practice in learning how to please one authority person. For boys, there may be special problems of living in a female-dominated world. The lower-class child thus can be uncertain of his identity, ambivalent about authority, and can find it difficult to subjugate himself to the control of an adult person whom he tends not to trust.

Opportunities to acquire status are also limited for the lower-class child. Within his immediate family, he finds that status is uncertain and difficult to come by. Many matters poorly understood to the child seem to absorb the parents' attention, and he is forced to be excessively resourceful in gaining their interest. Even if he is able to identify with his family, he quickly learns that they are demeaned and degraded for no apparent reason. In some instances, his efforts to gain respect may encounter the added rebuff of discriminatory and segregation practices as a response to situations he cannot change. Only the peer group seems to hold a place for him where there is some semblance of recognition, and to this haven he turns. In making the move, he carries with him feelings of frustration, bitterness, and counterrejection.

Each culture tends to sanction certain types of behaviors. This is one of the distinguishing features of a culture, and it involves two types of opportunities for behaving, the kinds of demands confronting the person, and the rewards available. Parents and authority persons in control of the culture are likely to promote their own standards and values and to feel threatened by any deviations. They are inclined to disapprove of excessive ambition and to reward an acceptance of one's "place in life." They actually have a minimum of resources, moreover, for the real support of ventures into the business and professional world. The child soon learns not to ask for much, not to count on his parents financing a college education, for example. Early manifestations of independence are encouraged. At least, the child's "getting out of the parent's hair" also gets the parent out of the child's hair. The outcome is one favoring a facade of compliance and subjugation while taking covert urges of a hostile nature to the peer group for expression.

A final important ego-development process is the acquisition of motivational components. Prospects for the culturally disadvantaged person incorporating a pattern of high achievement are bleak. From the first, important persons seem to care very little about what he does. So long as he is not bothersome to them, his parents are not likely to inquire or check up on what he has been doing. Casting about, he sees his own kind getting very little of the material benefits of life even though they may work very hard. Contacts with the middle-class culture may serve to sharpen rather than to invite ways to change this disparity. Attendance at school all too frequently proves to be anything but his cup of tea and may only enhance a nucleus of doubt as to his competence, even when he tries very hard to please. The final blow can well come when he is fed up and leaves school to test the vocational world. There he finds more doors closed than opened. Little choice remains but to succumb to low aspirations although high attainments may be verbalized in the "right" places.

TREATMENT PROGRAMS

Efforts to deal with the problems of the socially disadvantaged have been as numerous as are the manifestations of the difficulties. Physical and mental health services, dietary and housing improvements, recreational and cultural opportunities, and vocational and educational offerings are among the major approaches. Each of these lines of assistance has particular possibilities, and each has shown a degree of success. While acknowledging that all of these services are essential in dealing with the problem, our discussion will emphasize those programs which, if not educational in the traditional sense, have had close association with the schools. The choice is not dictated by a belief that an educational approach is the only solution to the problem, although this contention can be defended. It cannot be overlooked that there are unique and real contributions, for example, from the fields of medicine and community planning in addition to the important function which all of these services may do in reinforcing and maintaining changes effected by an educational program. The emphasis on educational programs in this discussion of treatment approaches is simply a reflection of the basic educational orientation of the text, the belief that all treatment programs for children are most effective when integrated, and the recognition that the school can and should be the most appropriate coordinating center.

Interest in applying educational solutions to alleviate the problems of the socially disadvantaged originated in resident corrective institutions but quickly moved into the regular school program. These provisions are more likely to be found in large metropolitan school systems where there are greater numbers of all types of pupils, including the socially disadvantaged. There has, in any case, been very little systematic effort to identify the socially disadvantaged and to refer these pupils for service. The programs have generally been loosely planned with some form of remediation available in the elementary grades and a gradual separation and placement into special classes, or even entire schools, with a "vocational" orientation at the secondary levels. Recent interest in the problems of the socially disadvantaged has led to a more intense concern for remediation and to an extension of usual school experiences to involve parent contacts and to fostering attitude changes by educational processes. A review of current attempts to deal with the socially disadvantaged has been compiled by Weikart (1967). Weikart's article is the major source of the discussion in the following section.

PROGRAMS FOR ACADEMIC DEFICIENCIES

Most attempts at educational intervention for remedying the problems of the socially disadvantaged have been directed to the correction of specific deficits in motor, language, or general experiential areas. The deficit is often more assumed than assessed. Educational procedures are involved on the premise that such disabilities are correlated with environmental deficiencies and can be compensated for by providing an enriched or an adjusted environment. A certain amount of justification for such programs, especially if intervention takes place in the pre-school years, is provided by experimental studies of "sensory deprivation" and "critical periods" in infrahuman animals.[1] Weikart has identified three basic educational approaches used in preschool programs for correcting cognitive disabilities of socially disadvantaged children.

Traditional Nursery Schools. The traditional nursery-school approach is probably most directly related to the child-development orientation. Nursery schools are, in fact, often staffed by someone who has been trained in a child-development program rather than in a curriculum for regular teachers. Nursery-school directors, then, are characterized by an air of permissive watching and waiting for the child's "needs" to emerge. The manifestation of these needs becomes the cue for arranging and timing the nursery-school activities.

The traditional nursery school has the objective of promoting optimal social, emotional, and motor growth for the child by providing those experiences required for development. According to Weikart, Operation Head Start programs have typically exemplified the tradi-

---

[1]For a discussion of the concepts of sensory deprivation and critical periods, the reader is invited to consult J. P. Scott, Critical periods in the development of social behavior in puppies. *Psychosom. Med.,* 1958, 20, 42-54.

tional nursery-school program. While emphasizing social development, Head Start programs also have the objectives of increasing language facility, developing positive attitudes toward learning, and extending the general realm of experiences for the child. Attendance has varied from intensive full-day programs for 6 weeks to part-day programs for as much as 24 weeks.

Structured Nursery Schools. Weikart describes this approach as one using the traditional nursery-school materials and methods, but the activities are carefully preplanned according to some specific developmental theory. The teacher is more likely to be trained in a customary teacher-training curriculum. Goals and objectives center about fostering cognitive and language skills as hoped-for outcomes from the controlled sequence of classroom activities. While stress is on the acquisition of good work habits and the achievement of selected academic goals, the basic teacher-pupil relationship is maintained and the learning occurs within the social organization of the class-room. The teacher carries out continual diagnostic evaluations of each child's progress in attaining the predetermined goals. Attendance in these programs has varied from part-time over three months to full-time over three years. Dawe's Institutional Training Program, Kirk's Early Education of the Mentally Retarded Project (1958), and Gray and Klaus' Early Training Project (1965) are cited as some examples of structured nursery-school programs.

Task-Oriented Nursery Schools. According to Weikart, task-oriented nursery schools maintain the emphasis on carefully sequenced presentations for the attainment of specific academic goals in the areas of reading, arithmetic, and logical thinking. The accomplishment of these objectives is promoted by the use of new activities and materials specifically designed for the task and unlike those methods and materials employed in the traditional nursery school. The academically oriented curriculum follows a businesslike schedule. Work sessions in which there is direct teaching of reading, arithmetic, and language are alternated with an activity session which provides refreshments, singing, and a short play period. Motor and socialization skills are not a part of this program, which focuses on the mastery of specific academic tasks. Teachers are trained in depth in a particular instructional area, and the entire arrangement is said to bear more resemblance to the secondary-school organization than to the elementary school. Weikart cites the project for teaching disadvantaged children in the preschool directed by Bereiter and Engelmann (1966) as typifying the as-yet rare task-oriented approach.

Parent-Oriented Preschool Programs. A frequently observed preschool program for the socially disadvantaged not included in Weikart's review has concentrated on working with parents. These programs seek to capitalize on the influence of the parent as a source of attitudes about school and to train the parent to become an effective "teacher" in the home. Although the children of such parents may be in preschool programs, school attendance is essentially a way for establishing contact with the child's home and parents. Training with the parent is carried out by visiting teachers who make regular home visits and in small-group classes which mothers may be paid to attend or some combination of these methods. Instruction given the mothers ranges from pointing out the advantages of continued and regular school attendance to ways of improving auditory, visual, and work-habit skills of children. Care is taken to see that needed materials are available for the parents. Examples of preschool programs geared for working with parents are Radin and Weikart's Preschool Intervention through a Home Teaching Project (1967) and Karnes, Studley, Wright, and Hodgins' (1968) project for working with mothers of disadvantaged preschool children.

PROGRAMS FOR CHANGING RACIAL ATTITUDES

Pursuing a course concentrating on correcting academic deficiencies may be in part a consequence of the school not wishing to highlight controversy. Although it can be maintained that repairing these deficits is dealing directly with the problem of the disadvantaged, there are other contentions that such an approach is in reality sidestepping the main issue: the resolution of social and cultural conflict. Earlier discussion in this chapter indicated that the problems of the disadvantaged can be interpreted as cultural conflict about as justifiably as cultural disadvantage. In any case, it seems logically advisable to consider how the several large groups of persons making up our society are going to get along with one another since it is unlikely that any one group is going to be able to live in isolation, exclusive of the others. This issue immediately poses questions as to the possibilities for bringing about attitude changes by educational experiences.

Since the schools have been reluctant to engage directly in teaching to change attitudes, studies investigating potential attitude change have had to rely on indirect data. In one such study, Chesler and Segal (1968) assessed attitude changes reported by a random sample of Negroes after the pupils had attended integrated high schools in Alabama. Several possibly highly significant findings were tabulated. Of the pupils sampled, 90 per cent indicated that they would repeat their decision to attend an integrated school because of perceived better facilities generally. Another finding was that while 63 per cent of the Negro pupils had believed that the white students would be superior intellectually to them, only 21 per cent reported that this expectation was confirmed. Furthermore, 80 per cent of the Negro pupils stated that white classmates had changed in a positive way toward them, but on analysis the "changes" cited were frequently minor and superficial. After one year of attendance in integrated classes, 37 per cent of the Negro pupils indicated that they trusted white classmates more, but 41 per cent said they trusted the whites less.

Data from a report of the United States Commission on Civil Rights (1967) also reflected attitudes associated with attendance in desegregated and segregated Southern schools. Of Negro pupils attending integrated schools, 70 per cent stated that they planned to live in integrated neighborhoods, whereas only 50 per cent of Negro pupils attending segregated schools expressed such plans. A trend toward desegregation or segregation preference seemed discernible and was related to previous experiences; that is, attendance in desegregated elementary schools fostered enrollment in a desegregated high school and encouraged residence in a desegregated neighborhood. Initial experiences of segregation seemed to favor choosing a continuation of segregated situations.

Although carried out on relatively small numbers of pupils (four classes of approximately 25 students each), the study reported by Jansen and Gallagher (1966) is one of the most direct efforts to investigate the influence of school integration on racial relationships. Pupils were assigned to these fourth-grade classes on the basis of being above average in measured intelligence and of coming from disadvantaged homes. Negro pupils comprised from two-fifths to about one-half of the total pupils in any one class. No effort was made to either encourage or discourage interracial relationships. When sociometric choices were analyzed for three situations (person you would choose to sit with, play with, work with), significant interracial choice was found in only one of the possible situations. In two other instances, significant racially limited choices were found, with whites choosing whites and Negroes choosing Negroes. Jansen and Gallagher felt that their findings were inconclusive as to the possibility for promoting favorable interracial relationships by attendance in an integrated classroom.

THE ROLE OF THE SCHOOLS RECONSIDERED

Evaluation of Academic-Deficiencies Approaches. In his review of preschool programs, Weikart (1967) concluded that the traditional nursery-school approach has proven ineffective in dealing with problems of the disadvantaged. This conclusion was based on the consistent finding that there were no statistically significant differences on standardized measures of intelligence and achievement attained by pupil participants in such programs. Participation in either structured or task-oriented preschool programs was associated with significant gains in measured IQ and achievement-test scores. Increases in IQ scores ranged from about 5 to 15 points and persisted over the entire two-year study period of one of the projects. Similar gains have been obtained with parent-oriented preschool programs. In addition to these demonstrable gains, all the preschool programs discussed in the academic-deficiencies approach claim similar gains in varying degrees of liking for school, more interest in school tasks, and difficult-to-measure personality variables.

Effectiveness of Attitude-Change Approaches. Prospects for attitude changes as a result of school experiences remain largely speculative since, as was previously pointed out, this possibility has not been directly explored. Currently available studies relevant to the problems of the disadvantaged, moreover, are typically concerned with attitudes of racial bias, which is only part of a larger problem. The only warranted conclusion on the basis of these data has been suggested by Jansen and Gallagher (1966): that attendance in integrated schools can influence interracial relationships in some situations and under certain conditions, but not in other situations or conditions. The sparse findings thus far available indicate favorable attitude changes for as many as 70 or 80 per cent of Negro pupils in integrated schools. On analysis, the changes are often discouragingly shallow and hardly more than manifestations of what could be termed "civil decencies." From 30 to 50 per cent of the pupils in the same situations report no changes in attitudes. Attitudes are known to be exceedingly durable and deeply ingrained in the individual personality. Therefore, projects for changing attitudes would likely be more successful with young children than with adolescents or adults. The relatively slight changes in attitudes reported for older children may be of considerable significance, although doubted by Proshansky (1966), who felt that the contacts and relationships possible in integrated classes were necessary but not guaranteed conditions for the development of favorable racial attitudes.

PRESENT STATUS OF EDUCATIONAL APPROACHES

A careful review of the gains demonstrated by present educational programs indicates that traditional programs are ineffectual for dealing with the problems of the disadvantaged. This same conclusion was voiced by Weikart (1967). It makes little difference whether the ineptness can be attributed to programs put together more on enthusiasm than on technical knowhow, to training periods which were too brief, or to training presented too late in the developmental period to be effective.

The reputed "gains" credited to regular preschool programs which have been slightly modified to be more appropriate for the disadvantaged have been widely acclaimed by many educators. Bloom (1964), for example, sees the demonstrated possibility of increasing IQ by 10 points as having great significance. Even if it is assumed that these gains are durable—a fact which has not been conclusively demonstrated—there is some question as to their worthwhileness in view of the fact that disadvantaged children in some studies have shown similar gains after one or two years of usual school attendance. These gains are demonstrable even when the children have not attended any preschool program but have passed the time in "unfavorable" home situations (see Kirk's [1958] project, Early Education of the Mentally Retarded). The gains in IQ scores are also produced by a variety of programs and techniques which raise a question of some underlying Hawthorne effects. Although an increase of 10 IQ points is a respectable change, and one to be appreciated, a hard-nosed consideration of what predictions can be made based only on a person's IQ forces a conclusion that such a view takes into account only a small part of the total picture.

SUGGESTED IMPROVEMENTS IN EDUCATIONAL APPROACHES

Modifications of Existing Programs

Admittedly, the school is confronted with an enormous problem in attempting to correct the problems of the socially disadvantaged. Alterations in existing educational programs such as the emphasis on vocational rather than academic skills, the continual identification and remedy of academic deficiencies, the acquisition of teachers trained in the educational programs of the disadvantaged, the introduction of new and appropriate instructional methods and materials, and the systematic inclusion of work with parents are techniques which have a certain amount of demonstrated effectiveness. They have been tried out on a small-scale basis, but must become a part of all school programs if they are to reach all disadvantaged children. The prevailing atmosphere of caution which has governed the actions of the public schools may dictate such a conservative course in dealing with the problem.

Continued Investigation of the Problem

Research investigating the outcomes of human behavior undoubtedly ranks high on the list of difficult endeavors. Newcomers to the field of education are often shocked by the lack of systematic provision for evaluation and research as a way of finding answers to pressing problems. This situation is changing somewhat, but there is an especially critical need for long-term and followup studies of outcomes of particular educational programs and practices.

As mentioned above, there is a possibility of Hawthorne effects underlying gains in IQ and in achievement measures reported by a variety of preschool programs. The implication is that the particular programs and associated instructional methods and materials were inconsequential in fostering the changes found. If this is the case, there may be other common factors which should be identified so as to increase the effectiveness and efficiency of the schools in correcting the problems of the socially disadvantaged. Studies carried out by Blank and Solomon (1968), Pitts (1968), and Zigler and Butterfield (1968) have suggested that a preschool program does not increase a pupil's intelligence. Any gains as a consequence of participation in such programs are related to the pupil's learning to become involved in a task, to his satisfaction from being successful, and to his acquisition of good work habits. The change is, then, in the area of being more efficient in the use of the individual's abilities.

There is a respectable amount of research indicating that socioeconomic status is highly related to academic ability and achievement (Coleman, Campbell, & Mood, 1966; Tulkin, 1968). Socioeconomic staus, as a global index, includes many possible sources of influence on behavior. Even if the school does not wish to undertake the job of changing cultural values, anticipated rewards, levels of aspiration, and motivational strivings, or to intervene into existing parent-child interactions, a more specific picture of how these factors influence school adjustment seems essential at least for keeping all children in school.

Although such a possibility is generally discounted by educators, evidence indicating a definite relationship between genetic factors and academic achievement has been compiled by Nichols (1966) and Jensen (1968). Rather than disregarding such a possibility, educators would be well advised to give close consideration to these analyses. Such influences, if operative, need not threaten the educational system in any way, for the individuals would still have to undergo some set of experiences by way of realizing their genetic potentials. Knowledge of the makeup of the genotype could, however, greatly increase the effectiveness of school programs geared to realistic possibilities.

Speculation on Future Trends

Evaluation of educational approaches for dealing with the problems of the socially disadvantaged child indicates that, to date, the schools have been rather ineffectual in dealing with the problems. The picture is not entirely bleak, however, for the schools' efforts have been held back by public opinion, by the prevailing influence of the family group, and by attitudes and practices present in the community. Programs have been hastily put together and expected to deal with topics which are complex and controversial. The schools will be extremely limited in making any changes unless there is public acceptance of the need for changes.

Athough many reports of program evaluation have cited gains in specific measures such as IQ scores, reading ability, and vocabulary, there is nowhere definitive evidence that deficits in these areas are critical to the later adjustment of the culturally disadvantaged. They may have a positive or a negative influence, but to be really effective, a program must change attitudes. The same can be said for technical job-skill training. Most people lose their jobs because of their attitudinal deficits not because they lack technical skills. Essential aspects of educational programs may not have been introduced on a systematic basis or at early enough points. Many pupils drop out of school long before the curriculum offers subjects that might appeal to the pupils' abilities and inclinations. When offered, corrective programs frequently have been deficit-oriented and overlook the pupil's strengths. To be effective, experiences must be those which deal with realistic materials and objectives. The girls would not likely have the impressive array of classroom gadgets available in their homes, and the boys may not easily find work as electricians even when they are skilled in this area.

The most promising consequences are those effected by programs which deal with the real problem—attitudinal changes. These programs are identifiable by admission of the child to the program at a very early age, preferably by age 1 or 2, by systematic training in selected middle-class values, and by continual involvement of the home and parents. The programs can be very successful even when the values of the parents are not greatly changed by the contacts of the caseworker or by the parents' participation at school (Radin & Weikart, 1967).

Future innovations will witness an emphasis on attitude change in preschool programs, whether this change be accomplished by strengthening present preschool programs, by expansions such as using the poor to help the poor, or by some intensive program in communal living.

SUMMARY

Making decisions and planning for the alleviation of the problems of the culturally disadvantaged raises many ethical and practical questions which must be considered and eventually resolved. There is relatively little information regarding genetic contributions to the problem. Jensen (1968) has suggested that the role of genetic factors warrants additional investigation, and Dunn (1968) has cautioned against educational programs which deny constitutional factors. The implication is that the objective of rendering everyone middle-class may be a genetic impossibility, although changes within limits would be tenable. The development of a program for inducing changes must also recognize that the subculture of the disadvantaged is a learned, universal, and persistent phenomenon which holds a certain amount of success and satisfaction for its members.

Assuming for the moment that the culturally disadvantaged could be changed, we encounter ethical problems associated with the instituting of a program for such change. There is no scale by which we can measure which of the cultures is the better, and even if such a scale is devised, it would not touch on the more fundamental problem: Which is the better culture for which type of person and for what life objectives? Accurate predictions of the specific social order of the future cannot be made at this time; that is, today's goal may not be tomorrow's goal. Middle-class standards have worked well for some people for some problems; it is unlikely that these values are appropriate for all persons and for all problems.

Whatever approaches may be agreed upon, it is obvious that a more careful evaluation of all the data must be made. Stated perhaps simplistically, what is to be accomplished is either to teach two differing groups to live together or to make all persons alike, thus eliminating the cultural conflict. Those who believe a change of this magnitude is guaranteed by an increase of IQ scores by 12 or even 30 points may have a tragically limited perception of the problem. Changes yet unanticipated may be forced or carried out by unknown technological developments in the future, just as part of the current problem can be related to automation with the consequent reduction of unskilled jobs. In any event, the matter of making lasting changes will proceed only with the participation of all persons. Middle-class persons must understand that many traits and characteristics ascribed of an ethnic basis of being Negro, Indian, or Mexican are in reality manifestations of a lower-class culture where a substantial number of such persons are to be found. Those traits which make a significant difference in adjustment must be differentiated from those which are unimportant. On the other hand, the culturally disadvantaged child must be willing to involve himself in change. He cannot, for example, continue to fall back on the excuse that he doesn't want to read because the material is not to his liking.

SUGGESTED READINGS

Deutsch, M., Katz, I., & Jensen, A. R. *Social class, race, and psychological development.* New York: Rinehart & Winston, 1968.

Environment, heredity, and intelligence. Reprint Series. Cambridge: Harvard Educational Review, 1969.

Lewis, O. L. *La Vida: a Puerto Rican family in the culture of poverty.* New York: Random House, 1965.

Riessman, F. *The culturally deprived child.* New York: Harper, 1962.

REFERENCES

Ausubel, D., & Ausubel, P. Ego development among segregated Negro children. In A. H. Passow (Ed.), *Education in depressed areas.* New York: Teachers College Press, 1963. Pp. 109-141.

Barber, B. *Social stratification.* New York: Harcourt, Brace, 1957.

Bereiter, C., & Engelmann, S. *Teaching disadvantaged children in the preschool.* Englewood Cliffs, N.J.: Prentice-Hall, 1966.

Bernstein, B. Language and social class. *Brit. J. Psychol.,* 1960, **11**, 271-276.

Blank, M., & Solomon, F. A tutorial language program to develop abstract thinking in socially disadvantaged preschool children. *Child Develpm.,* 1968, **39**, 379-389.

Bloom, B. S. *Stability and change in human characteristics.* New York: Wiley, 1964.

Chesler, M., & Segal, P. Southern Negroes' initial experiences and reactions in school desegregation. *Integr. Educ.,* 1968, **6**, 20-28.

Cloward, R. A., & Ohlin, L. E. *Delinquency and opportunity: a theory of delinquent gangs.* New York: Free Press, 1960.

Coleman, J. S., Campbell, E. Q., & Mood, A. E. *Equality of educational opportunity.* Washington, D.C.: Government Printing Office, 1966.

Davis, A. *Social class and influences upon learning.* Cambridge: Harvard Univer. Press, 1948.

Dawe, H. C. A study of the effect of an educational program upon language development and related mental functions in young children. *J. exp. Educ.,* 1942, **11**, 200-209.

Dunn, L. M. Special education for the mildly mentally retarded—is much of it justifiable? *Except. Child.,* 1968, **35**, 5-22.

Durkin, D. Children who read before grade one. *Reading Tchr,* 1961, **14**, 163-166.

Gerber, M. The psychomotor development of African children in the first year and the influence of maternal behavior. *J. soc. Psychol.,* 1958, **47**, 185-195.

Gray, S., & Klaus, R. A. An experimental preschool program for culturally deprived children. *Child Develpm.,* 1965, **36**, 156-172.

Haggard, E. A. Social status and intelligence. *Genet. Psychol. Monogr.,* 1954, **49**, 141-186.

Herzog, E., & Sudia, C. Fatherless homes—a review of research. *Children,* 1968, **15**, 177-182.

Jansen, V. G., & Gallagher, J. J. The social choices of students in racially integrated classes for the culturally disadvantaged talented. *Except. Child.,* 1966, **33**, 221-226.

Jensen, A. R. Social class, race and genetics: implications for education. *Amer. educ. Res. J.,* 1968, **5**, 1-42.

Karnes, M. B., Studley, W. M., Wright, W. R., & Hodgins, A. S. An approach for working with mothers of disadvantaged preschool children. *Merrill-Palmer Quart.,* 1968, **14**, 174-184.

Kirk, S. A. *Early education of the mentally retarded.* Urbana: Univer. of Illinois Press, 1958.

Lewis, O. L. *La Vida: a Puerto Rican family in the culture of poverty.* New York: Random House, 1966.

Lindgren, H. C. *Educational psychology in the classroom.* (3rd ed.) New York: Wiley, 1967.

Miller, D. R., & Swanson, G. E. *Inner conflict and defense.* New York: Holt, 1960.

Nichols, R. C. Schools and the disadvantaged. *Science,* 1966, **154**, 1312-1314.

Pasamanick, B., & Knobloch, H. Epidemiological studies on the complications of pregnancy and the birth process. In G. S. Caplan (Ed.), *Prevention of mental disorders in children.* New York: Basic Books, 1961. Pp. 74-94.

Pitts, V. L. An investigation of the relationships between two preschool programs in the adjustment and readiness of disadvantaged pupils. *Childh. Educ.,* 1968, **44**, 524-525.

Proshansky, H. M. The development of intergroup attitudes. In M. L. Hoffman & L. W. Hoffman (Eds.), *Review of child development research.* Vol. II. New York: Russell Sage Foundation, 1966. Pp. 311-372.

Radin, N., & Weikart, D. P. A home teaching project for disadvantaged children. *J. spec. Educ.,* 1967, **1**, 183-190.

Riessman, F. *The culturally deprived child.* New York: Harper, 1962.

Tulkin, S. R. Race, class, family and school achievement. *J. Pers. soc. Psychol.,* 1968, **9**, 31-37.

U.S. Commission on Civil Rights. *Racial isolation in the public schools.* Washington, D.C.: Government Printing Office, 1967.

Weikart, D. P. Preschool programs: preliminary findings. *J. spec. Educ.,* 1967, **1**, 163-181.

Witmer, H. L. Children and poverty. *Children,* 1964, **11**, 68-72.

Zigler, E., & Butterfield, E. C. Motivational aspects of changes in IQ test performance of culturally deprived nursery school children. *Child Develpm.,* 1968, **39**, 1-49.

7

Juvenile Delinquency

Delinquency remains one of the critical social problems in the United States. It is by no means a new problem in American society. Nor is it a problem confined to this country. It appears that delinquency is an intrinsic part of modern industrialized societies. In short, when we speak of delinquency, we are dealing with a historically chronic problem which has not yet yielded easily to preventive and treatment efforts.

DEFINITION AND INCIDENCE

One difficulty that arises in discussing the concept of delinquency is a matter of definition. Delinquency is an imprecise term. Its meaning is vague not only from a legal viewpoint but from a psychological and sociological viewpoint as well. Even among psychologists, there have been a variety of meanings attached to this term. For some psychologists, delinquency is viewed as a moral deficiency; for others, it is an underactivity of the central nervous system; and for still others, it is a score on a personality test (Wirt & Briggs, 1965). The diversity of meanings has been well illustrated by Carr (1950), who lists the following six terms which have been applied to the delinquent behavior of juveniles.

Term Applied	Population
Legal Delinquents	All deviates committing antisocial acts as defined by law.
Detected Delinquents	All detected antisocial deviates.
Agency Delinquents	All detected antisocial deviates reaching any agency.
Alleged Delinquents	All apprehended antisocial deviates brought to court.
Adjudged Delinquents	All court antisocial deviates legally "found" delinquent.
Committed Delinquents	All adjudged delinquents committed to an institution.

Incidence figures will vary with the definition used. The list above is arranged hierarchically, with the highest-incidence figure associated with the "legal" criterion and the lowest-incidence figure associated with the "committed" criterion. For our discussion of prevalence, the "alleged" definition (antisocial deviates brought before the court) will be used, since the Children's Bureau prepares its annual report on the basis of juvenile-court cases. The incidence figures yielded by the number of court cases falls somewhere between the incidence figures yielded by the "legal" and "committed" criteria.

Before proceeding to the incidence figures for court cases, we must caution the reader against accepting these data at face value. For one thing, the number of cases reported will be affected by differences between states as to whether a given activity is criminal, for example, drinking under the age of 18. Second, states vary as to the type of case and ages of children over which the juvenile court has juris-diction. Third, the number of court cases is significantly affected by the availability of other child-welfare agencies in the community. If these agencies are present, they might handle cases similar to those seen by juvenile courts in less well-to-do communities. The reader should bear in mind that juveniles brought before a court represent only about one-half of those juvenile offenders apprehended by the police (Federal Bureau of Investigation, 1963). Furthermore, a report by the President's Crime Commission (Phillips, 1967) concluded on the basis of a national survey covering 10,000 households that about half of those who had been victims of crime during the past year never reported these crimes to the police. We will talk more about this problem—that of "undetected" delinquency—shortly. It is sufficient to note at this time that we know a reasonable amount about the behavior and distribution of official delinquents, but we know far less about the occurrence of actual delinquent behavior and its distribution (Short, 1966).

With the foregoing cautions in mind, we will turn directly to some statistical reports. According to the data based on a representative sample of the nation's juvenile courts, there were 697,000 cases handled by juvenile courts in 1965 (U.S. Children's Bureau, 1966). This figure represents 2 per cent of all children aged 10 through 13. This figure also represents an increase of 2 per cent over the previous year's number of court cases. The upward trend in court cases which has been noticeable each year since 1949 cannot be adequately explained away by the increase in the general child population. For example, between 1957 and 1965, there was an increase of 58 per cent in the number of court cases—a figure almost double the rise of 32 per cent in the general child population (U.S. Children's Bureau, 1966). Thus, the rise cannot be attributed solely to the recent increases in the child population since the increases in both police arrests and court delinquency cases have far surpassed the increases in child population.

Is delinquency really increasing in terms of the actual number of cases and in terms of rate (per 1,000 juveniles, for example), or are the rising figures a statistical artifact of better reporting procedures, greater public awareness, and increased law enforcement and technology? It is difficult to answer this question since no one really knows how many delinquents there are. The factors mentioned above definitely have contributed to the rise observed in incidence figures. Yet, by no stretch of the imagination can all of the increase in delinquent activity be explained by these factors (Teeters & Matza, 1959). Even the more hard-nosed researchers point out that there does seem to be some real increase in delinquency in both the number of cases and the rate (Wirt & Briggs, 1965). It has been estimated, moreover, that given no change in the conditions conducive to crime, there will be 44 per cent more crime in the next decade than at present in the age group 15 to 19 simply because of the general population increase in this age group (Lohman & Carey, 1966). The emergence of new forms of delinquency among new participants has also added to our concern (Freedman, 1966).

FACTORS INFLUENCING INCIDENCE

Age

Delinquency is an age-bound phenomenon. It often starts relatively early in life. As Glueck and Glueck (1950) reported, almost 60 per cent of delinquents commit their first offense before age 10. Though delinquent conduct has an early onset, it is most common during the adolescent period. Eaton and Polk (1961), for example, pointed out that adolescents accounted for nearly 2 of every 3 referrals to the Los Angeles probation department. Among the variables studied, age was found to be the most significant one with respect to incidence. Similarly, Short (1966), quoting FBI statistics, noted that 17-year-olds constituted the largest number of arrests. Then came the 18-year-olds, followed by the 16-year-olds. For boys, the incidence doubled from age 11 to 12 and tripled between age 12 and 17. For girls, the incidence peaks at age 15 (Bell, Ross, & Simpson, 1964).

Kvaraceus (1966) speaks of a "delinquency curve"—a notion consistent with the above data. He pointed out that delinquency reaches a high point around age 17, then begins to level off. Kvaraceus also noted that the majority of juvenile delinquents become law-abiding citizens in adult life. Ausubel (1965) noted that forty years of research unequivocally refutes the uninformed contention that juvenile delinquents eventually became adult criminals. The more severely antisocial child might well, however, continue in his wayward manner. Robins

(1966), for instance, on the basis of a followup study of gang-member delinquents, concluded that individuals who were persistent and dangerous adolescent offenders became even more serious adult offenders. This finding is consistent with other research cited in Chapter 1 suggesting that serious acting-out behavior in children is predictive of adult maladjustment.

It is also instructive to look at age trends from the standpoint of the FBI's specific categories of crime. Analysis of the FBI reports (Pilcher, Stern, & Perlman, 1963) indicated that larceny, burglary, and property offenses (which accounted for nearly one-third of all arrests) declined with age. Arrests for auto theft leveled off after age 15. Offenses against persons, such as assault, murder, and forcible rape, increased with age in both urban and rural areas. These offenses are relatively infrequent, however, accounting for only 4 per cent of all arrests.

Sex

The sex of the offenders is also related to the frequency of arrest. Juvenile delinquency remains largely a male phenomenon despite the increasing rate of female arrests. The percentage for youthful male offenders, for instance, was five times greater than that for girls, even though the number of males is not appreciably different from that of females in the general childhood population (U.S. Children's Bureau, 1966). Another study likewise found that male offenders outnumbered female offenders by a ratio of 4 to 1 (Eaton & Polk, 1961).

The types of crime for which the sexes are arrested also differs. FBI statistics indicate more than 40 per cent of boys but only 25 per cent of girls were arrested for offenses against property. Larceny was the most frequent single offense for both sexes. In cases of burglary and theft, however, offenses by males far exceeded those by females. Arrests for murder and manslaughter by negligence, though rare, were even more uncommon for girls than for boys. About an equal number of offenses were committed by the sexes with respect to liquor-law violations, drunk driving, disorderly conduct, gambling, and vagrancy. Sex offenses, excluding forcible rape, constituted the basis for arrest in 4 per cent of offenses for girls but only 1.5 per cent of arrests for boys. This latter finding can most likely be attributed to the double standard applied to sexual behavior in our society. Sexual offenses are perceived as being of a more serious nature when committed by girls than by boys, whereas stealing and aggressiveness are handled more sternly by authorities when committed by boys (Wirt & Briggs, 1965). In support of this hypothesis, it is interesting to note that more girls than boys are brought before the courts for sexual misbehavior despite the fact that more boys are involved in such violations. Moreover, girls are referred more than 50 per cent of the time for misbehavior not ordinarily considered criminal—ungovernable behavior, curfew violations, running away, and truancy. Stealing and property destruction, on the other hand, constitute a primary basis of court referral for boys (U.S. Children's Bureau, 1966). Interestingly, girls are more frequently referred to courts by their mothers, whereas boys are more typically apprehended and referred by the police (Conger et al., 1960).

Family Stability

Rates of delinquent behavior have also been found to vary with the stability of the home situation. The research literature indicates that children from broken homes, as compared with those from intact homes, do contribute more than their share to delinquent activities. Eaton and Polk (1961) found that more than 50 per cent of all delinquents came from homes broken by death or marital discord. Following a review of studies which used control groups and adjusted for age, ethnic, and neighborhood factors, Monahan (1957) concluded that children, especially girls, from intact homes have a distinct advantage over those from broken homes. The home of the delinquent was found to be much more "defective," "immoral," or "inadequate" than were homes in general. Nye (1958) asserts that the broken home fosters the type of delinquency broadly classified as "ungovernability." Truancy, running away from home, expulsion from school, and driving without a license are illustrative of offenses classified in this category.

Perhaps certain cautions are in order. First of all, Monahan (1957) warns against the danger of overgeneralization. We must not lose sight of the fact that only a small minority of youngsters growing up in broken homes become delinquents. Second, while no critical age has been established, it appears that older children are less adversely affected by broken homes than are younger children. Third, research indicates that delinquents are as likely to come from disorganized but structurally unbroken homes as they are from broken homes (Nye,

1958; Browning, 1960). In other words, the fact that the home is a happy one may be more important than the fact that it is structurally intact.

Turning to intact families, we find that family organization and relationship has a definite role in generating delinquency. Craig and Glick (1963, 1964) found three factors related to delinquency: (1) careless or inadequate supervision by mother or mother substitute; (2) erratic or overstrict discipline; and (3) cohesiveness of the family unit. Bandura and Walters (1959) obtained similar findings using 26 delinquents and 26 nondelinquents matched on social class and IQ range. According to these researchers, the parents of the delinquents were found to be more rejecting and less affectionate than those of the nondelinquents. The boys' relationships with their fathers were considered more important than their relationships with their mothers. Generally speaking, there was an aura of ill will between father and son. McCord, McCord, and Zola (1959), in their reevaluation of the Cambridge-Somerville youth study, found a higher incidence of delinquency among boys who experienced paternal rejection and neglect and little maternal affection. A higher incidence of convictions was found where the mother was rated as "nonloving" than "loving." The incidence was lowest where mothers were both "loving" and used consistent means of discipline.

The current literature suggests that the relationship of the father to the son is an especially critical factor in the production of delinquent behavior. From a theoretical standpoint, Miller (1959a) argues that the lower-class child engages in gang delinquency in an attempt to establish his masculinity—something he cannot do within the confines of a female-based, father-absent household. Empirical support demonstrating the effect of impaired father-son relationships is reasonably abundant. For example, Siegman (1966) reported that father-absent boys were more delinquent than father-present boys. Like Miller, he hypothesized that father-absent boys rebel against a feminine identification by engaging in exaggerated masculine behavior. Likewise, Hurwitz, Kaplan, and Kaiser (1962), using a sample of 100 male delinquents, reported that boys who had been manhandled, especially by their fathers, tended to get into more difficulty than boys whose parents had more desirable coping patterns.

Theorists are now questioning the supremacy of maternal deprivation as a significant etiological factor in delinquent behavior (Andry,

1960) and are recognizing the importance of an adequate male model as a significant ingredient in the socialization process (Nash, 1965).

Socioeconomic Status

Viewed socioeconomically, delinquency appears to be a predominantly lower-class phenomenon. Reiss and Rhodes (1961), studying 9,238 white boys registered in the junior and senior high schools of Davidson County, Tennessee, reported that the largest proportion of delinquency tended to be in the lower-status areas and in the high delinquency-rate areas. In 1963, Reiss and Rhodes expanded their findings to include the fact that official delinquency rates vary inversely with socioeconomic status. These investigators hypothesized that the lower-class adolescent compares his life unfavorably with that of the higher class. Eventually he experiences feelings of frustration and deprivation which, in turn, generate feelings of aggression and a higher rate of delinquent behavior. Perlman (1963) tried to explain this general relationship by use of several economic and social trends which, operating together or separately, could produce delinquency among the dissatisfied lower-class youths. Certain postwar conditions—the emphasis on success and false values, poor housing, the breakdown of the family, and violence—were social factors intrinsically involved. Socioeconomic trends, such as population growth, increased urbanization, unemployment, and automation, were also regarded as factors contributing to the frustration and inadequacy of lower-class youth.

Despite the above data, some workers are not convinced that delinquency is basically a lower-class phenomenon. First of all, the higher rates of delinquency among the lower classes are found only in large cities. Studies conducted in small cities and towns have not found greater delinquent involvement among the lower classes (Erickson & Empey, 1965; Nye, Short, & Olson, 1958). Clark and Wenninger (1962), using a total of 1,154 public-school students from four different types of communities, also noted that social-class differentiation is unrelated to the incidence of illegal behavior within small communities. These investigators advanced the notion that there are community-wide norms within these smaller towns which are related to illegal behavior irrespective of social class.

Second, studies of "undetected" delinquency also fail to substantiate the notion of greater delinquent involvement on the part of lower-class youth. Some investigators, concerned about the inadequacy of official court records as a criterion of illegal youthful behavior, have attempted to bridge the gap between official and unofficial delinquency rates by studying the extent of unrecorded delinquency. Short and Nye (1958), using student questionnaires on a 25 per cent sample of all boys and girls in grades 9, 10, 11, and 12 in three medium-sized towns (10,000 to 30,000), found that there was no significant difference in the delinquent behavior of boys and girls in the different socio-economic strata. Differences that were found indicated greater delinquent involvement within the highest socioeconomic category than was previously considered. Other studies (Dentler & Monroe, 1961; Empey & Erickson, 1966), using the anonymous-questionnaire procedure, have also substantiated the finding that the number of violations differs little from one status level to another. Thus the traditional assumption of higher incidence of behavior problems in the lower socioeconomic stratum has been called into question. It must be noted, however, that these studies were carried out in small cities or towns, where community-wide norms rather than socioeconomic factors are related to delinquent pursuits. Clark and Wenninger (1962), who also used an anonymous self-report scale, found that although adolescents from various social strata had very similar over-all delinquency rates, the more serious offenses were more likely to be committed by lower-class urban youth.

While we are unable to make any definitive statement as to the relationship of "undetected" delinquency to socioeconomic status, it is clear that the relationship between social class and illegal behavior is by no means a simple one. In addition to further investigations on lower-class delinquents, we sorely need more research on the delinquent conduct of middle- and upper-class youth in order to clarify the role of socioeconomic factors in delinquency.

Racial and Ethnic Factors

There is often considerable variation in reports of delinquency rates among various racial and ethnic groups. Jewish children, for example, contribute far less than their expected share of the delinquency statistics (Robison, 1957). Whereas in 1952, Jewish children comprised 15 per cent of the general population in New York City, they accounted for only 3 per cent of the juvenile-court cases. Japanese-Americans also have a very low rate of delinquency, perhaps because of their tradition of compliance, their emphasis on education, the intactness of their families, and the importance of family honor (Eisner & Tsuyemura, 1965).

On the other hand, several studies indicate high delinquency rates for Negroes, Puerto Ricans, Mexicans, and American Indians. Negro delinquency rates are two or three times higher than those of whites (Douglass, 1959). Differences in rate as to the type of offense have also been noted, with a higher proportion of Negro boys committing offenses against persons or property as contrasted to a higher proportion of white boys violating important social norms (Segal, 1966).

Studies on the Negro problem point out a number of factors conducive to the production of antisocial behavior. These include a mother-centered family, the lack of a suitable male model, freer sexual behavior, illegitimacy, poverty, and an emphasis on physical combat. These delinquency-prone children, according to Cavan (1959), develop a concept of being deviant which is fostered by the parents. Clark (1959), analyzing the effects of minority status on personality patterns, concluded that the Negro child because of racial discrimination develops a self-concept that is negatively distorted, thus giving rise to hostile, aggressive, and antisocial responses. Hill (1959) expands this idea further, asserting that deviant behavior is a manner of adjusting to a segregated society in which many opportunities for recognition and accomplishment are unavailable.

Urban-Rural Differences

The rates of delinquency are about three times higher in urban areas than in rural areas. In fact, courts in urban areas handle more than two-thirds of all delinquency cases in the country. Clark and Wenninger (1962) found that rates for delinquent activity increase as one moves from rural farm to upper-class urban to industrial city and lower-class urban communities. This trend is especially true with regard to the more serious violations and to those involving a high degree of social organization. The greatest differences in rates of illegal activity occur between the lower-class urban and the upper-class communities. Upper-class urban youngsters are more prone to pass dirty pictures, gamble, and trespass, whereas their lower-class urban counterparts are more apt to steal major items, drink, carry weapons, and destroy property. There were no differences among the four communities with regard to the more minor misbehaviors. Consistent with the above findings, Ferdinand (1964) concluded that urban delinquents exhibited a much stronger preference for offenses against authority than did rural or village delinquents. Rural delinquents committed 1 offense against authority for every 13 property violations, whereas the urban offense ratio was 1 to 3.5.

Although juvenile delinquency remains largely an urban problem, juvenile-court statistics reveal that youth in rural areas show an even greater proportional increase than youth in the large urban areas. Thus, increases in delinquency are not limited to congested areas but are taking place in rural areas.

Intelligence

Interest in the relationship between intelligence and juvenile crime has had a long and polemical history. While most of the early research indicated a 15-20 point difference in IQ score between delinquents and the general population, later research consistently reports a difference of only 8 IQ points. Moreover, when socioeconomic status is controlled, there seems to be even less difference in intellectual status between delinquents and nondelinquents (Caplan, 1965). Even if this 8-point difference were valid, such a difference would not warrant postulating low intelligence as a major cause of delinquency. Low intelligence, though in and of itself unrelated to delinquency, can predispose youngsters in certain instances by increasing suggestibility, the tendency to take imprudent risks, the probability of being caught, and the possibility of academic failure (Ausubel, 1965).

Constitutional Factors

Interest in the area of constitutional factors has ranged from speculative discussion concerning hereditary factors to more rigorous studies on physiological factors. Early in this century, Lombroso (1918) advanced the notion that the criminal is biologically unable to behave in a responsible manner. He investigated the physical correlates associated with the presumed inborn antisocial traits. Later studies revealed that delinquents and nondelinquents did not differ with respect to recognizable physical stigmata. However, several studies continue to reveal a greater incidence of abnormal brain waves (EEG) among sociopathic delinquents, a group we will discuss shortly. There is further evidence to suggest that sociopaths, because of an inadequate constitution, are less able to respond with anticipatory anxiety to what are ordinarily tension-provoking stimuli. Without denying the possible etiological ramifications of these biological findings, especially in regard to certain delinquent subgroups, we must bear in mind the fact that many delinquents are free from such biological deviations and that similar abnormalities can be found in nondelinquent populations.

Much interest has also centered around the relationship between body build and delinquency. In their classic study comparing delinquent and nondelinquent youth, Glueck and Glueck (1956) reported a much higher proportion of muscular, big-boned, broad-shouldered boys (mesomorphs) among the delinquents. Conversely, the chunky, stocky boys (endomorphs) and the tall, thin boys (ectomorphs) were less apt to become delinquent. Has this relationship any causal significance? At this time, most authorities contend that physique most likely plays a predisposing role rather than a causal one. Given a mesomorphic build, a youngster with delinquent inclinations is better able to actualize his antisocial leanings through gang-type crimes. But this is not to say that his physique caused his delinquency. It must also be noted that 40 per cent of the delinquents in the Gluecks' sample did not fit the mesomorphic category. Moreover, most husky youths are not juvenile delinquents. Certain select cases of delinquency might be accounted for by physical constitution. Though future research might prove otherwise, most authorities today find even the more modern versions of the "bad seed" hypothesis untenable and prefer to seek the roots of delinquent behavior in the environmental and psychological forces which influence behavior.

PSYCHOLOGICAL DIMENSIONS

Despite the fact that delinquents and nondelinquents sometimes come from the same general family and socioeconomic backgrounds, have similar levels of intelligence, and are comparable in body build, they often differ with respect to personality characteristics. Studies using the Minnesota Multiphasic Personality Inventory indicate that such characteristics as impulsivity, aggressiveness, and irresponsibility are commonly found among those who engage in delinquent activities. On the other hand, people who score high on scales measuring social introversion, depression, and masculinity-femininity tend to have a lower-than-average rate of delinquency (Quay, 1965).

To the unsophisticated observer, the surface behavior of delinquent youth may appear very similar. Closer inspection reveals, however, the desirability of investigating differences in personality structures among subgroups within the general delinquent population. Indeed, the failure of earlier investigators to find meaningful personality differences between delinquents and nondelinquents (Schuessler & Cressey, 1950) can be attributed not only to the use of invalid psychological tests and unsophisticated research designs but also to the failure to seek differences in personality makeup within the subgroups of the total delinquent population (Quay, 1965).

Different investigators (Reiss, 1952; Quay, 1964, 1966), using a variety of research methodologies, have identified three broad personality dimensions among delinquents. The terminology varies but there is basic agreement among authorities as to the existence of these three categories: the psychopathic delinquent, the subcultural delinquent, and the neurotic delinquent.

THE PSYCHOPATHIC DELINQUENT

The first dimension represents a basic *deficiency in the socialization process.* Delinquent youngsters scoring high on this dimension have been given various labels: the psychopath, sociopath, unsocialized aggressive, defective-superego delinquent, and so forth. These youths are usually the products of rejecting homes. Professional workers generally regard this form of delinquency as the most severe and as having the poorest prognosis. Consequently, some form of residential treatment is apt to be employed. Clinicians are reluctant to diagnose a youngster as a sociopath since this label connotes incorrigibility. As mentioned in the earlier discussion on the stability of deviant behavior, Robins (1966), on the basis of a thirty-year follow-up study, reported that 2 out of 3 unsocialized aggressive youths persisted in their antisocial ways. What surprised most professional workers is the fact that 1 in 3 did show some improvement.

From the standpoint of clinical experience, those so labeled manifest many of the following behavioral characteristics:

1. Inadequate moral development is perhaps the most salient characteristic. While unsocialized aggressive children are intellectually able to distinguish between right and wrong, they frequently fail to observe such distinctions in their everyday behavior. Stealing, lying, drinking, and sexual misbehaviors are typical norm-violating activities on their part.

2. Associated with the deficiency in conscience development is the

superficiality of guilt and anxiety. Though such youngsters often verbalize such feelings when in a tough situation, they seem incapable of experiencing these emotions to a degree typical of normal youth. Since these youngsters are generally not bothered by their misbehaviors, they have little motivation to change their ways. Consequently, they fail to learn from experience, continuing in their old acting-out ways. Being poorly motivated with respect to behavioral change, they make poor candidates for traditional forms of psychotherapy.

3. Rebelliousness and impulsivity are also commonly seen. Typically these youngsters will be in trouble both at home and at school. One way to detect such individuals is to check their case histories. A long history of frequent involvement with law-enforcement agencies and/or educational authorities is very much the rule. They have considerable difficulty in accepting any constituted form of authority and frequently try to escape from rather unpleasant situations by becoming truants or going AWOL.

4. Their egocentricity is also readily apparent. While they often appear outgoing, gregarious, and optimistic, they tend not to form close interpersonal ties with others. In general, their emotional ties and loyalties are extremely shallow even with their own families. Their sense of responsibility is quite poorly developed.

5. Their extrapunitiveness and inability to postpone pleasurable activities also lead them into difficulty. One delinquent boy told the author, when queried about why he was incarcerated at a youth camp, that he did not have any problems until he got "a damn social worker." Likewise, a sexually provocative, blond high-school girl stated that she wanted to quit school and go to California "where things are happening." Striving toward long-range goals is usually out of the question. The smaller immediate pleasures of the present are perceived as better than the greater but more distant goods of the future. Such youths become easily bored, desire a frequent change of scenery, thrive on excitement, and want to be constantly on the go.

6. They often make a favorable impression on others and can, at times, be excellent manipulators. On one occasion a nice-looking, curly-haired delinquent adolescent escaped from a mental hospital at which the author worked. As was customary in such cases, the sheriff was notified and a search was undertaken. When, after several hours, neither the sheriff nor the delinquent returned, another phone call was placed to the sheriff's office. It was then learned that the adolescent

youth had "conned" the sheriff into writing a letter to the governor regarding his unjustified incarceration. Once this adolescent boy's long history of repeated criminal activity was revealed and his exploitation of others noted, the sheriff willingly returned him to the institutional setting.

THE SUBCULTURAL DELINQUENT

A second dimension that has been consistently uncovered represents a case of *deviant socialization*. But such an adjustment is deviant only in the sense that the asocial or antisocial values of the child's subculture are in conflict with those of the larger, middle-class society. A delinquent youth scoring high on this dimension is referred to as subcultural delinquent, socialized aggressive delinquent, sociologic delinquent, or integrated delinquent. Delinquent youngsters so designated typically come from a stable lower-class home in a deteriorated area of the community in which delinquent conduct constitutes an approved tradition. Their encounters with law-enforcement agencies stem from their prolonged daily exposure to behaviors which violate the legal norms of the larger society.

It should be noted that these youngsters are not emotionally disturbed. Aside from their delinquent pursuits, they are essentially normal youngsters. The prognosis is generally favorable, in that the vast majority grow up to be law-abiding citizens. They are not extremely anxious, as are neurotic children; nor do they experience a lack of personal identity, as do psychotic children. They differ from the sociopath in that they are able to experience guilt when they violate the standards of their own subculture and to form close emotional attachments and loyalties to others. Although able to identify with others, they usually select models that the larger community considers undesirable. For example, they are much more apt to identify with the "con" man or with an aggressive buddy than with the policeman or with a conforming peer, since identifications of the former kind lead to prestigious behaviors which offer him status within his own particular peer group.

What are some of the central values which are cherished by the lower-class peer culture? A partial listing would include the ability to dupe or outsmart others, physical prowess (such as the ability to take it and dish it out), a rebelliousness toward any form of constituted authority (the "no one is going to push me around" philosophy), a strong desire for excitement and thrill-seeking activities, and a strong belief in luck as a vital force in determining one's destiny (Miller, 1959a). This type of delinquency represents more of a cultural than a psychological problem. Kvaraceus and Miller (1959) assert that 75 per cent of delinquency is due to cultural factors and 25 per cent to psychological factors. In other words, these investigators would view the overwhelming majority of delinquent activities as emanating from normal lower-class youngsters who reflect the patterned deviancy of their lower-class culture. Since many of their crimes are committed in groups, the preferred method of treatment involves placement of the offender in a group setting where he is given a chance to identify with the more appropriate models afforded him.

THE NEUROTIC DELINQUENT

The third dimension along which delinquents might vary involves acting-out behaviors which stem from *neurotic-like conflicts*. That is, beneath a facade of violence and aggression, certain delinquents are anxious, unhappy, insecure, and in conflict. This youngster is commonly referred to as the solitary delinquent, the neurotic delinquent, the disturbed delinquent, or the weak-ego delinquent. There are at least four basic differences between the youngster scoring high on this dimension and those on the previously described dimensions:

1. Unlike the subcultural and the unsocialized delinquent in particular, in whom guilt tends not to be a component, the neurotic delinquent often experiences pangs of conscience and remorse over his transgressions.

2. The motivations underlying the antisocial behavior are presumed to be more unconsciously based in contrast to those of the subcultural delinquent, who more unconsciously opposes the larger social order. The clinical observations of the late Adelaide Johnson (1959) suggest that much of the individual delinquent's behavior is unconsciously fostered by defects in his parent's conscience. Hence, the child comes to adopt the antisocial attitudes which his parents convey to him in subtle ways. Presumably, these parents reinforce their offspring's antisocial conduct in order to obtain vicarious gratifications of their own needs.

3. The neurotic delinquent tends to come from a middle-class home and neighborhood. Sometimes the home atmosphere is characterized

by hostility and lack of love. On other occasions, there is the unconscious fostering of delinquent activities on the part of parents, as noted above.

4. This delinquent is more inclined to engage in criminal activities by himself in contrast to the subcultural delinquent, who seems to prefer a gang type of delinquent activity.

The youngster scoring high on this dimension might well engage in unlawful acts so that he will be caught and punished, presumably to satisfy deep-rooted feelings of guilt. Not uncommonly, his offenses seem purposeless and compulsive in nature. Lippman (1962) cites the case of an adolescent boy who obtained money by forging a check. As the adolescent was well known to the local merchant, the boy was easily apprehended by police. Shortly after being placed on probation, this boy committed the same offense in much the same manner on three more occasions. Again, he was quickly arrested. This boy's measured IQ was 170. Subsequent interviewing suggested the presence of a strong unconscious need to be punished.

The repetition of stupid errors occurring in conjunction with the commission of the crime often leads one to suspect the existence of a neurotic component in the delinquent pursuits. In short, the disturbed delinquent commonly manifests many of the basic characteristics of a neurotic-like condition, with the exception that his conflict assumes the form of behavior directed against society. Although the neurotic delinquent's responsiveness to treatment is not considered by clinicians to be as favorable as that of the subcultural delinquent, he is seen as reacting positively to probation and casework procedures.

PERSONALITY INSULATORS

The preceding discussion pertained to personality factors associated with the production of delinquency. By now, the reader may well have asked himself, "Are there any personality factors which insulate children against delinquency?" We have already mentioned the Minnesota studies, which indicate that individuals with high scores on the depression, social-introversion, and masculinity-femininity scales are less apt to become involved with law-enforcement agencies. It was also found that subjects who had delinquency-prone personalities but resisted delinquency differed from those with similar personality dispositions who did become delinquent in coming from economically better homes, having better socially adjusted parents, and having better relationships within the family (Wirt & Briggs, 1959).

Perhaps the best-known studies in this regard have been conducted by Reckless, Dinitz, and Kay (1957) on nondelinquent boys living in high-delinquency areas. Using a group of 125 "good" boys (those thought to be insulated against delinquency) and a group of 101 delinquency-prone boys, Reckless and his associates studied their personality differences from personal interviews, interviews with teachers and parents, the administration of a self-concept scale, and the California Personality Inventory. The results indicated that the good boys came from stable homes which kept them isolated from the delinquent patterns of the neighborhood. Close maternal supervision in the context of a harmonious family setting was thought to play a prominent role relative to the inhibition of delinquent activities. The good boys also scored significantly higher on the responsibility and socialization scales of the California Personality Inventory. They also seemed to have a more socialized self-concept in comparison to the delinquency-prone group. A followup study indicated that only 4 per cent of the insulated group had become known to the police (Scarpitti et al., 1960) in contrast to almost 27 per cent of the vulnerable group (Dinitz, Scarpitti, & Reckless, 1962). A trend toward poorer socialization and a more impaired self-concept was also noted in the vulnerable group, whereas the good boys maintained favorable attitudes toward the law, school, their parents, and themselves. The authors concluded that one's self-concept can serve as either an inhibitor or an excitor relative to participation in unlawful activities. Later research by Scarpitti (1965) has confirmed the role played by a negative self-concept as a crucial predisposing factor toward delinquency.

INTERACTION OF PSYCHOLOGICAL VARIABLES

Most of the research on characteristics has examined the relationship between delinquency and such variables as social class, IQ, and selected personality variables independently of one another. The interaction of the variables as antecedents of delinquent activities has for the most part been neglected. That the study of interactive effects among such variables as personality factors, neighborhood factors, IQ, and delinquency might well constitute a more valuable and true-to-life approach is seen in recent research efforts by Conger, Miller, and Walsmith

(1965). These authors caution that, though delinquents as a group show less acceptable social behavior, experience more academic difficulties, and have more emotional problems, the extrapolation of these findings to delinquent subgroups was precluded by the marked variations in relationships of various personality traits to delinquency from one social class—IQ group to another. In brief, these findings indicate that it is misleading to speak of personality differences between delinquents and nondelinquents on the basis of over-all average differences. To convey the marked variation existing among the subgroups with respect to personality, it is necessary to take into account the intellectual and socioeconomic levels from which these youngsters derive. For example, within the "below-average IQ—nondeprived" subgroup, the nondelinquents earned higher mean scores on a delinquency scale than did the delinquents themselves.

Studies of this nature illustrate the complex interactions among variables related to delinquency and point out the dangers associated with research which considers these variables separately. Aside from their norm-violating behavior, delinquents are anything but a homogeneous group. The translation of this awareness into more complicated research designs represents a methodological advance in the field of delinquency, an advance which should assist in casting into sharper relief the factors contributing to delinquency.

ETIOLOGICAL CONSIDERATIONS

Like any complex and multidimensional problem, delinquency can be attacked on different levels. We can, for instance, approach it from a biological, sociological, or psychological vantage point. It is virtually impossible from a practical standpoint, however, to investigate all aspects of this problem simultaneously. Consequently, various disciplines have approached the problem, with each professional specialty stressing certain determinants of the problem.

Most theories of etiology can be subsumed under two broad categories. On the one hand, there are those which emphasize the importance of the attitudes and emotions of individual delinquents. This theoretical position is predicated on the assumption that delinquency results from the emotional problems of individual youngsters. The earliest child-guidance clinics working with delinquents received their theoretical support (rationale) from individual psychology and later from psychoanalytic or other psychiatric viewpoints (Wheeler,

Cottrell, & Romasco, 1967). In brief, the clinical model focuses primarily on the pathology of the individual.

The other major approach views delinquency as sociogenic in nature. Advocates of this theoretical position stress the importance of the broader social environment as the source of delinquent conduct. The sociologist, accordingly, searches for causative factors in the social processes in the delinquent's environment. The treatment implications of these two major applications will be amplified later in the chapter.

SOCIOLOGICAL THEORIES

Within the limits of our present discussion, we will consider only three of the current sociological theories which emphasize the origin and effects of delinquent subcultures. The first two theories view the rise of these subcultures as a consequence of socially induced frustrations sustained by the working class at the hands of the middle class.

Status Deprivation. The first person to develop a theory of gang delinquency was Cohen (1955), who advanced the "status-deprivation theory." According to this position, the lower-class child is exposed to middle-class pressures for success through his contacts with teachers, playground directors, ministers, and so on. The lower-class child, though sensitive to the appraisals of various middle-class representatives, is experientially hindered in his ability to conform to middle-class standards. Postponement of gratification, for example, is less common among the working class than it is among the middle class. Cohen suggests that a loss of status results from social devaluation which, in turn, leads to rebellion. The lower-class child accordingly redefines the yardstick of status so that his own antisocial behavior constitutes the earmark of prestige. Thus, lower-class youth, confronted with a common loss of status, form a delinquent subculture which values the breaking of middle-class values. While lower-class delinquency is seen as an inability to compete successfully with the dominant and prestigious middle class, middle-class delinquency is viewed as an attempt to achieve masculinity.

Opportunity Structure. A second major social theory which views gang delinquency as emanating from blockages in the attainment of highly valued middle-class success goals is Cloward and Ohlin's (1960) opportunity-structure theory. Whereas Cohen stressed the lower-class child's inability to measure up to middle-class standards,

Cloward and Ohlin emphasize the unjust availability of opportunity among the lower classes. The lower-class child, in response to the limited opportunity afforded him, blames the social order. Alienation subsequently expresses itself in the development of various types of delinquent subcultures which offer illegal patterns of conduct as a source of status. This theory has had an important impact on action programs of prevention and treatment. Indeed, as we will discover later in the chapter, most treatment and prevention programs strive to offer delinquent and predelinquent youth an opportunity to develop skills which will enable them to participate meaningfully in adult society.

Focal Concerns. Miller (1959a) has proposed an alternative theory which challenges the two preceding formulations. Objecting to the reactive nature of gang culture, Miller views the life style of gang delinquency as a manifestation of lower-class culture. In other words, gang delinquency among lower-class youth is an expression of the values and thoughts pervading lower-class culture rather than a reaction against middle-class expectations and devaluations. What are the concerns around which lower-class life is patterned? The focal concerns, Miller postulates, are trouble, toughness, smartness, excitement, fate, and autonomy. The lower-class delinquent thus becomes acculturated to a way of life that is consistent with these focal concerns but at odds with, or antithetical to, dominant norms and values.

Despite the fact that we have presented only skeletal outlines of these social theories, their relevance to the school's role in delinquency is readily evident. There are at least two major implications emanating from theoretical positions which view delinquency as a result of blocked goal success (Schafer & Polk, 1967). First, poor school performance might well constitute a *common* form of frustration, for example, poor grades and nonpromotion. Second, academic failure leads these lower-class youths to believe that desirable jobs might be unavailable to them. As a consequence of these thwartings, lower-class students are more prone to delinquent activities. As for the educational implications of Miller's views, Schafer and Polk suggest that the school itself may be contributing to a lack of acceptable commitment or at least may not seize the opportunity to establish such a commitment when it is lacking. To offset the above-mentioned consequences, many schools have modified educational programs for lower-class youth. We will talk about one such *application*— work-experience programs—later in the chapter.

PSYCHOLOGICAL THEORIES

Most sociological theories fail to account for the middle-class delinquent as well as the large majority of lower-class youth who lead law-abiding lives. As Bandura and Walters (1959) note, the sociological variables may not play a causative role but may simply provide conditions promoting the existence of psychological factors which produce antisocial conduct.

Emotional Disturbance. As implied earlier, advocates of the psychological approach assume that antisocial acts have meaning to the individual delinquent in that his conduct represents either a reaction to frustrations within the family and/or peer group or an effort to meet unfulfilled needs, such as recognition. While the majority of delinquents are not emotionally disturbed, there remains a significant minority of delinquents for whom this designation is warranted. The psychological approach to delinquency is well illustrated by the classic study of Healy and Bronner (1936), in which case-study data were collected on 105 delinquents who had nondelinquent siblings near their own age. Despite similar environmental backgrounds, the delinquents differed markedly from their nondelinquent siblings in their personality traits, attitudes, and interpersonal relationships. The most noticeable difference between the two groups was in the area of family attitudes and emotional experiences. More than 90 per cent of the delinquents were very unhappy with their life circumstances or extremely disturbed because of life experiences. In contrast, inner stresses were found in only 13 per cent of the control subjects. Common emotional problems experienced by the delinquents included sharp feelings of rejection, inadequacy, insecurity, jealousy, and unhappiness.

Adult-Youth Alienation. Ausubel (1965) has proposed a refreshing view, which, contrary to many of the psychological approaches, does not hold that the basic causal factor in juvenile delinquency resides in a pathological personality structure. It inheres, instead, in the developmental-cultural phenomenon of adult-youth alienation which adolescents experience. According to Ausubel, adolescents alienated from adult society become immersed in a peer culture which provides them with status-giving activities, norms of behavior, and distinctive training institutions of their own. At the same time, however, participation in the peer culture reinforces their feelings of alienation from adult society and promotes compensatory antisocial modes of conduct which sometimes take the form of juvenile delinquency. Adult-youth alienation varies in accordance with such contributing and precipitating factors as sex, social class, parental attitudes, temperament, personality characteristics, and intelligence. Alienation from adult society, for example, is greater among boys than among girls and more pronounced among adolescents in minority groups than in middle-class groups. Middle-class delinquency is viewed as the result of a serious deterioration in the moral values of middle-class adults since the end of World War II.

PREDICTION

The problem of prediction is basic to any discussion of programs of prevention and treatment. There are now available a number of instruments designed to predict delinquency although few of these have been subjected to rigorous before-and-after tests of validation (Kvaraceus, 1966). The usual approach has been to administer a set of items to a group of delinquents and a group of nondelinquents. A comparison of their respective responses to these items is then conducted in an attempt to delineate the specific characteristics of the delinquent youth. Nondelinquent youth who possess the attributes characteristic of the delinquent sample are accordingly considered delinquency-prone. Finally the predictive value of the scores is ascertained through a followup study. While instruments for predicting delinquency have hardly received wide acclaim from either theorists or practitioners, few would deny the need for and value of a valid scale. What follows is a brief review of three of the more valid scales for predicting delinquency.

GLUECK PREDICTION TABLES

The first major effort to develop instruments for predicting delinquency was reported in 1950 by Sheldon and Eleanor Glueck (1950), who matched 500 delinquents and nondelinquents in the Boston area on the basis of age, ethnic origin, intelligence, and place of residence. Three tables were developed for distinguishing between these two groups. Table 1 dealt with five social factors: (1) discipline of the boy by the father, (2) affection of the mother for the boy, (3) affection of the father for the boy, (4) supervision of the boy by the mother, and (5) cohesiveness of the family. Table 2 dealt with personality traits as revealed by the Rorschach Inkblot Test. Table 3 dealt with personality characteristics as revealed through psychiatric interviewing. Of these three tables, only the social-factor table has been subjected to followup evaluation. The Gluecks recommend that delinquency prediction be made at the time the child enters school, around age 6.

To date, there has been only one major study which tested a group of youngsters at age 6 and then followed them up to determine the predictive validity of this instrument. In 1952-1953 the New York City Youth Board selected a sample of 224 first-grade boys from high-delinquency neighborhoods. Ratings on social factors were obtained through interviews conducted by social workers in the home setting. The investigators, in an effort to refine the social-factor table, devised a three-factor scale (supervision of the boy by the father, supervision of the boy by the mother, and family cohesiveness) and a two-factor scale (supervision of the boy by the mother, and family cohesiveness). After nine years of comprehensive followup, Craig and Glick (1964) concluded that the scale was a good differentiator between serious and persistent delinquents and nondelinquents. The results indicated, for example, that the three-factor scale predicted accurately 70 per cent of delinquents and 85 per cent of nondelinquents.

These findings seem encouraging, but objections raised by critics (Briggs & Wirt, 1965; Kvaraceus, 1966) cannot be lightly dismissed. The chief objections center around the subjectivity of the social workers' ratings, questionable statistical analysis, the nonapplicability of certain variables (for example, supervision by the father in fatherless homes), the cost in time and money of administering these scales, and the use of this scale with the general population. Glueck (1966b) has added two additional traits—nonsubmissiveness to authority, and destructiveness—in an effort to produce a more discriminative instrument. Although it is suggested (Glueck, 1966a) that these two new predictive instruments will be more accurate than the previously validated scales, the need for additional testing is also pointed out.

MINNESOTA MULTIPHASIC PERSONALITY INVENTORY

The MMPI is perhaps the best known of the structured personality inventories. It consists of 550 true-false items and yields scores on 10 clinical scales. Over the years, a sample of more than 15,000 ninth-grade students in Minnesota have been given this inventory in an effort to predict who will become delinquent. A followup study involving a search of police and juvenile-court records was made two years after the initial testing (Hathaway & Monachesi, 1953, 1957). Boys whose profiles on this inventory were most "normal" have the lowest delinquency rates. Elevations on certain scales, however, were found to be more closely related to the prediction of delinquency than others, with peaks on the psychopathic deviate and mania scales being most predictive of antisocial, acting-out forms of behavior. Those exhibiting a combination of characteristics associated with the psychopathic personality (such as impulsivity, rebelliousness, minimal guilt, and inability to learn from experience) and characteristics associated with mania (such as expansiveness, outgoingness, insufficient inhibitory capacity) were most likely to be known to the police and the juvenile courts. Certain neurotic indicators, on the other hand, such as a tendency to worry and to be anxious, were seen as favorable signs in that they seemed to have an inhibiting effect on potentially delinquent behavior. Wirt and Briggs (1959) found that delinquency could be more accurately predicted when social-agency contact was combined with the personality pattern than when either was used singly. These findings indicate the desirability of combining social factors and personality variables in the prediction of violative behavior.

This instrument has proved useful in differentiating between delinquent and nondelinquent groups but, despite what might be the most rigorous research to date on a predictive scale, it is generally inadequate for purposes of individual prediction. As far as school personnel are concerned, this inventory has additional limitations. It is not designed for use with elementary-school children, it uses language which may be objectionable and upsetting to many pupils and their parents (for example, "My sex life is satisfactory"), and it requires an experienced clinician for interpretation.

KD SCALES

Kvaraceus (1953, 1956) has devised a scale which consists of 75 multiple-choice items designed to differentiate delinquents from nondelinquents. Differences in personality makeup, in home and family backgrounds, and in school experiences are explored. Kvaraceus has also developed a KD proneness scale and check list for use by teachers and other professional workers concerned with the prediction of delinquency. This list consists of 70 items concerning family, home, school, and personal factors.

There is also a nonverbal scale (Kvaraceus, 1961) which has received the most extensive validation of all the KD prediction scales (Kvaraceus, 1966). Administration of the scale consists in the presentation of 62 circles each of which contains 4 pictures designed to differentiate delinquents from nondelinquents. The child is asked to select the picture that he likes the most and the one that he likes the least from each set. A three-year followup study conducted on almost 1,600 junior-high-school students indicated that there was a correspondence between the scores on this instrument and norm-violating behavior. The inconsistency in the findings suggested, however, that the instrument should not be used for predictive purposes on a "routine and perfunctory basis" (Kvaraceus, 1966).

SHORTCOMINGS OF PRESENT PREDICTIVE SCALES

Despite concerted efforts to predict delinquency, we have not as yet been successful in devising an instrument with high predictive power. Kvaraceus (1966) notes that we might well have to develop separate scales for middle-class and lower-class delinquent youth. He also points out that we might be more effective in identifying subcultural delinquents as opposed to emotionally disturbed delinquents. Briggs and Wirt (1965) assert that researchers must attend to a number of pragmatic concerns heretofore neglected if we are to know the actual value of a prediction system. To mention a few of the neglected concerns, we have to determine the cost of errors in prediction, for example, the cost of professional treatment for a child who probably would not have become delinquent anyway, the cost and availability of treatment facilities, and the cost of obtaining the predictive information. We must also specify what we consider acceptable rates of predictive success. Until we have dealt with such illustrative utilitarian matters, we will not be in a good position to know the real worth of any given predictive system. At present, it appears that teacher nominations provide as reliable a basis for the prediction of antisocial behavior as do the best psychometric instruments (Kvaraceus, 1966).

PREVENTION AND TREATMENT

How one attempts to treat or prevent juvenile delinquency depends to a large extent on how he conceives the problem. Those who see this phenomenon as having a sociological base are much more inclined to influence social processes in the delinquent's surroundings. The sociological stance, as translated into treatment efforts, thus tends to focus on various types of environmental changes. Inherent in this approach is a concern over such sociological phenomena as family instability, social organization in the community, the role played by gang membership, and the difference in value systems among members of various socioeconomic strata. To implement their concerns, sociologists have traditionally relied on some form of social action. In some cases, the total environment is changed, for example, institutionalization. On other occasions, rehabilitation programs are attempted within the child's existing environment, for example, supervised youth organizations or settlement houses. In any event, treatment is centered around some kind of cultural or social alteration. Consistent with this orientation has been a corresponding emphasis on the development of either community programs or responsive group environments to facilitate the acquisition of socially appropriate behavior.

In the psychological approach, delinquent behavior is usually regarded as a symptom of some underlying problem. Though meaningless to the outside observer, the delinquent activity is presumed to be meaningful to the offender in that it represents an effort on his part to meet needs for status, security, acceptance, and so forth. The delinquent child, in response to thwarting and in an attempt to fulfill such unmet needs, thus resorts to illegal activities. In the implementation of this clinical orientation, treatment is generally focused on the individual, and reliance is accordingly placed on the skills of caseworkers or psychotherapists.

As we will see below, even though the treatment methods of the psychological and sociological approaches sometimes overlap or are used in combination, there remains a basic difference in viewpoints—a difference which is translated into noticeable differences in the objectives and methods of action programs.

Sociological Approaches

The sociological approaches attempt to change the individual through community or group programs. In this sense, sociological interventions generally have a more comprehensive base than do psychological interventions. In this section we will review some of the better-known studies and indicate recent trends in the treatment of delinquent youth.

Total-Community Approach

Perhaps the best-known community-center program is the Chicago Area Project, which was initiated by Shaw and his associates (Kobrin, 1959). The first area project was developed in 1932, and by 1959 similar projects had arisen in twelve Chicago neighborhoods. These projects are predicated on the philosophy that the adults who live in these slum areas must become better motivated to accept greater responsibility in promoting socially acceptable behavior among the children in that area. The central aim is to involve local youngsters in various activities so that they will adopt conventional rather than delinquent modes of conduct.

Translating this philosophy into action was initiated by having a staff member identify leaders in the community and by enlisting their support for a strong local movement to combat delinquency. These natural leaders then formed organizations, directed the communities in establishing a program, and raised the funds necessary to support the program. In other words, the primary responsibility for the maintenance and effectiveness of the program lay with indigenous members of the low-income community. Outside professional direction, though given a definite role, was secondary. The area projects differed with respect to the specific contents of the programs, but all programs had three common elements: (1) the establishment of recreational programs, (2) the campaign for community improvement, and (3) direct work with gangs and individuals. The use of prestigious community leaders was to serve the dual purpose of attracting both other adults and youth members in the area as well as offering models for emulation.

As is the case with most projects of this nature, there has been little in the way of objective evaluation. It does appear, however, (1) that the residents of low-income areas can organize themselves effectively in developing welfare programs, (2) that these organizations are enduring, well administered, and adapted to the needs of the local situation, and (3) that such plans utilize leadership which would otherwise remain untapped (Witmer & Tufts, 1954). Whether or not these programs lower the incidence of delinquency is another question, however. Data based on the rate of delinquency between 1930 and 1942 in three of the four then existing project areas indicated a deceleration of delinquent activities, but whether such differences were a direct outcome of project efforts or due to other community factors is debatable. In any event, no spectacular claims have been made, and the subjective reactions have ranged from favorable to skeptical.

Group-Centered Approach

Another approach, which began in the 1920's and was given impetus by Thrasher's work with gangs, is becoming increasingly popular, especially in large urban areas. This is the use of the detached-worker approach. We have already noted that most delinquency occurs in the presence of other delinquents. Bearing this in mind, caseworkers evolved methods which reached beyond the child and his family and were extended to predelinquent or delinquent peer groups.

One of the most widely quoted group-work programs is Miller's Boston Delinquency Project (1962). This project, designed to counteract delinquency in a lower-class Boston area, ran for a period of three years (1954-1957). Unlike some group projects which simply encourage the child to become a member of an organized club (for example, a baseball team), this program attempted to influence the value systems of lower-class street gangs which lead them into conflict with law-enforcement agents. (Miller, as noted earlier, views lower-class delinquency as emanating in the mores of lower-class culture.) This project also differed from others in that all workers were professionally trained, each worker except one was assigned to a single group, and regular psychiatric consultation was available.

During the three-year treatment span, 205 youngsters in seven corner groups were given intensive service. By "intensive" we mean approximately 18 to 21 hours of actual contact per week, with contacts ranging over a period of 10 to 34 months. Of the seven groups, four were white males (mostly Irish), one was Negro male, one was Negro female, and one was white female. The control subjects consisted of seven groups which had received only superficial assistance. The ages of the subjects ranged from 12 to 18 at the start of the program. There were three major phases to the project. Specifically, professional staff sought (1) to establish personal relationships;

(2) to modify behavior through organized group activities, through direct influence, and through serving as intermediaries between the youth and the adult institutions, for example, setting up job interviews; and (3) to terminate the relationship in a therapeutic manner.

Did the project succeed in reducing violative behavior? To answer this question, three separate measures of change were used: (1) the incidence of disapproved forms of customary behavior (immoral behavior); (2) illegal behavior (unofficial crime); and (3) court appearances. While two earlier reports (Miller, 1957, 1959b) might lead us to believe that a "limited but definite" diminution in delinquent activities had occurred, later statistics based on all three of these criteria indicated that the project had a "negligible impact" on the incidence of violative behavior. This negative-impact finding seems most applicable to those treatment methods which were most extensively employed and hence most fully tested in the study. These included the use of organized recreational activities, the establishment of local citizens' councils, the identification and contacting of adolescent corner gangs, the establishment of relationships with gang members, the provision of access to adult institutions, and the availability of more socially acceptable adult models. The authors concluded that the incentives provided for engaging in antisocial behavior were more powerful than any counterpressures which the project could bring to bear.

Institutional Approach

The Highfields Project (Weeks, 1958) illustrates a short-term community-therapy approach for youthful first offenders aged 16-17. Highfields, a specialized facility where not more than 21 boys reside at any one time, uses an open approach to treatment. For example, there are no guards and the boys are allowed to visit local villages to pursue activities of interest to them. A serious attempt is made to let the adolescents lead as "normal" lives as possible. There is no formal schooling, but supervised work experiences are provided. Group sessions designed to help the youngsters understand the motivations underlying their behavior and to modify certain undesirable attitudes are also conducted five nights a week.

What were the results of this study? First of all, there was little evidence that the Highfields boys modified their attitudes toward law and order, toward life, or toward their families. Second, there appeared to be little change in basic personality structure as a consequence of treatment. Finally, followup data gathered over a 12-month period after release indicated a significantly lower recidivism rate among 229 Highfields boys when compared with boys from a more traditional type of reform school. Further analysis of the data indicated that the better parole record was accounted for by a greater number of Negro boys in the Highfields facility than in the control group; that is, Negro boys from Highfields responded more favorably following release. White boys from both institutions had similar rates of recidivism, however. Also of interest is the cost of this short-term treatment, which was approximately one-third that of the more traditional program. In large measure, the differences in cost can be attributed to the fact that boys in the more traditional school had been incarcerated for a longer period of time. Though research of this particular type is certainly needed and has merit, it is unfortunate that the research design was not a particularly tight one. Replication using more rigorous controls is indicated.

Institutional treatment has generally produced little positive effect (Caditz, 1959). In fact, there is substantial evidence indicating that the longer the youngster spends in a "correctional" setting, the more apt he is to fail when released on parole (Weeks, 1958). Several factors most likely are operative in the production of such results: the size of the patient population in the institution, the staff-inmate ratio, the shortage of professionally trained personnel, the inappropriateness of treatment efforts, and the return to an unhealthy environment upon release. A recent report on three studies (Buehler, Patterson, & Furniss, 1966) has documented what might be an even more important factor, namely, the reward system of the institution itself. According to the results, the social living system of a correctional institution tends to reinforce delinquent behavior (often through nonverbal communications) and to punish socially conforming behaviors. Such findings, if representative, constitute a severe attack on institutional treatment and call for an overhaul in the scheduling of reinforcers within this type of social system.

Evaluation of Sociological Approaches

We have accumulated over the years a vast body of findings about the control of delinquent behavior. The conclusions which can be drawn have been aptly stated as follows:

Indeed, as of now, there are no demonstrable and proven methods for reducing the incidence of serious delinquent acts through preventive or rehabilitative procedures. Either the descriptive knowledge has not been translated into feasible action programs, or the programs have not been successfully implemented; or if implemented, they have lacked evaluation; or if evaluated, the results have usually been negative; and in the few cases of reported positive results, replications have been lacking.

At the same time, there are systematic and plausible sets of ideas about delinquency that find at least partial support and that may be converted into systematic action strategies. These ideas deserve careful development and refinement, for in the absence of hard evidence they remain our best guide to action, and it sometimes takes years of planning and effort before programs can be successfully launched (Wheeler, Cottrell, & Romasco, 1967).

CLINICAL APPROACHES

Few delinquents are enthusiastic about psychotherapy. To most delinquents, the therapist is an outsider—an enemy not to be trusted. Delinquents are typically suspicious, fearing that the therapist has ulterior motives. Moreover, this population is not a particularly introspective group. They do not see themselves as having problems, but tend to put blame on factors external to themselves. When we recall the characteristics of the unsocialized and socialized aggressive delinquents, we have some idea of their lack of readiness for conventional treatment procedures. Consequently, delinquents are extremely difficult to get into treatment and if they are coerced, they have difficulty forming a positive relationship with the therapist.

Employer-Employee Approach

To circumvent many of the difficulties associated with the "doctor-patient" relationship in the treatment of unreachable lower-class delinquents, Slack (1960) cleverly substituted an "experimenter-subject" or "employer-employee" relationship. In this approach the delinquents were asked if they would be willing to work an hour or two a day. The prospective employer explained that the work was not hard and that they could quit any time they wanted. During their first visits to the laboratory, the subjects were told that the employer's job was "to learn about the kids in the neighborhood" and that he was willing to pay them if they were willing to talk about themselves and to take psychological tests. Material rewards such as food, cigarettes, and candy were made available to the subjects. Periodic bonuses were also given. Provided with this nurturant atmosphere, the subjects eventually came to have confidence in the therapist and to develop a therapeutic relationship with him. Once the youngster realized that he no longer was coming only for the sake of the material gains but because of the relationship itself, he was involved in a more conventional form of treatment.

The results of this study were positive in terms of initiating a positive relationship with unreachable delinquents. The small number of subjects (seven), the absence of a control group, and the presentation of only qualitative results are some of the more obvious shortcomings of the study. All in all, it would appear, however, that Slack did achieve his objective of devising a technique for introducing hard-core cases to treatment. Though a successful introduction to therapy is not a sufficient condition in itself, its accomplishment nonetheless represents considerable movement, as anyone who has worked with such cases will testify.

More recently, Schwitzgebel and Kolb (1964) continued Slack's employer-employee method. These investigators used 20 boys between the ages of 15 and 21 in the experimental group. All had been imprisoned at one time. A control group matched in type of offense, age of first offense, nationality, time imprisoned, and place of residence was used for comparison purposes. The subjects received $1.00 an hour for interview sessions. The approach was a problem-oriented one as opposed to a theory-oriented one. The subjects were seen approximately three times a week for about nine months with a store being used as a meeting place. After fifteen appointments, attendance became dependable for 90 per cent of the subjects.

A followup study three years later showed that the number of arrests and the length of incarceration of the experimental group was approximately one-half that of the control group. There were no statistically significant differences in recidivism rates, although the trend was in the expected direction. This latter negative finding may be due to the different definitions of crime employed by the two groups, however. Unofficial crime rates were used as a criterion for the experimental group, whereas official crime rates—a less rigorous criterion—was used for the control group. Schwitzgebel concluded that the modification of delinquent behavior is more effectively achieved by the development of competing socially acceptable behaviors through operant-conditioning techniques (giving of money, cigarettes, food, and the like) than by direct attacks on delinquent behaviors per se. In accordance with this interpretation, Schwitzgebel's (1967) later research has been based primarily on an operant-conditioning paradigm.

Behavior-Modification Approach

Schwitzgebel's later work provides a nice introduction to the present topic, namely, behavior-modification or learning-theory approaches to the treatment of delinquent behavior. For most learning theorists, antisocial behavior is learned, maintained, and modified by the same learning-theory principles as are other learned behaviors. Given this assumption, Burchard (1967) created an experimental residential environment where consequences for one's behavior were programed according to learning-theory principles. The program was a standardized one which involved mostly nonprofessionals.

As is characteristic of behavior-modification approaches, specific target behaviors were selected for modification. These included maintaining a job, staying in school, buying food and meals, cooperating with peers and adults, budgeting money, and buying and caring for clothes—behaviors which would facilitate adjustment in the community. Tokens which could be exchanged for such things as an hour of recreation with female residents and a trip to town were used as rewards for desirable behavior. Conversely, undesirable target behaviors (fighting, lying, stealing, property damage, and so on) were punished. Punishment took the form of time-outs and seclusion, during which time tokens could not be earned. Moreover, when a staff member said "Time out," it cost the delinquent four tokens. When a staff member had to say "Seclusion," a charge of fifteen tokens was assessed. Within this context, Burchard completed a series of illustrative experiments with quite favorable results.

Psychoanalytically Oriented Approach

The behavior-modification approach has utilized as subjects what we have termed the sociological or subcultural delinquent. The late Adelaide Johnson (1959), who is known for her work with individual or neurotic delinquents, took a quite different tack, emphasizing the need to involve parents in treatment since the child's delinquent activities are presumably initiated and maintained by the parents. In her psychoanalytically oriented therapy sessions with parents, she stressed the need for frankness, making very clear their involvement in the child's problems.

There were two main drawbacks to this approach. First, intensive treatment efforts require involving the family which rendered this approach impractical for most child-guidance clinics since parents are typically not available for more than one visit per week. Second, the danger of intensifying an already emotionally upset parent through direct confrontation must be also weighed. This circumstance could be especially unfortunate in those instances where we wrongly ascribe the child's acting-out to deficiencies in the parent's conscience.

Evaluation of Clinical Approaches

Much remains to be learned about the treatment and prevention of delinquency. As indicated above, intervention outcomes are far from being wholly satisfactory. We have no sure-fire techniques that will reduce delinquency appreciably. Commonly employed approaches such as casework, counseling, psychiatric therapy, and recreational programs most likely have an ameliorative effect in certain cases, but they have not kept the rate of delinquent activity from climbing. Yet, despite the rather disappointing findings, it behooves workers to continue to evaluate the effectiveness of their endeavors. Though some clinicians and theorists still appear to think otherwise, it is encouraging to note that we are becoming more and more appreciative of the necessity for objective appraisal of our intervention efforts. We can no longer afford to assume romantically that our attempts and idealistic desires to reduce delinquent activities are being magically fulfilled.

Bearing in mind the limited results of achievement efforts and the transitory nature of most delinquent activity, Miller (Kvaraceus, 1966) questions whether the huge expenditures for treatment are worthwhile. But although this questioning attitude deserves more consideration than most workers are apt to give it, it seems quite clear that treatment efforts will not be deterred by the negligible results reported in evaluative studies. We will continue to train more psychiatrists, psychologists, social workers, and school counselors to fulfill their established roles. Since this is the case, it behooves us to ask why our results have been so limited and to inquire as to what we must do to better our therapeutic record. First of all, we must face the possibility regarding the inappropriateness of traditional treatment strategies. Empirical support for this hypothesis is seen in a study by Gottesfeld (1965), in which a list of 65 different treatment methods were sent in questionnaire form to 235 professional workers and 332 gang-member delinquents. The professionals were instructed to rate the usefulness of these methods, and the delinquents were asked to indicate their preferences among the various methods. The results indicated some very basic differences in orientation between the two groups. Whereas the professionals believed that the worker should be nonjudgmental and nonauthoritative in his role, the delinquents seemed to express a need for a mature parent substitute who would teach them how to relate better socially and help them to find a place in adult society.

Many authorities now recognize that we have used psychotherapy on many delinquents who were not in need of this type of treatment. This is especially true of the sociological delinquent, who is a basically sound youngster from the standpoint of mental health. Furthermore, we have not geared our treatment methodologies, by and large, to those who externalize their problems. Instead, we have focused most of our energies on the development of treatment strategies suited to those who internalize their problems. We expect delinquents, whose adjustive behaviors are already suspect, to adapt to our treatment methodologies, whereas we—as rigorously trained professionals—seem to feel little need or obligation to gear our treatment techniques to their level of readiness. Can you imagine a medical doctor expecting a patient to adapt his biochemistry so that it will respond more readily to the prescribed drug? Just as we have hard-core delinquents, it also appears that we have hard-core professionals. Researchers who use the employer-employee model and behavior-modification procedures deserve recognition for their more functional, straightforward, and down-to-earth approach. They have devised rewards and incentives which are sociologically consistent with the delinquent's subculture and which are apparently sufficiently powerful to lead or entice these youngsters to establish more legal modes of meeting their needs.

One of the more divergent approaches involves the use of former delinquents as nonprofessional workers. Since peers can inhibit the norm-violating activities of others, it might well be that the ex-delinquent peer has certain advantages as a therapist. For one thing, there is less social distance between him and the client than usually exists between the middle-class professional and the lower-class patient. Moreover, the indigenous nonprofessional is typically seen as "one of us." He is also able to give help with present reality crises, and he can offer this help within the confines of the client's daily surroundings. In other words, the client does not have to go to the therapist's office or to the community agency. The nonprofessional is thus able to give help in an informal manner. Anyone who has had experience with lower-class delinquents readily recognizes their aversion to the formal, futuristic atmosphere that is characteristic of conventional forms of therapy. While it is still too early to evaluate the effectiveness of such approaches, it does appear on a-priori grounds that they have considerable merit. Conceivably, the use of indigenous nonprofessionals could not only lead to more effective intervention approaches, but also help to alleviate the existing manpower shortage in the mental-health fields. Let us hope that the professionally trained workers will not become too threatened if these paraprofessionals achieve results which have thus far eluded us.

We must also devote greater consideration to gearing our intervention approaches to the child's sex, developmental level, socioeconomic status, and "type" of delinquency. Thus, for example, an employer-employee type of therapy might fit well with the older adolescent offenders but would be inappropriate for younger delinquents. It might well prove that the type of intervention is a more important determinant of effectiveness than the earliness of intervention. For example, finding a delinquent a job which offers him adult status and recognition and thus removes him from his poor environment might be more effective than doing intensive casework with a much younger child who is living in the slums with his parents. Or, with respect to the various dimensions of delinquent activity, we might do well to concentrate treatment efforts on those who are most apt to continue in their wayward manner. Unfortunately, those with the most unfavorable prognoses are the very youngsters who are least apt to receive help since they do not fit our traditional treatment model. Hopefully, however, the emergence of more innovative approaches will serve to remedy this state of affairs.

EDUCATIONAL APPROACHES

As authorities have become increasingly concerned about the close relationship between academic failure and delinquency, schools today have been given appreciably more responsibility for socially malad-justed youth. This association between antisocial behavior and difficulty in school continues to be supported by current research. Burke and Simons (1965), for instance, find that among institutionalized delin-quents, 90 per cent were reported as truants or had made poor adjust-ments to school, about 75 per cent had repeated two or more grades or had dropped out of school before the legal age, and 67 per cent were reading below the sixth-grade level. Similarly, noting that low academic achievement, absenteeism, and impulsivity differentiate de-linquents from nondelinquents in both white and Negro popula-tions, Miller (1959a) optimistically hypothesized that the incidence of delinquency would decrease as educational achievements increase.

The growing conviction that juvenile delinquency is partly height-ened by certain other widespread conditions in American education is reflected in a report prepared by the Task Force on Juvenile Delin-quency (1967). According to Schafer and Polk (1967), there are four basic ways in which school experiences can contribute to delin-quency:

1. By stressing the need for educational success and yet simul-taneously insuring educational failure, the schools block legitimate means of entering the mainstream of American life.

2. Educational activities often seem meaningless in relation to the students' needs. Hence, because school tasks and rewards are perceived as unrelated to the students' future role in life, education becomes a rather empty activity. Consequently, illegitimate alternatives assume greater attractiveness.

3. The school is often unable to elicit a strong degree of commit-ment to conformity and legitimate achievement from students. A sense of alienation results which renders students more susceptible to delin-quent pursuits.

4. The manner in which the school handles student misconduct is also relevant in this connection. For example, overly punitive sanc-tions of a degrading nature can serve to push the student toward illegitimate forms of commitment.

Since the conditions which give rise to these unfortunate debilitating effects are deeply rooted in existing notions and organizations of our educational system, Schafer and Polk argue that education must do more than adopt stopgap measures which deal solely with surface problems. Adding more counselors and social workers, for example, constitutes a rather myopic viewpoint which ignores broader dimensions of the school's role in delinquency. These authors stress the need for such things as fostering a belief in the educability of all pupils, expanding preschool educational facilities, developing meaningful and relevant instruction, innovating more appropriate teaching strategies, using flexible grouping, continuing reeducation of teachers, providing alternate career-oriented programs, increasing the accessibility to higher education, reintegrating dropouts, and so forth. Unless fundamental and radical educational changes are made in the schools, these authors declare, schools will continue to contribute significantly to delinquency.

Despite the relationship of such factors as educational retardation, truancy, and school adjustment to delinquent pursuits, teachers receive little training in the area of delinquency (Eichorn, 1965). A survey of 260 educators in graduate courses revealed that about half of them had no more than one or two class hours devoted to this topic. The same criticism might well be leveled with respect to the management of aggressive students in general, namely, that teachers are given only minimal instruction in how to cope with acting-out youth, despite the fact that these youngsters are the very ones who are most disruptive to effective classroom functioning. In this section, we will focus primarily on special classes, work-experience programs, and behavior-modification techniques, although passing reference will be made to other modifications in educational strategies for delinquent youth. The classroom management of aggressive students will be treated in Chapter 11.

Educational Provisions

In view of the educational retardation of delinquents, there have been numerous attempts to modify the educational provisions provided socially maladjusted youth. Kvaraceus and Ulrich (1959) have done an admirable job of surveying the various ways in which school districts throughout the country have tried to meet the educational needs of these youths. The approaches included identification procedures, provisions within the classroom, curricular adaptations, special classes, and closer relationships with families, law-enforcement agencies, and community agencies. Their work, though nonevaluative, nonetheless provides a valuable resource for educational practitioners in that it delineates general principles and examples of specific action programs.

Special Classes

Evidence that the schools can occupy a strategic position in coping with juvenile delinquency is seen in the results of a study conducted in Quincy, Illinois (Bowman, 1959). Several traditional approaches were initially utilized with semidelinquent and delinquent adolescents in an effort to mobilize the talents of youngsters in the community. Foster-home placement was used but found to be unsuccessful, especially with the children between the ages of 12 and 14. Intensive casework was also attempted but proved to be too time-consuming. No community agency was sufficiently staffed to undertake such an intensive program on any sort of extensive basis. Recreational programs were also tried but found to be wanting. These programs, it was concluded, provided an excellent means for contact between children and the community but could not be relied upon to effect any significant changes in acting-out children.

Finally, an approach was tried which would permit intensive contact with target groups and yet be available to the typical community, namely, school intervention. Sixty youngsters who were doing poorly in their eighth-grade schoolwork were selected for intensive study. Of these subjects, nearly all were discipline problems and 41 per cent had police or court records. The subjects were randomly assigned to three groups of 20 each. Thus, there were two experimental groups and one control group. Teachers were assigned on the basis of their interest in working with acting-out pupils. As such, these teachers had no special training in handling delinquent youths. Pupils in the experimental programs spent from one-half to three-fourths of their school day with one teacher who was sympathetic toward them. Instructional methods and materials were adjusted to the child's interests and level of functioning in order to make school activities more pleasant. Practical materials were stressed more than textbooks, and the pace of instruction was slowed. During the first two periods of the morning the focus was on academic subjects with the third period being devoted to discussion and films on general and social problems. For some subjects the afternoon session consisted of study periods, small-group discussions, handwork, and special projects. For others, outside employment constituted the main activity during the afternoon. Written reactions to the special classes by the students were favorable. As might be expected from the slowed pace, differences in academic performance between the experimental and control subjects were only slight. There were also no significant differences between the two groups in the number of school dropouts. It appears, however, that youngsters in the experimental group achieved a greater job success as reflected by employer ratings and job stability. The experimental subjects also seemed to have a greater interest in school as inferred from their better attendance records. Of most significance, however, were their respective delinquency rates. Whereas the rate for the control subjects more than tripled, the rate for the experimental subjects decreased by more than one-third. Furthermore, there were fewer serious offenses among the students in the special classes. While the number of subjects is too small to permit widespread generalization, the findings do suggest the benefits which can accrue from the use of special classes, where the pupils are provided with interested teachers, a revised curriculum, and freedom from competition with more advanced students.

Work-Experience Program

Work-experience programs are becoming increasingly popular as a form of educational therapy for delinquent youth. Recognizing that treatment of delinquents in the usual clinic setting had not been highly successful, Massimo and Shore (1963) sought to determine the effectiveness of a comprehensive vocationally oriented treatment program. This experiment included 20 adolescent boys of normal intellectual ability. All had histories of antisocial behavior and were out of school at the time of the study. They either had been suspended by school authorities or had voluntarily withdrawn. The subjects were randomly assigned to either an experimental or a control group. Those adolescents in the experimental group received the services of a detached worker who provided, over a ten-month period, three types of services: intensive psychotherapy, remedial education, and employment. It was hypothesized that this treatment program would lead to positive changes in ego functioning as evidenced by changes in academic skills, personality attitudes, and overt behavior.

All three hypotheses were confirmed. Educational-achievement test scores favored the experimental group at a statistically significant level. Three dimensions of personality in terms of attitudes—toward the control of aggression, toward the self, and toward authority—all improved for the experimental subjects. Overt behavior as reflected in the work-history records also favored the experimental group. At the end of the ten-month period, seven members of the experimental group were still on the job, with the other three members having returned to school. On the other hand, three of the control group were unemployed throughout the ten-month period, and a fourth was unemployed at the end of this period. Further, only one of the control group returned to school. Probation officers, who did not know whether a child belonged to the experimental or the control group, also rated members of the treatment group as improved in overt behavior. An informal followup study seemed to indicate that those who did well on the program had been able to maintain their gains, while the adjustment of control subjects continued to deteriorate over time. Three members of the control group, for example, are presently institutionalized, while none of the experimental subjects find themselves in this circumstance.

Though the number of subjects was quite small and the therapeutic variables difficult to disentangle because of the comprehensive nature of this program, the results are sufficiently promising to encourage further investigation along these lines. It should certainly be cautioned, contrary to the belief of some educators, that school programs of this nature are probably not suitable for all deviant youth. The psychotic youngster and the hostile sociopath are examples of those who might be too disturbed to profit from interventions of this kind. The interested reader can find additional descriptions of current work-experience programs for delinquent youth by consulting Schreiber (1966).

While work-experience programs are becoming more numerous, they have not been in existence long enough to permit adequate evaluation. Hence, for the present the findings must be regarded as tentative. Nevertheless, it would appear, as Schreiber (1966) declares, that school-based work-study programs do provide a second chance for alienated youth to join the achievement-based mainstream of American life. These programs, while differing considerably from one another, do possess common therapeutic elements which have been succinctly stated by Schreiber as follows:

[These programs] (1) encourage and permit alienated youth to improve their self-images and self-concepts; (2) enable them to learn and exercise self-discipline and to develop proper work habits and work attitudes; (3) enable them to maintain at least minimum levels of education and work skills which are marketable; (4) offer alienated youth opportunities to relate themselves with and to other persons and encourage them to do so; and (5) give direct and indirect satisfaction to the individual in knowing that he can both undertake and complete a job satisfactorily.

Behavior-Modification Approach

A fascinating investigation of remedial reading by Staats and Butterfield (1965) combined the use of two emerging approaches to the mental-health problems of children, namely, behavior-modification principles and the use of nonprofessionals. The subject for this study was a 14-year-old culturally deprived juvenile delinquent who had a long history of delinquency and maladjustment. His difficulties in school were, in part, attributable to his lack of academic skills and to his failure to respond to traditional classroom reinforcers. He had a full-scale IQ of 90 on the Wechsler Intelligence Scale for Children. His Verbal Scale IQ was 77, however, which would indicate a slow rate of school-learning ability. The method of treatment relied on an extrinsic token reinforcement system, with three types of tokens being used: a blue token was worth one-tenth of one cent; a white token was worth one-third of one cent; and a red token was worth one-half of a cent. Correct responses on the first trial yielded a token of high value, whereas correct responses made following errors yielded tokens of lower reinforcement value. The tokens could be used to purchase a variety of items; that is, the child could choose his own reward. Materials from the Science Research Associates' reading kits were adapted for use in the study. Vocabulary words were typed on separate 3×5 cards. Oral reading materials of paragraph length were typed on separate 5×8 cards, so that each story could be presented individually. Comprehension questions were typed on $8\frac{1}{2} \times 13$ sheets of paper for use in promoting the understanding of silent reading materials. The objective was to develop remedial reading procedures that could be applied in a standard manner by nonprofessionals trained in this procedure. The tutor in the study was a probation officer.

Forty hours of remedial reading spread over a 4½-month interval yielded considerable success. For example, the boy's reading ability rose from a beginning second-grade level to a fourth-grade level. This gain might not seem impressive except for the fact that this boy accomplished more in reading during this 4½-month period than he had in all of his previous 8½ years of schooling. Moreover, he passed all of his courses in school for the first time, his misbehavior became less frequent, and his general attitude toward school improved. Some other points of interest include the fact that the subject received only $20.31 worth of tokens and that reading itself became reinforcing, so that more reading responses were made per reinforcer as time went on. The most important educational implication stemming from this case study is that standard reading materials can be adapted to a relatively uniform type of presentation by training nonprofessionals in the context of reinforcement principles. Later research (Staats et al., 1967) based on mentally retarded, culturally disadvantaged, and emotionally disturbed subjects of junior-high-school age provided a more general test of these procedures and, by and large, confirmed their practical value. High-school students and adult volunteers served as the tutors in this later research project.

Another impressive illustration of the behavior-modification approach has been carried out at the National Training School for Boys by Cohen (1966). The project was entitled CASE (Contingencies Applicable for Special Education). The specific target behavior in this study—academic performance—was shaped through the use of programed instruction. Once a student successfully completed 90 per cent of a unit, he was eligible to take an examination on which he could earn points worth one cent each. These points could then be spent for Cokes, potato chips, items from Sears Roebuck, entrance into the lounge to visit with friends, book rentals, time in the library, and so forth.

Cohen reported that the systematic contingent application of reinforcement yielded best results when it took place in a highly structured environment that increased the likelihood of prosocial behaviors and decreased the likelihood of antisocial behaviors. To this end, a special environment was prepared, consisting of classrooms, study booths, control rooms, a library, a store, and a lounge. The results reflected a gradual shifting away from material reinforcers, like Cokes, toward more educationally relevant rewards, like new programs. Aside from the enormous surge in educational activities, there were also favorable changes in the social behavior of the subjects. In fact, there were no discipline problems or property destruction during a 4½-month period.

The findings of these two studies bear considerable significance in light of the shortage of mental-health specialists and remedial teachers. The authors know of no school district which has a sufficient number of remedial reading specialists or, for that matter, the enabling funds to employ them in the needed quantities. The tendency for gains to spread beyond the cognitive and academic areas into the social and emotional realms also merits close attention for it speaks to one role that the school can legitimately and apparently successfully assume relative to mental health. Like work-study programs, remedial programs offer students a reality-based therapy that is not typically achieved during the insulated "talk-therapy" sessions in the clinician's office.

SUMMARY

Delinquency continues to constitute an urgent social problem, especially in industrialized countries. Strictly speaking, delinquency is a legal term, although it carries no uniform meaning even in this restricted usage. Incidence figures indicate that juvenile delinquency has increased over the past decade or so. The rates of delinquency are influenced by a multitude of factors—the child's age, sex, family stability, social class, racial and ethnic membership, urban-rural residency, intelligence, and physical constitution.

Research studies reveal three psychological dimensions of delinquency: the psychopathic delinquent, the subcultural delinquent, and the neurotic delinquent. Psychopathic delinquency is regarded as the most severe and as having the poorest prognosis. Subcultural delinquency probably has the most favorable prognosis of the three "varieties."

There are two broad theories as to the causes of delinquent activity. Psychological theories of delinquency generally stress the pathology of the individual, for example, his feelings of rejection. Sociological theories, on the other hand, emphasize broader aspects of the social environment, for example, community disorganization. Psychologically oriented theorists generally use a clinical approach, such as community programs. The outcomes of both types of treatment strategies have been critically appraised. With respect to the prediction of norm-violating conduct, teacher nominations fare as well as the best psychometric instruments. The school's role in relation to delinquency has been examined, and educational provisions for acting-out youth (special classes, work-study programs, and behavior-modification approaches) have been discussed.

SUGGESTED READINGS

Giallombardo, R. *Juvenile delinquency.* New York: Wiley, 1968.

Kvaraceus, W. C., & Ulrich, W. E. *Delinquent behavior.* Vol. 2, *Principles and practice.* Washington, D.C.: National Education Association, 1959.

Peterson, D., & Becker, W. Family interaction and delinquency. In H. C. Quay (Ed.), *Juvenile delinquency.* Princeton, N.J.: Van Nostrand, 1965. Pp. 63-99.

Redl, F., & Wineman, D. *Children who hate.* New York: Free Press, 1951.

REFERENCES

Andry, R. G. *Delinquency and parental pathology.* London: Methuen, 1960.

Ausubel, D. Psychological factors in juvenile delinquency. Paper read at seminar on juvenile delinquency, Marylhurst College, Oregon, October, 1965.

Bandura, A., & Walters, R. H. *Adolescent aggression.* New York: Ronald Press, 1959.

Bell, J. C., Ross, A., & Simpson, A. Incidence and estimated prevalence of recorded delinquency in a metropolitan area. *Amer. sociol. Rev.,* 1964, **29,** 90-92.

Bowman, P. H. Effects of a revised school program on potential delinquents. *Ann. Amer. Acad. polit. soc. Sci.,* 1959, **322,** 53-61.

Briggs, P. F., & Wirt, R. D. Prediction. In H. C. Quay (Ed.), *Juvenile delinquency.* Princeton, N.J.: Van Nostrand, 1965. Pp. 170-208.

Browning, C. J. Differential impact of family disorganization on male adolescents. *Soc. Prob.,* 1960, **8,** 37-44.

Buehler, E., Patterson, G., & Furniss, J. The reinforcement of behavior in institutional settings. *Behav. Res. Ther.,* 1966, **4,** 157-167.

Burchard, J. D. Systematic socialization: a programmed environment for the rehabilitation of antisocial retardates. *Psychol. Rec.,* 1967, **17,** 461-476.

Burke, N. S., & Simons, A. E. Factors which precipitate dropouts and delinquency. *Fed. Probation,* 1965, **29,** 28-32.

Caditz, S. Effect of a training school experience on the personality of delinquent boys. *J. consult. Psychol.,* 1959, **23,** 501-509.

Caplan, N. S. Intellectual functioning. In H. C. Quay (Ed.), *Juvenile delinquency.* Princeton, N.J.: Van Nostrand, 1965. Pp. 100-138.

Carr, L. *Delinquency control.* New York: Harper, 1950.

Cavan, R. Negro family disorganization and juvenile delinquency. *J. Negro Educ.,* 1959, **28**, 230-239.

Clark, J., & Wenninger, E. Socio-economic class and area as correlates of illegal behavior among juveniles. *Amer. sociol. Rev.,* 1962, **27**, 826-834.

Clark, K. B. Color, class, personality and juvenile delinquency. *J. Negro Edu.,* 1959, **28**, 240-251.

Cloward, R. A., & Ohlin, L. E. *Delinquency and opportunity: a theory of delinquent gangs.* New York: Free Press, 1960.

Cohen, A. *Delinquent boys.* Glencoe, Ill.: Free Press, 1955.

Cohen, A. *Deviance and control.* Englewood Cliffs, N.J.: Prentice-Hall, 1966.

Conger, J., Miller, W., Gaskill, H., & Walsmith, C. *Progress report.* NIMH Grant No. M-3040. Washington, D.C.: U.S. Public Health Service, 1960.

Conger, J., Miller, W., & Walsmith, C. Antecedents of delinquency: personality, social class and intelligence. In P. H. Mussen, J. J. Conger, & J. Kagan (Eds.), *Readings in child development and personality.* New York: Harper, 1965. Pp. 442-468.

Craig, M. M., & Glick, S. J. Ten years' experience with the Glueck Social Prediction Table. *Crime & Delinq.,* 1963, **9**, 249-216.

Craig, M. M., & Glick, S. J. *A manual of procedures for application of the Glueck Prediction Table.* New York City Youth Board, 1964.

Dentler, R., & Monroe, L. Early adolescent theft. *Amer. sociol. Rev.,* 1961, **26**, 733-743.

Dinitz, S., Scarpitti, F., & Reckless, W. Delinquency vulnerability: a cross group and longitudinal analysis. *Amer. sociol. Rev.,* 1962, **27**, 515-517.

Douglass, J. H. The extent and characteristics of juvenile delinquency among Negroes in the United States. *J. Negro Educ.,* 1959, **28**, 214-229.

Eaton, J., & Polk, K. *Measuring delinquency.* Pittsburgh: Univer. of Pittsburgh Press, 1961.

Eichorn, J. R. Delinquency and the educational system. In H. C. Quay (Ed.), *Juvenile delinquency.* Princeton, N.J.: Van Nostrand, 1965. Pp. 298-337.

Eisner, V., & Tsuyemura, H. Interaction of juveniles with the law. *Publ. Hlth Rep.,* 1965, **80**, 689-691.

Empey, L. T., & Erickson, M. L. Hidden delinquency and social status. *Soc. Forces,* 1966, **44**, 546-554.

Erickson, M., & Empey, L. Class position, peers, and delinquency. *Sociol. soc. Res.,* 1965, **49**, 268-282.

Federal Bureau of Investigation. *Uniform Crime Report,* 1963. Washington, D.C.: U.S. Department of Justice, 1963.

Ferdinand, T. N. The offense patterns and family structures of urban, village and rural delinquents. *J. crim. Law, Criminol. Police Sci.,* 1964, **55**, 86-93.

Freedman, M. Background of deviancy. In W. W. Wattenberg (Ed.), Social deviancy among youth. *Yearb. nat. Soc. Stud. Educ.,* 1966, **65**, Part I. Pp. 28-58.

Glueck, E. T. Distinguishing delinquents from pseudodelinquents. *Harv. educ. Rev.,* 1966, **36**, 119-130. (a)

Glueck, E. T. A more discriminative instrument for the identification of potential delinquents at school entrance. *J. crim. Law, Criminol. Police Sci.*, 1966, **57**, 27-30. (b)

Glueck, S., & Glueck, E. *Unraveling juvenile delinquency.* New York: Commonwealth Fund, 1950.

Glueck, S., & Glueck, E. *Physique and delinquency.* New York: Harper, 1956.

Gottesfeld, H. Professionals and delinquents evaluate professional methods with delinquents. *Soc. Prob.*, 1965, **13**, 45-59.

Hathaway, S. R., & Monachesi, E. D. *Analyzing and predicting juvenile delinquency with the MMPI.* Minneapolis: Univer. of Minnesota Press, 1953.

Hathaway, S. R., & Monachesi, E. D. The personalities of predelinquent boys. *J. crim. Law, Criminol. Police Sci.*, 1957, **48**, 149-163.

Healy, W., & Bronner, A. F. *New light on delinquency and its treatment.* New Haven: Yale Univer. Press, 1936.

Hill, M. The metropolis and juvenile delinquency among Negroes. *J. Negro Educ.*, 1959, **28**, 277-285.

Hurwitz, J. I., Kaplan, D., & Kaiser, E. Parental coping patterns and delinquency. *J. Offender Ther.*, 1962, **6**, 2-4.

Johnson, A. Juvenile delinquency. In S. Arieti (Ed.), *American handbook of psychiatry.* New York: Basic Books, 1959. Pp. 840-856.

Kobrin, S. The Chicago area project—a 25-year assessment. *Ann. Amer. Acad. polit. soc. Sci.*, 1959, **322**, 19-29.

Kvaraceus, W. C. *KD proneness scale and check list.* New York: World Book, 1953.

Kvaraceus, W. C. *Forecasting juvenile delinquency.* New York: World Book, 1956.

Kvaraceus, W. C. Forecasting delinquency: a three-year experiment. *Except. Child.*, 1961, **27**, 429-435.

Kvaraceus, W. C. Problems of early identification and prevention of delinquency. In W. W. Wattenberg (Ed.), Social deviancy among youth. *Yearb. nat. Soc. Stud. Educ.*, 1966, **65**, Part I. Pp. 189-220.

Kvaraceus, W. C., & Miller, W. B. *Delinquent behavior.* Vol. 1, *Culture and the individual.* Washington, D.C.: National Education Association, 1959.

Kvaraceus, W. C., & Ulrich, W. E. *Delinquent behavior.* Vol. 2, *Principles and practice.* Washington, D.C.: National Education Association, 1959.

Lippman, H. S. *Treatment of the child in emotional conflict.* (2nd ed.) New York: McGraw-Hill, 1962.

Lohman, J., & Carey, J. Rehabilitation programs for deviant youth. In W. W. Wattenberg (Ed.), Social deviancy among youth. *Yearb. nat. Soc. Stud. Educ.*, 1966, **65**, Part I. Pp. 373-397.

Lombroso, C. *Crime: its causes and remedies.* (English trans. Henry P. Horton) Boston: Little, Brown, 1918.

McCord, W., McCord, J., & Zola, I. *Origins of crime: a new evaluation of the Cambridge-Somerville youth study.* New York: Columbia Univer. Press, 1959.

Massimo, J. L., & Shore, M. F. The effectiveness of a comprehensive vocationally oriented psychotherapeutic program for adolescent delinquent boys. *Amer. J. Orthopsychiat.,* 1963, **33**, 634-642.

Miller, W. The impact of a community group work program on delinquent corner groups. *Soc. Sci. Rev.,* 1957, **31**, 390-406.

Miller, W. Lower class culture as a generating milieu of gang delinquency. *J. soc. Issues,* 1959, **14**, 5-19 (a)

Miller, W. Preventive work with street-corner groups: Boston Delinquency Project. *Ann. Amer. Acad. polit. soc. Sci.,* 1959, **322**, 97-106. (b)

Miller, W. The impact of a "total-community" delinquency control project. *Soc. Prob.,* 1962, **10**, 168-191.

Monahan, T. P. Family status and the delinquent child: a reappraisal and some new findings. *Soc. Forces,* 1957, **35**, 250-258.

Nash, J. The father in contemporary culture and current psychological literature. *Child Develpm.,* 1965, **36**, 261-297.

Nye, F. I. *Family relationships and delinquent behavior.* New York: Wiley, 1958.

Nye, I., Short, J., & Olson, V. Socio-economic status and delinquent behavior. *Amer. J. Sociol.,* 1958, **63**, 381-389.

Perlman, R. Juvenile delinquency and some social and economic trends. *Welfare Rev.,* 1963, **1**, 12-20.

Phillips, E. Crime, victims, and the police. *Trans-action,* 1967, **4**, 36-44.

Pilcher, D., Stern, L., & Perlman, R. Juvenile delinquency. *Hlth, Educ. Welfare Indic.,* 1963, pp. 5-18.

Quay, H. C. Dimensions of personality in delinquent boys as inferred from the factor analysis of case history data. *Child Develpm.,* 1964, **35**, 479-484.

Quay, H. C. Personality and delinquency. In H. C. Quay (Ed.), *Juvenile delinquency.* Princeton, N.J.: Van Nostrand, 1965. Pp. 139-166.

Quay, H. C. Personality dimensions in preadolescent delinquent boys. *Educ. psychol. Measmt,* 1966, **26**, 99-110.

Reckless, W., Dinitz, S., & Kay, B. The self-component in potential delinquency and potential nondelinquency. *Amer. sociol. Rev.,* 1957, **22**, 566-570.

Reiss, A. J. Social correlates of psychological types of delinquency. *Amer. sociol. Rev.,* 1952, **17**, 710-718.

Reiss, A. J., & Rhodes, A. The distribution of juvenile delinquency in the social class structure. *Amer. sociol. Rev.,* 1961, **26**, 720-732.

Reiss, H., Jr., & Rhodes, A. Status deprivation and delinquent behavior. *Sociol. Quart.,* 1963, **4**, 135-149.

Robins, L. N. *Deviant children grown up.* Baltimore: Williams & Wilkins, 1966.

Robison, S. A study of delinquency among Jewish children in New York City. In M. Sklare (Ed.), *The Jews: social patterns of an American group.* Glencoe, Ill.: Free Press, 1957. Pp. 535-550.

Scarpitti, F. Delinquent and nondelinquent perceptions of self, values, and opportunity. *Ment. Hyg.,* 1965, **49**, 399-400.

Scarpitti, F., Murray, E., Dinitz, S., & Reckless, W. The "good" boy in a high delinquency area: four years later. *Amer. sociol. Rev.,* 1960, **25**, 555-558.

Schafer, W. E., & Polk, K. Delinquency and the schools. In Task Force on Juvenile Delinquency, *Juvenile delinquency and youth crime.* Washington, D.C.: Government Printing Office, 1967. Pp. 222-277.

Schreiber, D. Work-experience programs. In W. W. Wattenberg (Ed.), Social deviancy among youth. *Yearb. nat. Soc. Stud. Educ.,* 1966, **65**, Part I. Pp. 280-314.

Schuessler, K., & Cressey, D. Personality characteristics of criminals. *Amer. J. Sociol.,* 1950, **55**, 476-484.

Schwitzgebel, R. Short-term operant conditioning of adolescent offenders on socially relevant variables. *J. abnorm. Psychol.,* 1967, **72**, 134-142.

Schwitzgebel, R., & Kolb, D. Inducing behavior change in adolescent delinquents. *Behav. Res. Ther.,* 1964, **1**, 297-304.

Segal, B. E. Racial perspectives and attitudes among Negro and white delinquent boys: an empirical examination. *Phylon,* 1966, **27**, 27-39.

Short, F. J., Jr. Juvenile delinquency: the sociocultural context. In M. L. Hoffman & L. W. Hoffman (Eds.), *Review of child development research.* Vol. II. New York: Russell Sage Foundation, 1966. Pp. 423-468.

Short, J. F., & Nye, F. I. Extent of unrecorded delinquency; tentative conclusions. *J. crim. Law, Criminol. Police Sci.,* 1958, **49**, 296-302.

Siegman, A. Father absence during early childhood and antisocial behavior. *J. abnorm. Psychol.,* 1966, **71**, 71-74.

Slack, C. W. Experimenter-subject psychotherapy: a new method of introducing intensive office treatment for unreasonable cases. *Ment. Hyg.,* 1960, **44**, 238-256.

Staats, A. W., & Butterfield, W. Treatment of nonreading in a culturally deprived juvenile delinquent: an application of reinforcement principles. *Child Develpm.,* 1965, **36**, 925-942.

Staats, A. W., Minke, K. A., Goodwin, W., & Landeen, J. Cognitive behavior modification: "motivated learning" reading treatment with subprofessional therapy-technicians. *Behav. Res. Ther.,* 1967, **5**, 283-299.

Task Force on Juvenile Delinquency. *Juvenile delinquency and youth crime.* Washington, D.C.: Government Printing Office, 1967.

Teeters, N., & Matza, D. The extent of delinquency in the United States. *J. Negro Educ.,* 1959, **28**, 200-213.

U.S. Children's Bureau. *Juvenile court statistics.* Statistical Series No. 85. Washington, D.C.: Government Printing Office, 1966.

Weeks, H. *Youthful offenders at Highfields: an evaluation of the effects of short-term treatment of delinquent boys.* Ann Arbor: Univer. of Michigan Press, 1958.

Wheeler, S., Cottrell, L. S., Jr., & Romasco, A. Juvenile delinquency: its prevention and control. In Task Force on Juvenile Delinquency, *Juvenile delinquency and youth crime.* Washington, D.C.: Government Printing Office, 1967. Pp. 409-428.

Wirt, R. D., & Briggs, P. F. Personality and environmental factors in the development of delinquency. *Psychol. Monogr.,* 1959, **73** (485).

Wirt, R. D., & Briggs, P. F. The meaning of delinquency. In H. C. Quay (Ed.), *Juvenile delinquency.* Princeton, N.J.: Van Nostrand, 1965. Pp. 1-26.

Witmer, H., & Tufts, E. *The effectiveness of delinquency prevention programs.* U.S. Children's Bureau Publication No. 350. Washington, D.C.: Government Printing Office, 1954.

8

Childhood Psychoses

Childhood psychoses have probably attracted more attention than
have any other childhood disorders because of their spectacular and
bizarre nature. Indeed, the history of emotionally disturbed children
has centered predominantly around these baffling disturbances (Kanner, 1962). Yet, despite the aroused concern and voluminous literature available on the subject, very little of a definitive nature is known
regarding the etiology or treatment of psychoses in children. We are
not even sure whether psychotic conditions in children are a manifes-

tation of the same basic disorder seen in adults or whether they are a special type of ego malfunction. While there are a number of theories on childhood psychoses, the present state of knowledge might well be termed fragmented and confused.

DEFINITION

Contributing to this confusion has been the lack of agreement among authorities in the field concerning the term to be used in describing or labeling this condition. By 1900, professional workers were willing to recognize and accept the existence of psychotic disturbances in children. Yet, it was not until the 1930's that systematic efforts were put forth to investigate seriously debilitating childhood emotional disorders with respect to diagnosis, etiology, course, and treatment (Kanner, 1962). While it was Bleuler who in 1911 introduced the term "schizophrenia," it was Potter (1933) who, some twenty years later, was apparently the first to employ the term with reference to children.

In the 1940's, Kanner (1962) observed two opposing trends emerged relative to terminology. On the one hand, there was a tendency toward an inexplicitness characteristic of the earlier pre-Kraepelin era. Beata Rank (1949), for example, coined the term "atypical child" to encompass a wide variety of serious disorders manifesting themselves in early childhood. The inexactness or vagueness inherent in this term is reflected, for instance, in the lack of differentiation between such conditions as childhood psychosis and mental deficiency. In a similar vein, Blau (1962) has written:

Much confusion arises from indecision and evasion regarding the name of the syndrome. To my mind the following designations are more or less synonymous: atypical, prepsychosis, ego deviant, seriously deviant child, infantile anaclitic depression, preschizophrenia, autistic, symbiotic, brain injured, incipient schizophrenia, pseudo psychoses, psuedo neurotic psychoses, abnormal child, schizoid personality, impulse ridden character, and oligophrenia. All conditions are of serious ego disturbance.

On the other hand, Kanner and others have stressed the need for more precise terminology rather than clumping an assortment or variety of "heterogeneous clinical entities" under a common rubric. In keeping with this philosophy, Kanner (1943) delineated early infantile autism as a distinct clinical entity. Mahler (1952) discussed symbiosis as a form of childhood schizophrenia, and Bender (1954) analyzed childhood schizophrenia into three basic subtypes: the pseudo-defective, the pseudo-neurotic, and the pseudo-psychopathic.

Kessler (1966) notes that general terms for childhood psychosis included schizophrenia (used by Bender and by Goldfarb), atypical child (Rank and Putnam's preferred term), and infantile psychosis. Among the more specific terms used to describe subcategories are autism (Kanner) and symbiosis (Mahler). The loose terminology continues to pose an obstacle to the undertaking of careful research in this field; some kind of terminological consensus is mandatory if the frontiers of knowledge are to be advanced. For purposes of discussion, this childhood disorder will be defined as a severe deviation in ego functioning which manifests itself in disordered thinking, affect, speech, perception, motility, and individuation (Committee on Child Psychiatry, 1966). In this chapter, we will restrict discussion to three forms of psychotic manifestation in children: childhood schizophrenia, infantile autism, and symbiotic psychosis.

INCIDENCE

As is true of most behavior disorders in children, it is extremely difficult to know the frequency of psychotic conditions in children. Estimates will be influenced by the definition used, the biases of the diagnostician, and the policies of the reporting agency. Despite the tremendous difficulties involved in obtaining epidemiological data, certain trends can be gleaned from available statistics. First, childhood psychoses appear to be relatively uncommon disorders. Data based on outpatient clinics in the United States for 1961 indicate that the rate is about 8 or 9 per 100,000 boys and just 3 per 100,000 girls in the age range 5 to 14 (Rosen, Bahn, & Kramer, 1964). Data based on first admissions to 284 state and county hospitals in the United States also reveal that childhood psychotics under 15 years of age constitute less than one-half of 1 per cent of all hospitalized patients (U.S. Dept. of HEW, 1964). Second, reported psychotic conditions in youth are most common during the 15–17 age range (23.6 per 100,000 males and 17.6 per 100,000 females) and least common in the category under 5 years of age (1.6 per 100,000 males and .7 per 100,000 females) (Rosen, Bahn, & Kramer, 1964). This increase during the stressful adolescent years is also reflected in data based on hospitalized patients (U.S. Dept. of HEW, 1964). For example, in 1964 there were less than 700 psychotic patients under

15 years of age in state and county hospitals, compared to more than 6,400 psychotic patients in the 15–24 age range. To some extent such increases may reflect a reduced parental tolerance as well as an inability to deal with serious overt pathology in older children, rather than an actual increase in incidence. It is doubtful, however, if such factors could account for the large differences reported above. Third, as the age trend implies, the frequency of psychotic conditions appears to be far higher in adults than in children. Finally, there are some interesting sex differences occurring with age. According to data based on state and county hospitals (U.S. Dept. of HEW, 1964) there were 2 females to every 3 male patients under 15 years of age, whereas there were 4 female patients to every 5 male patients in the 15–24 age range. Similarly, reports from community clinics (Rosen, Bahn, & Kramer, 1964) indicate that whereas the rates for psychotic youth under 18 years of age indicated a sex ratio of 3 boys to 1 girl, the rates in adulthood become equalized.

CHARACTERISTICS

CHILDHOOD SCHIZOPHRENIA

Childhood schizophrenia, a term generally reserved for psychotic disorders making their appearance after the first four or five years of life, manifests itself in many ways. The wide variety of symptomatology among children classified as schizophrenic has been very adequately described by Boatman and Szurek (1960), who list more than 100 different abnormal symptoms. The symptomatology apparently varies with the child's developmental level, the age of onset, the nature of early childhood experiences, and the type of defense mechanisms used (Rabinovitch, 1954). Despite the marked heterogeneity of symptomatology, there is a basic core disturbance, namely, the child's lack of contact with reality and his subsequent development of his own world. In addition to the central core disturbance, there are additional secondary characteristics, the major ones being represented in Kaufman's list of "clinical manifestations" (Kaufman et al., 1959):

1. Bizarre body movements, such as robotlike walking or fluid, graceful gyrations.

2. Repetitive, stereotyped motions, such as twirling objects and arm flapping.

3. Distorted use of body or body parts, such as the use of a body fragment to represent a totality or the use of the total body to represent a body part.

4. Conveying a nonhuman identity by posture, movement, or sound, for example, barking or rocking or calling oneself a windshield wiper.

5. Disturbances in speech structure and content, such as speaking in fragments of sentences; displaying asynchronism of affect, verbal content, and tone of voice; parroting; or expressing distorted identification by misuse of the personal pronouns.

6. Apparent denial of the human quality of people near one, such as attempting to use a nearby person as a stepladder when reaching for an object.

7. Inappropriate affect, ranging from flatness to explosiveness.

8. Hypertrophied interest in, or knowledge of, some special subject related to the child's pathology, such as detailed information of the city's transportation system.

9. Distorted time orientation, with a blending of past, present, and future; for example, the child may relate events which happened years ago such as his fantasied fears in a manner suggesting that they are part of his current existence.

In brief, it appears that a wide number of areas of development—cognition, perception, emotion, language, and physical motor—are impaired as a result of the child's basic disability. Since so many of these features are seen developmentally in children, it would be advisable to caution that probably no *one* of them is sufficient, in and of itself, to justify the label *psychosis*. Yet, since three of these characteristics—language disturbances, impaired interpersonal relationships, and inappropriate affect—appear so commonly in childhood schizophrenia, we will discuss them in greater detail in the sections that follow. Moreover, in keeping with the psychoeducational nature of this text, attention will also be focused on the classroom achievements of these atypical students.

Disturbed Language and Speech

One of the most widely noticed disturbances in childhood schizophrenia centers around the use of language and speech. Though there is a miscellany of linguistic distortions rather than a single pattern, the fact remains that many childhood schizophrenics do show peculiarities in this area. The language and speech disturbances are most likely symptomatic of fragmented and disintegrated thought processes. Consistent with this hypothesis is the finding that the presence of meaningful speech by age 5 is predictive of a more favorable later outcome. In an effort to uncover factors related to aberrant speech, Goldfarb, Goldfarb, and Scholl (1966) matched 23 schizophrenic children and their mothers with 23 normal children and their mothers. Comparisons of the speech and communicative abilities of the two groups supported the contention that mothers of schizophrenic children, as objects for emulation and as sources of reinforcement, constituted one factor in the production of aberrant language patterns in their offspring.

Some schizophrenic youngsters are mute or will only utter single words on rare occasions. For example, one schizophrenic boy in a state hospital would never say a word to anyone, although he would infrequently say an isolated word or two (*dog* or *blue*) when the teacher had her back turned. Those who do have speech often do not use it for communicative purposes. On the contrary, their idiosyncratic use of language commonly interferes with effective communication as much as it facilitates it. In fact, Kanner (1946) contends that their metaphorical language is designed to safeguard their autistic seclusion. Hence, language, instead of serving to maintain the child's contact with reality, enables him to become more detached.

Repetition of words in a parrotlike fashion is not uncommon. Obsessively focusing on certain events and evidencing this preoccupation verbally are another impressive feature often witnessed. Then again, language distortions sometimes manifest themselves in the development of a private language, with old words being given different meanings or with unusual word sequences being devised. Confusion in pronoun use, reflective of ego-identity problems, has also been noted. These youngsters not uncommonly refer to themselves as "you" and tend to avoid the use of "I." Play with words and sounds is seen in rhyming and alliterative speech.

In addition to an inability to use language as a means of effective interpersonal communication, speech disorders are often present. Goldfarb, Braunstein, and Lorgo (1956) reported on a study of speech disorders found in 12 schizophrenic children, based on clinicians' judgments after one year's observation of these children. Most characteristic of the speech problems noted was an absence of inflections, which resulted in a dull or wooden voice quality. Thus, whereas normals can effectively convey mood or emotion by means of their voices, many schizophrenic youngsters cannot. Nasality, denasality, breathiness, throatiness, and glottalization were also common. As has been noted by other clinicians, some schizophrenic children are characterized by very high-pitched voices. The authors recall one schizophrenic adolescent in a public-school class for the mentally retarded who would frequently talk in a high-pitched, squeaky voice, but who would return to a more normal pitch once he was instructed to "fix" his voice. Goldfarb and his associates (1956) also found that emphasis is placed on the syllables and words not essential to the meaning of the message. Further, there is little relationship between facial and body gestures on the one hand and spoken words on the other hand. In short, the individualized and sometimes bizarre patterns of language and speech result in an inability to use language for normal purposes of communication.

Impaired Interpersonal Relations

Impaired interpersonal relationships are also highly characteristic of the schizophrenic youngster. Whether this disability expresses itself in the form of an empty, symbiotic clinging or an autistic aloofness, a severe and enduring impairment of emotional interactions with other people is clearly evident. The symbiotic child, while attaching himself tenaciously to the mother, nonetheless manifests an absence of normal emotional relationships with others. Autistic youngsters, on the other hand, often give the impression that others are not around, reacting toward others as though they were inanimate parts of the surroundings. People seem to have little meaning for them. Their highly impersonal relations and aloneness have been described as "a noninvolvement" because of their nonresponsiveness to people.

In addition to the indifference and withdrawal which typify the schizophrenics' relations with adults as well as peers, their discomfort in the presence of others is seen in their inability to maintain eye contact with others. In marked contrast to their interpersonal isolation is their relationship with inanimate objects. One autistic child with whom the authors worked would invariably avoid contacts with others, remaining emotionally neutral in their presence. Furthermore, he would not associate with any agemates or adults in his cottage or classroom. Yet, when provided with tops or other objects to spin, he would immediately smile and show considerable fascination with the objects. Once the objects were put away, however, he quickly reverted to his characteristic state of detachment, manifesting no apparent positive affect. Selective reactions to his surroundings, as illustrated above, have led many clinicians to suspect that the autistic child, though conveying the impression that he is oblivious to his environment, is actually aware—perhaps painfully so—of what is happening around him.

Distorted Affect

Distortions of affect, while expressing themselves in a variety of ways, constitute another major symptom. The schizophrenic child may be extremely withdrawn or submissive at times and uncontrollably and viciously assaultive toward others and himself on other occasions. Seemingly insignificant changes in the routine or environment, which interfere with his rigid need for sameness, can precipitate excessive anxiety or rage. For example, certain schizophrenic youngsters sometimes become quite upset when they have a substitute teacher or when the classroom is rearranged.

Emotional expression, often described as flattened or wooden, becomes acutely heightened during the temper outbursts. The autistic child may show delight while watching a spinning object or spinning himself, but be emotionally neutral and noninvolved when adults or peers approach him. Teachers and parents often complain that they cannot reach these youngsters and that the children wall themselves off with their blank and unresponsive behavior.

Retarded Educational Performance

Another characteristic, one of central concern to teachers, has to do with the educational progress of such atypical pupils. That a large majority of schizophrenic children, whose contact with reality is markedly impaired, should experience difficulty in learning is not unexpected. Success in academic subjects, such as reading and arithmetic, requires concentration, assertiveness, and an interest in the external environment. Autistic withdrawal, individualized or idiosyncratic language patterns, and personal nonaccessibility—characteristics seen in varying degrees among most schizophrenic youngsters—obviously are not conducive to the effective utilization of a child's intellectual potential. Educational retardation is therefore a common finding in studies on schizophrenic children. From the standpoint of classroom performance, these atypical children often function much as educable mentally handicapped children do.

In certain instances, the teacher or psychologist may underestimate the academic accomplishments of a schizophrenic youngster because of his nonparticipation in classroom activities. Surprisingly, some schizophrenic pupils—despite their apparent unawareness of, noninvolvement in, or personal detachment from, the classroom environment —have mastered academic skills at their expected levels of achievement, as revealed by their performance on standardized achievement tests. This result often surprises teachers in that, although the child has mastered appropriate academic skills, he has not displayed any evidence of these accomplishments in his classroom performance. In other words, even though the pupil may have acquired skills at a level commensurate with his current level of mental ability, he fails to translate these learnings into meaningful classroom activities.

Schizophrenic youngsters sometimes mask their school learnings through the use of negativism. One 10-year-old schizophrenic girl, who was enrolled in a public-school class for the trainable mentally handicapped, would cooperate with the examining psychologist until she noticed that she was complying with his desires. At that point, she would become silent, pout, and sometimes lie on the floor, emitting guttural sounds. If coaxed or humored, she would read selections on a third-grade level during the testing, but in the special-class setting she gave no indication whatsoever of ability to read.

As is characteristic of their performance on psychological tests, the school performance of schizophrenic children is frequently erratic. They may on occasion successfully complete a complex academic assignment, only to fail simpler assignments. It is this kind of inconsistency which, in addition to frustrating or bewildering the teacher, alerts him to the fact that the child has more intellectual capacity than he is able to mobilize on any consistent basis.

While the majority of schizophrenic pupils are difficult for the teacher to reach, there are some who communicate verbally and who are more accessible. For this type of schizophrenic pupil, intellectual processes may be reasonably intact and academic accomplishment may well be commensurate with the expected level of achievement. In fact, some schizophrenic children may be precocious and mentally astute, excelling in abstract thinking and displaying special talents in language, graphic arts, and dancing. Hence, though the vast majority of schizophrenic children can be expected to encounter difficulty in school-learning activities, we should guard against the danger of overgeneralization and realize that some of these youngsters do learn despite their severe personality impairments.

INFANTILE AUTISM

While various workers differ in their classification of schizophrenic disturbances among children, two subcategories have received particular attention, namely, infantile autism and symbiotic psychosis. Early infantile autism was first described by Leo Kanner, when he reported the case histories of 11 youngsters whose behavioral abnormalities constituted a syndrome previously unknown (Kanner, 1944). The six characteristic features of this disturbance are (1) profound withdrawal of contact with other people, (2) an intense need to preserve the status quo, (3) skillful relationships with objects, as opposed to (4) an inability to deal with people, (5) an intelligent, pensive expression despite the extremely low level of intellectual functioning, and (6) severe disturbance of language functioning.

Because a primitive state of autism arises during the first three months of life, this disorder often goes unrecognized by the infant's parents. In fact, the infant is often viewed as quite healthy and alert in appearance. However, those experienced with babies may begin to notice signs of difficulty as early as the fourth month. From this point on, the severe symptomatology becomes more apparent. In addition to some of the characteristics mentioned above, there are persistent rocking motions and head banging. By the time the baby is 2 years old, the parents are typically quite concerned over the child's pattern of development, especially his self-insulation.

While Kanner views infantile autism as a variation of childhood schizophrenia, Rimland (1964) cogently argues that infantile autism is a unique disorder. He contends that the controversy surrounding these two disorders stems from (1) the infrequent incidence of autism so that many professional workers and writers have never encountered an authentic case, (2) the prevailing belief that childhood behavioral disturbances are psychological in nature, a belief which is somewhat incompatible with the specificity of this disorder (the more specific a given syndrome, the more some workers believe that it is physical in nature), and (3) the general inadequacy of current classification systems. Most European writers are in basic agreement with Rimland's position, which is based on a thorough review of current research.

After analyzing available evidence, Rimland postulated 15 points of contrast to discredit the view that infantile autism is simply one of the schizophrenias.

1. *Onset and Course.* The diagnosis of childhood schizophrenia involves symptoms occurring after a period of normal development, whereas symptoms of autism are present from the beginning of life. Evidence suggests that the autistic child remains unchanged in his early detachment, whereas a schizophrenic child eventually develops psychiatric symptomatology (delusions and hallucinations) of the adult schizophrenic.

2. *Health and Appearance.* Autistic children are routinely characterized by outstanding health, whereas schizophrenic children are typically characterized by "poor health from birth." Further, autistic children are often dark-complexioned and attractive in contrast to schizophrenic children, who are light-complexioned and thin.

3. *Electroencephalography.* Research indicates that more than 4 out of 5 schizophrenic youngsters have abnormal EEG recordings. Autistic children, on the other hand, tend to have normal EEG recordings.

4. *Physical Responsiveness.* Autistic children are generally physically unresponsive to adults, but schizophrenic children tend to mold themselves to adults.

5. *Autistic Aloneness.* The autistic child is known for his inability to adjust emotionally to adults. The schizophrenic child, however, is often far from being emotionally unresponsive and can elicit adult empathy.

6. *Preservation of Sameness.* This characteristic constitutes a cardinal symptom among autistic youngsters, but is uncommon among schizophrenic youngsters.

7. *Hallucinations.* There is an absence of hallucinatory activities in autistic children, whereas both visual and auditory hallucinations and delusional systems have been reported among schizophrenic children.

8. *Mode of Performance.* Autistic children appear to be much more skillful in gross and fine motor coordination than are schizophrenic children.

9. *Language.* Characteristic of autistic children, but not of schizo-

phrenic children, are the language patterns of affirmation by repetition, pronominal reversal, delayed echolalia, metaphoric language, and part-whole confusion.

10. *Idiot/Savant Performance.* Unusual abilities, such as phenomenal memories and musical and mechanical abilities, are frequently found in autistic children but only rarely in schizophrenics.

11. *Personal Orientation.* The autistic child seems to be more detached from, and indifferent to, his surroundings. Conversely, the schizophrenic seems more anxious and confused about his relationships to his surroundings. Whereas "frantic withdrawal and rejection" appear to describe the schizophrenic child's personal orientation, "aloneness and nonparticipation" seem to describe the autistic child's orientation.

12. *Conditionability.* For some unknown reason, schizophrenic children appear to condition much more rapidly than do autistic children.

13. *Twins.* Autism seems to be disproportionately more common in twins than is childhood schizophrenia. Furthermore, when schizophrenia does occur in twins, these sets usually assume the typical ratio of two or more dizygotic pairs for each monozygotic pair. Conversely, the preponderance of autistic twins are monozygotic.

14. *Family Background.* Parents of autistic youngsters are typically intellectual and highly educated, while parents of schizophrenic children are generally described as providing inadequate homes.

15. *Family Mental Disorder.* The families of autistic children (parents, grandparents, and siblings) appear to have a lower incidence of mental illness. The converse appears to be true of families of schizophrenics.

SYMBIOTIC PSYCHOSIS

Another commonly cited subcategory is that of symbiotic psychosis. This condition seems to have a later onset than autism, with symbiotic psychosis usually appearing between the ages of 2½ and 5. Kessler (1966) notes that symbiotic psychotics seem less strange than do autistic youngsters and they are frequently diagnosed as being borderline between neurosis and psychosis. An intensive case study will often reveal a normal accomplishment of developmental tasks followed by a regression at the time of a traumatic incident. The symptomatology associated with this disorder typically becomes apparent about the time the child fails to forgo the normal symbiotic relationship with his mother. With the advent of increased neuromuscular maturation, the normal child is able to separate himself from his mother and to distinguish between self and nonself. The symbiotic child's sense of differentiation remains in an infantile state, and he cannot function independently of the mother.

In psychoanalytic parlance, the child is unable to distinguish himself from his mother and he is living on a borrowed ego. Whereas the autistic child quickly avoids contact with people, the symbiotic child has an intense attachment to his mother from whom he cannot tolerate emotional separation. Mahler (1952), who first defined the syndrome, notes that intense anxiety is elicited by threatened separation from the mother. The child, through his symbiotic alignment with the mother, attempts to defend against the anxiety and insecurity associated with psychological differentiation. It is impossible, however, for the child to maintain an unthreatened relationship with his mother, for such events as the mother becoming ill or the birth of a sibling normally arise. The child is unable to fend against such traumas, however, and psychosis ensues.

Mahler, Furer, and Settlage (1959) list six primary symptoms of this disorder:

1. Panic reactions with violent rage.
2. Unpredictable outbursts of excitement and apparent pleasure, alternating with violence and destructiveness.
3. Confusion between inner and outer reality, a consequence of the fusion of self and nonself.
4. Inability to differentiate between animate and inanimate reality, and use of magical control over external stimuli.
5. A strong, but spurious, clinging attachment to adults.
6. Conspicuous presence of dereistic thinking, feeling, and acting.

Secondary symptoms develop as the psychosis lingers. These include panic in new situations, bizarre communication, and difficulties in habit-training areas. After a period of time, the symbiotic youngster often becomes indistinguishable from his autistic counterpart because of the similarity in symptomatology.

DIFFERENTIAL DIAGNOSTIC CONSIDERATIONS

As a general rule, a clinician relies on four sources of data in rendering a diagnosis of childhood psychosis: (1) case-history materials, (2) clinical observation, (3) medical findings, and (4) psychological test results. Differential diagnosis can be very difficult because the symptoms of psychotic conditions in children are sometimes similar to those of other aberrant conditions. It is extremely difficult and sometimes impossible to distinguish, for example, between a young mentally retarded child and an emotionally disturbed child who displays minimal speech and unresponsiveness to the environment. Another complex diagnostic problem is sometimes posed with respect to assessing the child's reality-testing. It is frequently no easy matter to distinguish between the active fantasy life characteristic of many young children with vivid imaginations and the blurring of reality characteristic of seriously impaired children. In such cases, there are no firm guidelines to follow. Rather, all of the adjustment characteristics, test data, and the history must be considered carefully. With somewhat older youth, the diagnosis of schizophrenia can frequently be made on the basis of pathological behavior which is more openly bizarre (White, 1964).

In essence, the diagnostic process is a sifting procedure in which the attempt is to rule out systematically those disorders with overlapping symptomatology. The disorders which most commonly require differentiation include mental retardation, brain damage, and severe personality disturbances. The problem of differentiation among the various classes of psychoses in children has been handled earlier in the chapter and, hence, will not be repeated here. In sorting out childhood psychoses, diagnosticians would do well to bear in mind the axiom that it is the entire diagnostic picture rather than a single pathological feature which differentiates the psychotic condition from other conditions.

MENTAL RETARDATION

Mental retardation is one condition for which childhood psychosis is sometimes mistaken. As noted earlier in the chapter, the severely disturbed child often functions below grade level, as does the mentally retarded child. In terms of their everyday academic performance, many disturbed children operate on a level much like that of a mentally retarded child. Such poor academic performance often raises questions in the teacher's and psychologist's minds as to the child's intellectual inadequacy.

Since many psychotic children do score in the defective range on intelligence tests, it sometimes happens that they are hospitalized and mistaken for mental retardates. One youngster, for example, spent eight years in a state hospital before it was realized that he was not mentally retarded. He was admitted at age 4 with a reported IQ score of 35 on the Stanford-Binet, a measuring scale which requires considerable verbal facility. Later measures, based on nonverbal tests of intellectual ability, revealed that he was essentially of normal intelligence.

Intelligence quotients, per se, are often not as useful as might be inferred from the case described, since youngsters characterized by both conditions often score below the average range. What clinicians regard as more revealing are the intratest variations and the quality of the subject's responses. For diagnostic purposes, it is sometimes helpful to distinguish between inconsistent and consistent unevenness of performance. On the one hand, clues as to hidden intellectual potential will often be suggested by inconsistent performance on a test of intelligence. The child may, for example, miss the answer to a simple question only to answer a much more difficult question of a similar nature. Such inconsistency would lead the teacher or clinician to suspect that the child might not be mentally retarded, as his over-all IQ score suggested. The presence of consistent unevenness, on the other hand, might lead one to suspect that a child is not emotionally disturbed, since emotionally based disturbances in thinking might occur on any type of test at any time rather than being restricted to specific mental functions (Des Lauriers & Halpern, 1947). In other words, consistent patterns of deviation and performance may lead one to suspect conditions like brain damage and mental retardation. Piotrowski (1937) found, for example, that schizophrenic children (aged 5 to 16), in contrast to high-grade congenitally defective children, consistently obtained higher scores on verbal tests than on nonverbal tests. Analysis of the answers given to specific items is also warranted because the nature of some responses not uncommonly conveys the bizarre thought disorders associated with psychotic conditions in children.

For purposes of differential diagnosis, clinicians generally regard projective techniques as being more useful than IQ tests. With the use of projective techniques, incoherence, contradictions, unusual verbalizations, and neologisms have been reported as characteristic of thought disorganization among psychotic children (Leitch & Schafer, 1947). The Rorschach Inkblot Test has revealed that the perceptual difficulties, poor reality-testing, lack of stable self-concept, and absence of meaningful identifications are common responses for schizophrenic children (Halpern, 1960).

Case-history materials and clinical observations are also helpful in distinguishing a mentally deficient child from a psychotic youngster. Children with infantile autism can be distinguished from mental retardates by virtue of their good intellectual potential—excellent memories and musical abilities—and certain physical characteristics— graceful movements and the absence of a dull appearance (Rimland, 1964). Moreover, the isolation, aloneness, and detachment typical of the autistic child stand in contrast to the repetitive activities of the retarded child (Kanner, 1949).

Though we have stressed how childhood psychoses can be mistaken for mental retardation, the reverse situation can also obtain, especially in those mentally retarded children who have met with severe sensory and social isolation and intense parental rejection. It must also be noted that some children can be both mentally retarded and psychotic.

BRAIN DAMAGE

Organic impairments constitute another set of conditions which sometimes simulate psychoses in children, especially with respect to young children having organically based language disorders. Isolated from others by their lack of communicative ability, these youngsters may develop an autistic-like existence of their own and thereby pose a particularly difficult diagnostic puzzle. Again, four kinds of evidence are helpful in rendering a differential diagnosis:

1. *Psychological tests,* especially those designed to measure specific mental functions, such as visual-motor coordination, can be informative, particularly when integrated with case-history material and clinical observation. One of the best-known tests for organic brain damage is the Bender Gestalt Test, which samples the child's ability to reproduce geometric figures. Intelligence tests like the Wechsler Intelligence Scale for Children and projective techniques like the Rorschach Inkblot Test have also been used to detect organic brain damage. Though sometimes helpful in individual cases, these tests certainly cannot be regarded as an open sesame to differential diagnosis.

2. *Medical tests* can be helpful in individual cases. By and large, however, their validity is probably overestimated by nonmedical

people. For example, Shaw (1966), a psychiatrist, notes that the electroencephalograph, which is one of the most common medical tools, is of "little or no value" in the diagnosis of brain damage in children.

3. *Case-history materials* often supply evidence suggestive of organic involvement. Obstetrical complications, aftereffects of childhood illnesses, head injuries, and prolonged high fevers are typical of information gleaned from a case history which can have relevance to differential diagnosis. Again, however, such evidence is rarely conclusive.

4. *Clinical observation* is quite revealing, generally speaking. Both the brain-injured child and the psychotic child may be hyperactive and distractible, but of diagnostic significance is the marked difference in how youngsters with these two conditions relate to others and organize their worlds of experience.

ETIOLOGICAL CONSIDERATIONS

Questions pertaining to the issue of etiology have met with a diversity of professional opinions. Although workers no longer view the causes of psychoses in children as strictly dichotomous, we will for purposes of discussion represent viewpoints as falling into two categories: the psychogenic and the somatogenic. Incidentally, it is interesting to note that even though many of the early workers were reluctant to admit the possibility of insanity in children, most of the probable causes of psychoses in children had already been discussed by 1900.

THE PSYCHOGENIC VIEW

Parent-Child Relations

In the early part of this century, emphasis was placed on the role played by congenital factors in the production of childhood schizophrenia. However, the advent of Freud's psychodynamic position ushered in a new era, stressing the role of parental attitudes as determinants of childhood psychopathology (Gianascol, 1963). Early workers, including Jung, Sullivan, Brill, and Klein, also implicated parental psychopathology as having a causal role. In recent years, mothers have been indicted to such an extent that a new term was coined—the schizophrenogenic mother—to indicate their causal role.

Two workers who are particularly well known for their descriptions of the parents of autistic children are Kanner and Eisenberg. The parents of autistic youngsters, according to these authors, are cold, distant, intelligent, sophisticated, obsessional, and highly impersonal and mechanistic in their life adjustments. Lacking in emotional warmth, they are said to rear their children in "emotional iceboxes." On the basis of their clinical experience and research with such youngsters, these authors concluded that autism stems from an innate inability to relate to people which is adversely influenced by the attributes of their parents.

In one particular study of 100 fathers of autistic youngsters, Eisenberg (1957) found that, in 85, there were serious personality difficulties which adversely influenced the fulfillment of a normal father-child relationship. This study suggests that consideration must be given to paternal as well as maternal inadequacies and also lends support to a psychodynamic explanation of schizophrenia. It should be noted, however, that other investigators have found that more than 15 per cent of parents are not of the "refrigerator" variety noted above. Bender and Grugett (1956), for example, point out the diversity of personalities among parents of such atypical youngsters. We must also remember that there are many frigid parents who do not produce schizophrenic children.

A revealing study by Klebanoff (1959), investigating the relationship between parental attitudes and childhood schizophrenia, indicates the need for a more cautious and careful appraisal of cause-effect relationships. Hypothesizing that parental attitudes might be the result rather than the cause of childhood schizophrenia, the investigator administered a parental-attitude questionnaire to 15 mothers of hospitalized schizophrenics, 15 mothers of hospitalized mentally deficient and brain-injured children, and 26 mothers of normal youngsters. Although there were differences in educational level among the mothers, the three groups were matched on age, religion, and socioeconomic status. The results showed that the mothers of schizophrenic children had less deviant attributes than did the mothers of the brain-injured and retarded children. This finding suggested that parents who have children with severe clinical conditions developed faulty child-rearing attitudes and practices as a consequence of their having to manage and care for difficult children and that their faulty attitudes did not cause the disability. The finding illustrates the complexities and the pitfalls involved in a search for causes.

Family Relations

In recent years, attention has shifted from the schizophrenogenic mother to the schizophrenogenic family as a unit of study. While there have been many investigations contributing to the analysis of family interaction patterns and their relationships to schizophrenia, three groups have been particularly influential in shaping the course of current opinion and research (Mischler & Waxler, 1965).

1. Lidz and Fleck (1960) contend that it is not the individual characteristics of the parents which create conditions conducive to schizophrenia, but the conditions of strife characterizing the family which are responsible. According to these theorists, there is a blurring of the age-sex structures in the family which prevents the child from learning appropriate forms of behavior. In other words, the child does not learn to behave appropriately because the parents themselves behave inappropriately for their age and sex with regard to each other and to the child. This theory depicts two types of family pathology patterns: the skewed and the schism. In the marital schism pattern there is chronic strife, discord, and threat of separation. Neither problems nor satisfactions are shared. The work of one partner is frequently devalued to the child by the other partner, and there is competition for the child's loyalty. This pattern has been found to be related empirically to the development of schizophrenia in male children. In the marital skewed pattern, the conflict is less open. While the marital relationship is not threatened, family life is dominated by the psychopathology of one partner over the other. This latter type of deviant family interaction has been found to be associated empirically with schizophrenia in female children. In brief, both types of environments expose the · child to a family irrationality which hinders the growth of a healthy ego.

2. The double-bind theory has been developed by Bateson, Weakland, and Haley. The basic ingredients of the double-bind situation are (1) an intense interpersonal relationship, (2) conflicting communications, and (3) an individual who is unable to comment on the message so as to clarify its meaning (Weakland, 1960). The child, dependent on the parent, has to try to make reasonable responses to the confused communications which he receives. The child's situation

is rendered more difficult in that he is not allowed to question a message or show that he perceives the inadequacy of the communications. With repeated exposures to such irrationality, the child either fails to develop or loses his hold on a rational existence. An experiment by Berger (1965) found that a 30-item scale designed to reveal inconsistency of the sort described by the double-bind hypothesis did differentiate between normals and schizophrenics. However, only 5 of the 30 items discriminated between schizophrenics and a maladjusted, nonschizophrenic group. These data would seem to suggest that the double-bind situation can lead to other forms of maladjustment besides schizophrenia.

3. The last of the family-interaction theories is Wynne's, which stresses the role of ego functioning as a link between the individual and the culture. The prerequisite for the formation of a healthy ego and adequate identification, according to Wynne and Singer (1963), is a stable and coherent environment which provides opportunities to reality-test a variety of roles during the course of development. That is, the healthy, well-organized ego requires a stable environment to test various roles. Families of schizophrenics, however, lack both of these attributes: stability and coherency. The instabilities at home, together with the too loose or too rigid or too ambiguous role relationships, hinder the development of a stable personal identity. In brief, the thought disturbances typically associated with schizophrenia are thought to be the consequence of disordered patterns of family interaction.

While it certainly seems reasonable that early experiences, especially those in the home, lead to the development of learned behavior patterns, normal as well as abnormal, a critical review of the research literature conducted over the past forty years has failed to uncover factors in parent-child relationships which can be identified as unique to the parents of psychotic children (Frank, 1965). Whether this finding is due to the absence of specific patterns or of inadequate research remains to be seen, but all of the theories of family interaction discussed above have yet to explain why some children who are exposed to the postulated pathological conditions fail to become schizophrenics. Moreover, we may ask why some children exposed to these particularly deviant family situations do not become neurotic delinquents instead of psychotics. Many questions remain to be answered; yet, in all fairness, it should be noted that these theories have served to alert us to what might be significant phenomena in family life which had been neglected by other theorists and researchers (Mischler & Waxler, 1965).

Learning Theory

Ferster (1961), using learning concepts, has offered a clear conceptualization of infantile autism. He attributes the two major and related characteristics of this disorder—limited responsiveness to social control and deficient linguistic facility—to parent-child interactions. In developing his theory, Ferster advances the notion of a critical age period, 1½ to 4, in the development of this severe ego disturbance. He reasons that parents, as the primary socialization agents, can readily extinguish the development of normal behaviors and positively reinforce the development of deviant behaviors by virtue of the amount of control they have over the child at this stage of life.

In an effort to answer the question as to what specific circumstances promote autism, Ferster examined parental behaviors which might be instrumental in this respect. He hypothesized that the inadequate speech development so characteristic of the autistic child has its origins in the absence of a positively reinforcing environment. The parents are described by Ferster as concerned with their own interests (for example, telephone conversations) and problems (for example, somatic complaints) to a degree that interference by the child in their daily affairs rapidly acquires an aversive quality. The parents, in an effort to minimize the child's nuisance value, ignore him whenever possible. The parent may respond to the child's verbal demands (for example, "Give me an apple"), but pays little attention to the child's other uses of language, such as description (for example, "Here comes the milkman"). If valid, this formulation helps to explain why language, when used by the autistic child, often takes the form of requests related to some deprivation (for example, "Candy"). Under such conditions, the child never learns to respond to the more verbal social reinforcers (for example, "Good boy"). Instead, he continues to respond to the more concrete rewards associated with the satisfaction (reduction) of his own primary needs, such as hunger and thirst. This hypothesis might well explain an observation based on therapeutic experience with psychotic children, namely, that the therapist must be directly useful to the child by providing immediate and material satisfactions (Kessler, 1966).

Since the child living under these conditions has no socially accept-able means of gaining attention, he resorts to temper tantrums, self-destructive activities, and other atavistic forms of behavior which the parent then, in turn, positively reinforces with personal attention. As a consequence of such child-rearing conditions, the child develops an narrow behavioral repertoire, meager linguistic facility, and only a limited responsiveness to social control; that is, he develops a syn-drome called autism.

THE SOMATOGENIC VIEW[1]

Evidence supporting the psychogenic viewpoint is not so conclusive as to rule out the possibility of a biological basis for psychotic condi-tions in children. In fact, despite the absence of crucial research data, most experienced workers seem to favor a constitutional viewpoint of etiology. As Shaw (1966) notes, many psychotic youngsters come from reasonably healthy and normal environments which could not have conceivably produced such severe disturbances. He also questions whether such "total absence of the integrative function of the nervous system" could be a learned phenomenon. Rimland (1964), in a similar vein, has advanced a neurological theory of infantile autism in which the basic disorder is related to the reticular formation of the brain stem.

One of the strongest proponents of the constitutional viewpoint is Loretta Bender. She regards childhood schizophrenia as a maturational lag which begins during the embryonic period. Maturational regulari-ties are upset with precocious development in some areas and obvious retardation in other areas. Because of the organic involvement of the central nervous system, the child is unable to organize his expe-riences in an orderly fashion. Although Bender regards the predisposi-tion toward childhood schizophrenia as hereditary in nature, she views the schizophrenic reaction itself as being precipitated by a physiological crisis, such as a trauma in the prenatal period, at birth, or during infancy. Studies on schizophrenic children do reveal de-ficiencies in activities related to nervous-system functioning, for

---

[1]In this section, no attempt has been made to report evidence pertaining to the role of biochemical research in schizophrenia. For a concise review of biochemical factors, see S. Kety, Current biochemical research in schizophrenia. In P. Hoch & J. Zubin (Eds.), *Psychopathology of schizophrenia.* New York: Grune & Stratton, 1966. Pp. 225-232.

example, visual-motor perception. Whether these deficiencies constitute an explanation of schizophrenia or are simply part of an elaborated secondary symptom complex is not altogether clear at this time.

Kallmann's (1938, 1956) research has provided perhaps the most commonly cited evidence supporting a genetic basis for schizophrenia. Studying the blood kin of all schizophrenics admitted to a Berlin hospital between 1893 to 1902, with followup to 1929, he found that:

1. Schizophrenia occurs in less than 1 per cent of the general population. If one parent is schizophrenic, however, the same disorder develops in about one-sixth of the offspring. If both parents are schizophrenic, more than two-thirds of the offspring are similarly affected.

2. Similar results were obtained for siblings of the patients. Schizophrenia was found in 85 per cent of the cases where the sibling was an identical twin of the patient, in about 15 per cent of fraternal twins and full siblings, and in about 7 per cent of half-siblings.

More recent data, based on 57 pairs of twins, one of whom was diagnosed as schizophrenic, likewise indicated a strong genetic basis. When an identical twin was schizophrenic, the other twin was found to be 42 times more likely to become schizophrenic than was an individual from the general population. With fraternal twins of the same sex, if one was schizophrenic, the other was at least 9 times as likely to develop schizophrenia as was someone from the general population (Gottesman & Shields, 1966).

Many psychologists and geneticists do not view schizophrenia as directly inherited in the same sense that eye color is inherited. Rather, they assume that some predisposing factor is inherited which renders the individual susceptible to environmental insult and to the subsequent development of particular sets of reactions. According to this view, the person would not develop the disorder unless exposed to damaging experiences. Most workers, including those who question the extent of genetic involvement, as implied by the studies discussed above, do concede that there is an inherited predisposition to this disorder. The method of inheritance is not understood, although it seems likely that the disturbance is polygenically based. Whether this predisposition takes the form of an innate, unresponsive passivity or a heightened sensitivity to fear and pain is still a moot issue.

Those who favor a more environmental viewpoint argue, with

some validity, that the finding of schizophrenia among other family members does not constitute conclusive evidence for a genetically based disorder, since twins, especially identical twins, have very similar learning environments. Unfortunately there have been very few recorded cases of schizophrenic twins who have been reared apart. Consequently, we lack studies which might provide more crucial evidence on this point. A further theoretical difficulty inheres in the fact that no one has yet identified the physical anomaly which is presumably inherited and which accounts for the genetic effects. Until such evidence is forthcoming, the genetic explanation of schizophrenia will remain a supposition, albeit a potentially fruitful one for future research.

THE MULTIPLE-CAUSATION VIEW

Some authorities do not conceive of childhood schizophrenia as a single entity which can be attributed to a single cause. Goldfarb (1961), rather than postulating a single cause, proposes a continuum of causal factors ranging from the purely somatic to the purely psychogenic. Thus, this worker, who prefers to classify childhood schizophrenia on the basis of etiology as well as on overt symptomatology, believes that such profound ego impairments can arise from organic inadequacies in the child or from psychosocial inadequacies in family relations.

Goldfarb's research with 26 schizophrenic children admitted for residential treatment lends support to his contention that organic and nonorganic subgroups do exist. Reasoning analogously, he argues that childhood schizophrenia, like mental retardation, can be the result of either hereditary or environmental factors or varied combinations thereof. It would certainly be premature at this time to accept his notions on etiology. Yet, his reasoning carries considerable appeal as it seems to reflect the complex realities of clinical experiences. Other theorists, while giving lip service to the role of dual etiological factors, tend to place greater emphasis on either one or the other in explaining all cases of childhood schizophrenia.

TREATMENT APPROACHES

The numerous approaches to the treatment of psychotic children have run the gamut from psychotherapy to physical therapy. By and large, the particular treatment approach is related to the clinician's view of etiology. Generally speaking, if the condition is regarded as psychogenic in nature, then psychological interventions will be prescribed. Conversely, if the condition is regarded as somatogenic in nature, then a variety of physical interventions might be attempted. Treatment plans, of necessity, are always contingent upon the facilities accessible. The available care plans may vary from weekly outpatient sessions to day-care centers to residential treatment centers, depending on the severity of the condition, the nature of the home environment, and the philosophy of treatment facilities. In the section which follows, we will discuss philosophies of and attempts at psychotherapeutic interventions with psychotic children. In the following sections, behavioristic approaches, educational therapies, residential treatment, and physiological interventions will be reviewed.

PSYCHOTHERAPEUTIC APPROACHES

Individual Therapy

By way of introduction, it may be instructive to see what happens to such atypical youngsters when they are referred to community agencies. In a study conducted by Bahn, Chandler, and Eisenberg (1962), data from 50 mental-health centers in Maryland were used to assess the degree to which psychiatric classification was a practically significant variable in determining the course of community clinic services for 5,000 child patients seen during an 18-month period (July 1958 through December 1959). The following findings pertain to child services afforded psychotic children by psychiatric clinics in the community:

1. Of four psychiatric classifications—neuroses, transient situational disorders, psychoses, and personality disorders—children with psychotic conditions (the most severe of emotional disorders) had the second-shortest clinic stay. Only those children with personality disorders were seen for a shorter period of treatment.

2. Psychotic children were the least likely of these four groups to receive outpatient treatment. Only 1 in 5 such youngsters was given outpatient treatment. Since these children had such a guarded prognosis, many community agencies (which can offer only limited help) declined to accept them. Typically, this diagnosis led to hospital referral. In fact, more than 1 in 2 were referred to mental hospitals. There were no immediate plans made for the future in 7 per cent of the cases.

3. This diagnosis was associated with the poorest rate of improvement. Despite the fact that only 1 of 5 was chosen for outpatient treatment, there were two unimproved patients for each improved patient. Such data convey the severity or seriously incapacitating nature of this disorder.

Mahler, Furer, and Settlage (1959) are quite specific with regard to therapeutic goals with psychotic children: (1) to establish greater body integrity and a sense of identity, (2) to develop object relationships, and (3) to restore missing or distorted maturational and developmental ego functions. These goals are accomplished by having the child go through the stages of normal development which he has missed. The therapist provides the child with a substitute ego, thus helping the child to progress through the autistic, symbiotic, and separation-individuation phases. The therapist helps to shelter the child from realities which may be too harsh. Yet, he assists the child in understanding various aspects of reality, such as body functions and social relationships. He also sets firm limits on destructive behaviors.

Individual treatment is seen by Mahler as a preferred method of treatment with autistic children. The detached autistic child who shies away from personal contacts must be drawn out and helped to test reality through the provision of satisfying, pleasurable forms of stimulation. Caution must be exercised against hastening reality contacts, however, lest the child be thrown into a state of panic and further withdrawal.

The symbiotic child, on the other hand, can benefit from the educational therapy afforded by the residential treatment school. Since he needs diversified parent substitutes to counteract his pathological attachment to the mother, the symbiotic child is given support by the numerous adults with whom he interacts in the residential treatment center. Only through living on the borrowed ego strength of other adults can he eventually develop sufficient ego strengths of his own. Although the child may come to function on a higher level, Mahler is quite pessimistic regarding the prospects for attaining a normal adjustment.

Bender, an advocate of the genetic viewpoint, suggests psychotherapy as an aid in adjusting to internal and external pressures. The child is helped to develop a tolerance for disturbance stemming from his basic disorder (Bender & Guerevitz, 1955). The formation of active defense mechanisms is supported, clearer conceptions of his body image and identity are attempted, and more effective relations to people and objects are sought (Bender, 1960). In brief, psychotherapy is designed to enable the child to live more effectively with the results of his genetically based disturbance by relieving anxiety, supporting ego defense mechanisms, and stimulating maturational processes (Bender, 1947).

Group Therapy

Group therapy has been used not only with parents of schizophrenic children to help them overcome such feelings as guilt, despair, and resentment, but also with schizophrenic children themselves. In one study (Speers & Lansing, 1964), group-therapy procedures were used with preschool autistic youngsters and their parents. The early results indicated that the children became more withdrawn as a consequence of their association with other atypical children. Panic reactions were evident and biting would sometimes occur. One interesting technique involved giving mirrors to individual children so that they might watch others in the group by turning the mirror at an angle and also alleviate anxiety over their own self-images by looking at themselves in the mirror occasionally. The investigators noted that the addition of a new child to the group often served as a catalyst for group formation, for the original group members then had a common enemy against whom they could unite. Gradually, with the passage of time, structured play activities became possible, speech became more communicative, children became capable of following directions, and established group members helped control the panic reactions of new members. In addition to the group-therapy sessions, considerable attention was given to these youngsters by staff nurses, psychologists, and occupational and recreational therapists. Prior to this experiment it was commonly believed that the treatment of young psychotic children must be restricted to individual treatment sessions.

Another study (Lifton & Smolen, 1966) also suggested the feasibility of group therapy with child schizophrenics. Basing treatment on the premise that childhood schizophrenia is a severe, multiply caused ego disturbance, the therapist assisted the children by explaining the child's behavior to him and by preventing self-destructive activities as well as activities harmful to others. Praise was given for improvements in social behavior. Warmth and personal support were available when needed. Higher levels of ego integration were achieved, withdrawal and isolation tendencies lessened, and bizarre behavior and irrational thought processes decreased. The authors were careful to point out, however, that the greatest behavioral changes occurred in children whose egos were most intact prior to treatment. Treatment was least successful with the very young severely disturbed children.

Parental Involvement

We again encounter divergent viewpoints when we broach the topic of parental involvement. Some therapists insist that the parents become involved in therapy on either an individual or a group basis before the child will be accepted for treatment. Mahler (1965), who stresses the importance of the child's symbiotic relationship to the mother, for instance, tries to treat mother and child simultaneously. Even Bender, who sees childhood schizophrenia as an essentially biological disorder, stresses the need for group-therapy sessions with parents to help them become more effective in dealing with their children's problems. In contrast, Bettelheim (1950) prefers not to deal with parents. He states that he has had little luck working with these parents and advocates that the child be separated from the home situation.

General Effectiveness and Prognosis

Of all the behavior disorders which children manifest, perhaps none has a more uniformly unfavorable prognosis than that of childhood psychosis. The only other severe disorder which rivals childhood psychosis in this regard is that of the sociopathic personality. Even the educable mentally retarded child seems to fare far better in adult life than does the childhood schizophrenic. Though some improvements in behavior are noted over time, the outlook for the schizophrenic child remains a gloomy one. The large majority of such youngsters will never live full, normal lives. In general, the research indicates that the probabilities of remission are at best 1 in 4.

A major longitudinal study was conducted by Bender and Freedman (1952) on 120 schizophrenic children seen at the Children's Psychiatric Service at Bellevue. Only a small segment of these youngsters, whose ages ranged from 3 to 11 at the time of initial diagnosis and from 17 to 26 at the time of followup, were found to be making an adequate adjustment to early adulthood. More than three-fourths were hospitalized in state institutions for the mentally ill or mentally defective. Less than one-fourth were living in the community, and even among these more than half were probably still schizophrenic.

Bennett and Klein (1966), who conducted one of the longest followup studies, examined 14 cases of childhood schizophrenia 30 years later; 4 of the subjects could not be located for additional study. These workers found that in adult life only 1 of the 14 was able to maintain himself outside of a hospital setting and 9 were in institutions. Of the institutionalized cases, 2 were at the same level of dysfunction and 7 had severely regressed.

Eisenberg (1956) followed the later adjustment of 80 autistic children seen at Johns Hopkins Children's Psychiatric Service. Of the 63 who were traced, he classified 46 of these youngsters as achieving a poor adjustment, 14 as having a fairly adequate adjustment, and only 3 as achieving a good adjustment. By combining these last two categories, we see that only 1 in 4 achieved a reasonably normal adjustment. Rimland (1964) states that no form of psychiatric treatment has been known to alter the course of autism.

Bettelheim (1967) is certainly one of the most optimistic authorities when it comes to the treatability of autistic youngsters. His views, which stand in sharp contrast to those of other experts on this topic, are based on the outcomes of 40 autistic youngsters treated at his Orthogenic School in Chicago. Applying Eisenberg's categories, 17 (42 per cent) were rated as having achieved a good adjustment, 15 (37 per cent) as having a fair adjustment, and only 8 (20 per cent) as having a poor adjustment. Differences between these findings and those of other studies were attributed by Bettelheim to the intensity of treatment given. He argues that infantile autism can be influenced by therapy if treatment efforts are sufficiently intense. Bettelheim stresses that it takes the schizophrenic child about as many years to recover as it requires for the average child to develop his personality, that is, some two to four years of uninterrupted living in an environment conducive to autonomous personality development.

Bettelheim aside, most authorities who have worked with psychotic children contend that psychotherapeutic treatment efforts have not cured the disordered thought processes which constitute the chief disturbance in these atypical children. While the child remains psychotic, much can be done to improve his adjustment, however. Ego disturbances that so seriously impair several aspects of functioning with their early onset in life appear to be long-lasting and severe in nature.

Certain specific behaviors, especially language, seem to be related to prognosis. Eisenberg (1956), for example, noted that the presence or absence of speech by age 5 was the most critical factor in forecasting the child's status in later life. Of those who had useful speech by age 5, half achieved a reasonably normal adjustment in adolescence. Conversely, of those 31 schizophrenic youngsters characterized by mutism at age 5, only 1 achieved a fair or good adjustment. In a later study, Brown (1963) also cited severe language impairments among schizophrenic children as predictive of poor later adjustment. Her data, however, suggested a cutoff age of 3 instead of 5 as suggested by Eisenberg's data.

While the findings differ as to the age of demarcation, perhaps because of differences in severity among the samples studied, it appears that adequate language usage during the preschool period is highly prodromal of adequate social adjustment in cases of childhood schizophrenia. In addition to basic language disturbances, Brown also found that inability to use objects for their intended purposes or functions, repetitive motoric play, and severe autism were associated with later adjustment difficulties. On the other hand, an expression of interest in one's surroundings, effective communication, and directed aggression were disclosed to be signs associated with a more favorable outcome.

Psychotherapy is a particularly slow and difficult process with psychotic children. Frequently they have difficulty in forming a close tie with the therapist because of their severe disturbances in ego functioning. Progress is often discouraging, and the dividends in improvement minimal in contrast to the patience, effort, and time invested. Yet, there appears to be an increasing consideration among clinicians of the role psychotherapy can play in the treatment of these children (Ekstein, Bryant, & Friedman, 1958). In the next section, we will discuss some of the more recent efforts stemming from learning theory which hold promise.

BEHAVIOR-MODIFICATION APPROACHES

As is evident from the foregoing, psychotic conditions in children have not proved amenable to traditional forms of psychotherapeutic interventions. A recent and radically different treatment approach which has stimulated interest, especially among psychologists, is that of behavior therapy. Rooted in Pavlovian classical conditioning and in various schools of learning theory which have since emerged, behavioristic therapy involves the application of learning-theory principles to the modification of behavior. The term *behavior therapy,* as such, refers more to an approach than to any particular technique. As a part of experimental psychology, behavioristic treatment has been applied to the alteration of extremely inappropriate behaviors, including those typically found in child psychotics. In this section, we will illustrate the general approach of behavior therapy as used in the treatment of childhood psychoses, and we will sample representative research studies.

The Use of Reinforcement

It was Skinner (1953) who provided the impetus for treating schizophrenic children by reinforcement techniques devoid of verbal instruction. Ferster (1961) later offered a conceptual analysis of childhood schizophrenia couched in a learning-theory framework. Ferster, in collaboration with his colleague DeMyer (Ferster & DeMyer, 1962), was successful in managing and expanding the behavioral repertoire of autistic youngsters in a controlled laboratory setting.

Additional research by Hingtgen, Sanders, and DeMyer (1963) indicated that social responses in a schizophrenic child can be shaped by making reinforcement contingent upon interpersonal associations. These investigators used 6 childhood schizophrenics, aged 3 through 8, who had not previously interacted socially with their peers. They were trained to operate a lever which released coins which could then be spent in vending machines for treats such as candy and food. Subjects were paired and given 30-minute training sessions daily. After an average of 23 training sessions, the results indicated that it was possible to establish social interactions between psychotic children by using the method of successive approximations—a procedure whereby approximations of the desired response are shaped gradually. The frequency of physical contacts between children (though not directly reinforced) increased, and both vocal responses and facial expressions directed toward partners were noted. This study and a later one (Hingtgen & Trost, 1966) suggested the feasibility of positive reinforcement as a therapeutic intervention technique designed to increase the social and vocal behavior repertoire of young schizophrenic children.

We, the authors, would be remiss in our duties if we failed to report the experimental studies done by Ivar Lovaas and his associates on childhood schizophrenia. One of the studies (Lovaas et al., 1963) dealt with the effects of presenting and withdrawing social reinforcers on the deeply ingrained self-destructive tendencies of a 9-year-old schizophrenic child. In addition to the self-destructive behaviors, self-stimulatory activities and stereotypic interactions with inanimate objects also constituted a major part of this child's behavior patterns. To minimize external distractions, therapy sessions were conducted in a room containing only tables and objects. Through the use of social reinforcements such as smiling and verbal approval, this 9-year-old girl was taught over a two-month interval certain physical responses, such as dancing and clapping her hands to music. During the period which followed, the acquired behaviors were extinguished by withdrawing reinforcement. Following this extinction period, successive acquisitions and withdrawal procedures were repeated. The researchers noted that self-injurious activities occurred when approval for physical responses was withdrawn. Similarly, musical behavior response was minimal when the self-injurious behaviors were at a peak.

The Use of Punishment

The use of mild punishment in conjunction with the use of positive reinforcement is also receiving considerable attention in the literature. Whereas punishment as a behavioral technique has been traditionally conceived as applicable primarily to acting-out behavior, this therapeutic technique has also been extended to extremely withdrawn youngsters, as is exemplified in the research by Lovaas and his associates (1965) on a schizophrenic girl who was administered mild electric shocks when she became uncontrollable. Being barefooted, she was given mild shocks through the floor when she began to stare bizarrely at her hand instead of attending to her reading assignment. After the shock, the teacher would then insist that the girl continue with her reading. After a while, the girl would again become unmanageable, and another mild jolt of electricity was administered. The verbal response "No" was paired with the presentation of the punishment in the hope that she would eventually be able to respond to the verbal stimulus alone. Lovaas and his associates (1966) have also conditioned autistic children to approach adults in order to avoid a painful electric shock.

As noted above, punishment has been most commonly used to combat hostile, antisocial behavior. One team of investigators (Wolf, Risley, & Mees, 1964) found a combination of mild punishment and extinction effective in alleviating certain annoying behaviors in a preschool psychotic boy. Among the target behaviors selected for modification were his bedtime difficulties, eating problems, and the throwing of his corrective lenses. His resistance at bedtime was handled by leaving the bedroom door open as long as he would remain in bed. When he got out of bed, however, he was instructed to return to his bed or told that the door would be closed. If he did not comply, the mild aversive consequence, namely, closing the door, was enforced. After the sixth night of such treatment, the boy seldom posed bedtime difficulties during the rest of his stay in the hospital or at home following his discharge.

This same boy's eating habits also posed problems for the staff. He would take food from other children's plates, refuse to use silverware, and commonly throw his food around the dining room. These problems were handled by removing his plate for a few minutes whenever he ate with his fingers and by removing him from the room whenever he snatched food from others or tossed his food about. After a few warnings and actual removal from the dining room, the boy's food-stealing and food-throwing behaviors were completely eliminated. He also learned to use eating utensils after his plate had been removed several times during one meal.

This boy's series of eye operations early in life necessitated the wearing of glasses. His glasses-throwing behavior, therefore, obviously, had to be controlled, especially since it proved to be moderately expensive. Consequently, he was isolated in a room for ten minutes following each glasses-throwing episode. When a temper tantrum developed in the course of the correction, he had to remain in isolation until it had ceased. Within five days, the boy stopped throwing his glasses.

The mother reported, some six months after her son's discharge, that he was still wearing his glasses, posed no sleep problems, and engaged in no more temper tantrums. In summary, by the removal of reinforcements for obnoxious behaviors and by the administration of mild aversive stimulation, this boy became a much more manageable and acceptable child. It is interesting to note that the concept of punishment which had earlier fallen into disrepute as a shaper of human behavior is now being reassessed by psychologists. More will be said about this concept in the chapter on classroom management.

Parental Involvement

One of the most encouraging aspects of behavior therapy has been the ability to train significant others in the child's life so that they can play a therapeutic part in the child's rehabilitation program. To date, undergraduate college students (Davidson, 1965), psychiatric nurses (Ayllon & Michael, 1959), teachers (Zimmerman & Zimmerman, 1962), and parents (Risley & Wolf, 1964) have been trained as behavioral technicians.

Risley and Wolf, realizing that the parents must be involved if the child's newly acquired behavior patterns are to persist, trained parents in the techniques of behavioral modification. In such cases, the parents generally observe the techniques used by the behavior therapist in establishing and maintaining the child's more desirable behaviors. Sometimes the therapist will also go into the home to observe the parents in action. Of the seven sets of parents so trained, all, according to Risley and Wolf, are assuming a major role in the rehabilitation of their disturbed children. This type of parental training serves to ensure gains made during therapy by facilitating the continuity of treatment efforts.

General Effectiveness and Prognosis

Lest the reader be misled by the encouraging results discussed above, it should be noted that behavioristic treatment has not to date transformed schizophrenic children into normal youngsters. Nevertheless, the improvements noted, though minute relative to the gains needed for a satisfactory adjustment, do represent substantial progress, considering the extreme inaccessibility of schizophrenic youngsters. Some critics complain that these youngsters are still psychotic following the treatment of specific target behaviors. While the criticism is valid, and readily admitted by the behavior therapist, such critics often fail to remember how disruptive and annoying these target behaviors were to those living with the seriously disturbed youngsters in question. The basic personality structures have not been reconstructed, true enough, but life has become more meaningful for them and a closer linking to reality has been established as consequences of such treatment. Further, these youngsters become more acceptable to their parents and their caretakers.

Bettelheim (1967) opines that conditioning therapies are too mechanistic and that behavioristic treatment intensifies the regarding of psychotic children as objects instead of as individuals capable of making their own choices. It may well be that we need mechanistic approaches to deal with these mechanical children, at least until such time as people can become social reinforcers for them. Moreover, it would seem that implicit in behavioristic treatment is the therapist's respect for the child's capacity to change. On the assumption that the therapist's attitude is conveyed to the child, behavior therapy therefore need not be the dehumanizing experience which many critics claim. While it would be rash to abandon traditional forms of psychotherapeutic intervention, it would be equally imprudent to overlook what appears to be a promising fresh approach to what has heretofore been an untreatable problem.

EDUCATIONAL APPROACHES

Psychotic youngsters are usually not encountered by teachers in the regular public-school classroom. When they are found in the regular class, they are most typically at the kindergarten or first-grade level or at preadolescence. Even public-school teachers of special-education classes for the disturbed do not encounter large numbers of psychotic pupils. According to the landmark survey of public-school classes for the disturbed, conducted by Morse, Cutler, and Fink (1964), only 1 in 10 pupils enrolled in these classes is considered psychotic. The large majority of such youngsters are in residential institutions or, having been excluded from school, at home. One of the serious drawbacks in caring for schizophrenic children at home is the shortage of community day schools which will accept them. Some of the more forward-looking organizations and states in the nation are currently putting forth efforts to provide such facilities.

Surprisingly little has been done in the area of educating severely disturbed pupils. By and large, educational programs have taken the form of "holding actions" or of quasi-therapy. In the former, the educational goal is to help the child maintain his earlier academic learnings rather than to stress the acquisition of new skills and concepts. In other words, the child is "marking time" until he is given some form of treatment or is released from the institution. The fact of the matter is that many such pupils are sent to residential schools which do not have sound educational or therapeutic programs. In other words, the "problem" is simply shifted from the public school to the residential school without the child being afforded any greater opportunity for rehabilitation. Conditions in the regular classroom might well improve, but at the child's expense. Altogether too common is the practice whereby a seriously disturbed child is declared uneducable and removed from school without any adequate consideration of those circumstances in which the child might be educated or treated therapeutically. The child simply does not "fit" what the school has to offer, so he has got to go. This practice seems even more common with senior-high-school students than with elementary-school pupils. Indeed, some of the states with the most advanced mental-health policies specifically exclude disturbed junior- and senior-high-school students from special-education classes (even if they are not psychotic).

Strangely enough, many residential institutions regard holding actions as a legitimate goal. The education of these youngsters has also been retarded by quasi-therapeutic philosophies which view educational programs as secondary to the treatment of the child's emotional problems. It is still widely believed, at least as reflected in the literature, that once the child achieves a more satisfactory personal adjustment, it will be relatively easy for him to catch up academically. Because adherents to this philosophy have emphasized the therapeutic aspects of the educative process, there has been a dearth of material forthcoming on curricula and teaching methods for seriously disturbed children. True, there are some rather broad philosophies regarding the education of emotionally disturbed children, such as those advanced by Bruno Bettelheim, Fritz Redl, Virginia Axline, and Clark Moustakas. But there is scarcely anything in the literature that deals with specific factors that enhance or interfere with academic achievement in schizophrenic youngsters. Fortunately, we are now witnessing a shift toward an educational philosophy which lays greater stress on the academic aspects of the school programs for the disturbed.

It is still too early to tell if it is a wise investment of the professional skills of teachers to continue to teach children who, as a group, seem to benefit so little from teaching. There is a definite need for teachers to share their experiences relative to teaching techniques and programs for severely disturbed youngsters (Johnson & Juul, 1950). Relatively controlled observations and measurements of improvement in learning are also badly needed. At present, descriptions of characteristic learning patterns of schizophrenic pupils are nonexistent. Research in this area is complicated by the fact that current psychiatric classification systems have, at best, only minimal educational significance. It has not been possible to establish anything approximating a one-to-one correspondence between the degree or type of personality maladjustment and the extent of educational attainment. More appropriate taxonomies are essential if the mental-hygiene fields are to aid the teacher for the role of therapeutic educator.

While the answer to this question as to educational benefits must, of necessity, remain indefinite at this time, some developments indicate that the situation is not altogether hopeless. Goldberg (1952), for example, conducted an experiment at Bellevue Hospital with schizophrenic children who had reading disabilities. One group was given only psychotherapy, and the other group was given psychotherapy plus individual tutoring in reading. This experiment demonstrated that an individualized remedial reading program was a valuable adjunct with schizophrenic children, not only for the reading gains involved, but also as an effective form of therapy. Goldberg believes that the approach to teaching emotionally disturbed children should vary somewhat from the conventional approach. She notes that schizophrenic children need a very concrete approach to the task. In teaching the mechanics of reading, Goldberg found clay to be a very helpful tool. Raised letters were formed with clay. Of all the teaching tools employed, clay was found to produce the least amount of anxiety. Emotionally neutral reading materials also seemed to work best with these youngsters. Through the use of such materials, the instructor is able to deal with conflict-free or safe areas of the child's makeup. To increase the feelings of achievement, books with few pages and short chapters were used. Of the utmost importance is the establishment of a positive relationship between the tutor and the child. Hirschberg (1953) has also cited the ego-building potential of education. An educational orientation toward reality, together with a focus on the development of skill and mastery, can go far in providing a source of self-esteem.

Bettelheim's Psychoanalytic Approach

One of the better-known approaches to the treatment and education of severely disturbed children is that developed by Bettelheim at the Orthogenic School for emotionally disturbed children. The school's basic aim is to satisfy the emotional needs of the children. To this end, extensive use is made of environmental or milieu therapy, which implies that treatment occurs throughout the child's day. Milieu therapy demands an ordered, controlled environment. Yet the permissiveness of the institution is also stressed, for assertive action on the child's part is needed to circumvent the danger of a passive automaton-like adjustment to institutional regulations (Bettelheim & Sylvester, 1948). The atmosphere may well be termed one of "structured permissiveness." As a child-centered institution, the Orthogenic School stresses a pleasant atmosphere so that the child will feel welcome. Ample gratification is afforded the child; for example, food is always available because it is regarded as symbolic of security and of all other gratifications.

In the milieu therapy, formal schooling is considered an integral part of institutional life (Bettelheim, 1950). A great deal of attention is directed to the child's emotional problems regardless of whether or not they are associated with academic matters. Considerably less attention is devoted to the child's academic accomplishments, and competition with oneself is substituted for competition with classmates. The criterion of teaching success rests more on the teacher's ability to foster a relaxed atmosphere in a tense classroom than on her students' scholastic gains. Further, of the 3½ hours spent in a classroom on a typical school day, considerable time is given over to nonacademic activities, such as drawing and caring for classroom animals (fish, turtles). Educational progress, it is reasoned, will come readily once the emotional problems have been resolved. In fact, the problem, according to Bettelheim, is not a student's slow rate of progress but a too rapid rate which might pose problems of adjustment once the youngster returns to a regular class in the community. Though classes are scheduled daily, the child is not kept in school against his will; he is free to leave if he so desires. Class size is small to facilitate individualized instruction, and the teacher is given considerable latitude in developing a program in the child's best interest. Whenever possible, the pupils are encouraged to set their own tasks. Teacher-parent contacts are generally discouraged since they are viewed as more harmful than beneficial. A parent, for example, may ask why his child has not progressed academically, with the result that the teacher might be made unnecessarily defensive.

Hewett's Learning-Theory Approach

An approach to the education of seriously disturbed youngsters, which is quite different from Bettelheim's psychoanalytic philosophy, comes from recent developments in learning theory. The use of operant-conditioning techniques is illustrated in a study which represents one of the few explicit attempts to teach reading to a 13-year-old autistic child who had not developed speech. Hewett (1964), noting the boy's interest in jigsaw puzzles, letters, and gumdrops, took advantage of these interests in setting up a simple operant-conditioning model. The six stages used in this boy's educational programing were:

1. Associating picture cards with concrete objects.
2. Matching picture and word symbols.
3. Building a 55-word sight vocabulary.
4. Classifying words and pictures.

(These four stages took up most of the first year of the educational programing. By then, the boy was interested in learning per se, and the teacher had taken on secondary reinforcement value.)

5. Learning the alphabet.

(This task was to promote his communication skills, although he still did not talk.)

6. Writing simple phrases.

(He would hold up the phrase cards to make his needs known.)

Hewett states that the acquisition of rudimentary reading and writing skills increased the boy's interest in his surroundings and rendered him more susceptible to control. Given ordinary instructional techniques, this youngster would have been considered unteachable—a backward case unfit for school even in a residential setting.

Autistic youngsters have also acquired speech through the use of conditioning models (Hewett, 1965; Lovaas et al., 1966). Although the acquisition of reading skills and speech does not constitute a cure for these severe disabilities, it does afford a significant means of social interaction and reality contacts.

Another recent development which bears on such germane issues as classroom discipline, educational sequencing, and pupil motivation is Hewett's engineered classroom. Based on a behavior-modification model, the engineered classroom is designed to implement Hewett's hierarchy of educational tasks, a hierarchy which takes into account the normal stages of psychoeducational development in which disturbed children are often deficient (Hewett, 1964, 1967a, 1967b). This theoretical framework for teacher-pupil interaction allows the teacher to adopt a developmental viewpoint and to set realistic educational goals for emotionally disturbed children with learning disabilities.

Each of the seven levels in this hierarchy (see Table 13) is concerned with the reciprocal tasks of the student and the teacher in the development of a working educational relationship. Whereas the average child has successfully mastered the first five levels in this hierarchy prior to school entrance, the majority of emotionally disturbed pupils have not. As Hewett (1967a) notes, many disturbed youngsters lack the readiness necessary for a successful school adjustment because they have difficulty in paying attention, following directions, getting along with others, and so forth. Hewett does more than simply enumerate the levels in the educational hierarchy through which disturbed pupils should progress. He goes on to describe the educational tasks, types of rewards, and degrees of teacher structure which correspond to the level at which the child is currently functioning.

Perhaps the main merit of Hewett's hierarchy is that it allows the teacher to assess the child's specific liabilities and to establish an educational program for a particular child on the basis of this assessment. For example, with a child at a primitive level of development, it would be necessary for the teacher to secure the child's attention through the use of concrete rewards before advancing to the response level, where the basic concern is to get the child involved in learning. Or, for an unruly pupil, it may be necessary to focus on the social level, in which social appropriateness is basic, before advancing to the mastery or achievement level.

Note that the nature of the rewards varies with the developmental readiness of the child. The diversity of rewards (concrete, social attention, task completion, sensory stimulation, task accuracy, and task success) used in this approach takes into consideration the complexity of human motivation and learning. It is certainly more than a narrowly conceived behavior-modification paradigm based on candy

TABLE 13. THE HIERARCHY OF EDUCATIONAL TASKS WITH EMOTIONALLY DISTURBED CHILDREN [DESCRIPTION OF THE HIERARCHY OF EDUCATIONAL TASKS – HEWETT, 1967]

Hierarchy Level	Attention	Response	Order	Exploratory	Social	Mastery	Achievement
Child's problem	Inattention due to withdrawal or resistance.	Lack of involvement and unwillingness to respond in learning.	Inability to follow directions.	Incomplete or inaccurate knowledge of environment.	Failure to value social approval or disapproval.	Deficits in basic adaptive and school skills not in keeping with IQ.	Lack of self-motivation for learning.
Educational task	Get child to pay attention to teacher and task.	Get child to respond to tasks he likes and which offer promise of success.	Get child to complete tasks with specific starting points and steps leading to a conclusion.	Increase child's efficiency as an explorer and get him involved in multisensory exploration of his environment.	Get child to work for teacher and peer-group approval and to avoid their disapproval.	Remediation of basic skill deficiencies.	Development of interest in acquiring knowledge.
Learner reward	Provided by tangible rewards (e.g., food, money, tokens).	Provided by gaining social attention.	Provided through task completion.	Provided by sensory stimulation.	Provided by social approval.	Provided through task accuracy.	Provided through intellectual task success.
Teacher structure	Minimal.	Still limited.	Emphasized.	Emphasized.	Based on standards of social appropriateness.	Based on curriculum assignments.	Minimal.

Source: F. Hewett. Educational engineering with emotionally disturbed children. *Excep. Child.*, 1967, **33**, 459-467. Reprinted by permission.

as the primary reinforcement. Note also that the degree of teacher structure varies with the developmental level of the child. In line with this learning-theory approach, the child is assisted along the educational hierarchy through the use of the principle of "shaping." Hence, rather than unrealistically demanding that the disturbed pupil perform the ultimate in desired classroom behavior—namely, the mastery level, which is characterized by self-motivation and successful achievement—the teacher guides the pupil toward that goal through a series of successive approximations. The child achieves some degree of mastery at one level before proceeding to the next level until ultimately he reaches the mastery level.

In implementing his hierarchical approach to the education of disturbed children, Hewett advocates that the physical environment of the classroom be divided into three sections which parallel the levels in the hierarchy. Thus, there are (1) a mastery-achievement center, where academic lessons are undertaken; (2) an exploratory social center, which is further subdivided into science, art, and communications areas; and (3) an order center, in which skills at the first three levels of the hierarchy are developed. Check marks are also given to the students in accordance with very specific standards. Thus, for example, two check marks are given for starting an assignment (a task which falls at the attention level of the hierarchy), and three check marks are given for completing the assignment (a task which falls at the response level). When maladaptive behavior occurs, for example, daydreaming, assignments are quickly altered.

Although Hewett provides a list of student interventions which correspond to the levels of the hierarchy, the teacher is allowed considerable latitude in the choice of intervention techniques when undesirable behavior occurs. For instance, a child who has become bored and restless at the mastery level might be given a pass to the exploratory center, where he can engage in an art, science, or communication activity. The teacher thereby offers the student an opportunity for motoric release of his tensions while minimizing the need for disciplinary action. Further, the pupil learns that certain types of behaviors are appropriate and specific to each of the designated areas of the classroom.

Hewett believes that, given a well-organized classroom, an aide to assist the teacher, and the use of concrete rewards at times, this design can be functional for the education of disturbed children in both institutional and public-school settings. Psychotic youngsters, when included in a public-school setting, would be working for the most part on the first five tasks in the hierarchy, although not always so.

How effective is this approach? Hewett, Taylor, and Artuso (1968) reported that emotionally handicapped children in engineered classrooms maintained a task-attention advantage of 5–20 per cent over pupils in control classrooms. Gains in arithmetic fundamentals were significantly associated with the use of the engineered design, but reading and spelling gains were not significantly different between the experimental and control conditions.

RESIDENTIAL TREATMENT APPROACHES

As was indicated earlier in the discussion of the study conducted by Bahn, Chandler, and Eisenberg (1962), the majority of psychotic children are referred for residential treatment. Although the schizophrenic child might be best treated at home (Bakwin & Bakwin, 1966), environmental change is necessary to treat certain psychotic children. Environmental change, which might entail sending the child to a residential treatment center or boarding school, affords the child new experiences with other adults and other children in a hopefully therapeutic milieu.

One experiment which studied the differential treatment of day-school versus residential treatment centers was reported by Goldfarb, Goldfarb, and Pollack (1966). This study, extended over a three-year period, involved 13 well-matched pairs from structurally intact homes. All subjects showed early signs of schizophrenia. In general, children from both treatment groups who showed a minimal degree of adaptive capacity at the start of treatment showed no improvement in ego status and remained unscorable on the Wechsler Intelligence Scale for Children. Among those children who were initially scorable on the Wechsler scale, the organically impaired schizophrenic children receiving day-care treatment showed progress that was not appreciably different from those receiving residential care. The non-organically deficient schizophrenic child in the residential treatment center, on the other hand, showed greater improvement, especially in the third year of treatment, than did the matched children in the day-care centers. The authors concluded that day-care facilities might well receive increasing usage for organically defective schizophrenic youngsters, whereas residential centers might be advised for maximum benefit to the nonorganically impaired schizophrenic children.

PHYSIOLOGICAL INTERVENTIONS

Convulsive Therapy

Since the clinical manifestations of childhood schizophrenia run the gamut from the psychological to the biological, it is not surprising that a variety of types of treatments has evolved. This section will focus on two of the physical methods of treatment: electroshock therapy and drugs. Electroshock treatment is used in some centers, particularly where large numbers of youngsters must be treated and processed quickly (Ekstein, Bryant, & Friedman, 1958). Bender (1947), who views the disorder chiefly as a biological phenomenon, has used both drugs and electroshock treatments with severely disturbed children. Bender has used electroshock treatments with numerous child patients, concluding that the treatments do lessen the child's anxiety and increase his manageability. Moreover, according to Bender, convulsive therapy is better tolerated by children than by adults, and there is no discernible intellectual impairment in the children. The ultimate prognosis, however, is not improved. Because of its controversial nature, convulsive therapy is much less widely used today than in the past.

Psychoactive Drugs

Clinicians now seem to favor the use of psychoactive drugs in coping with conditions which were previously treated by convulsive therapy. Psychopharmacologic treatment is considered not only safer but also more successful than convulsive therapy (Lucas, 1966). Bender (1960) notes that the psychoactive drugs seem to reduce anxiety, impulsivity, and disorganized behavior patterns while promoting more harmonious interpersonal relationships. While clinicians do not view these drugs as curative, they do regard them as a useful adjunct to other therapeutic interventions such as group therapy or play therapy.

Drugs used in the treatment of schizophrenic children fall basically into two categories: the tranquilizers and the antidepressants. Whether or not psychoactive drugs will be beneficial to a specific child is difficult to determine in advance. The drug's effectiveness depends on the child in question, the therapist's attitude when dispensing the drug (for example, enthusiasm or suggestion), and the child's environment (Lucas, 1966). Although psychoactive drugs are now accorded a definite place in the treatment plan, particularly in residential treatment centers, there have been few well-controlled studies evaluating their effectiveness. In general, these studies have suffered from personal bias, the absence of adequate control groups, and the limited use of statistical techniques of evaluation (Rosenblum, 1962). We still do not understand the chemistry of these drugs nor their loci of operation within the central nervous system (Mariner, 1967). All we know is that when dosages within specific ranges are administered, certain changes in psychotic behavior occur. Why they occur we do not understand at this time.

AIMS AND METHODS OF TREATMENT APPROACHES

To summarize this section on treatment, therapeutic efforts have generally centered about one or more of the following aims and methods:

1. To supply the missing basic needs—psychotherapy.
2. To remove stresses operating on the child—residential placement.
3. To assist in the development of more appropriate skills—behavior therapy or therapeutic education.
4. To compensate for organic deficits—medications.
5. To rehabilitate the child so that he is better able to accept and live with his disability—supportive counseling.

Which approach or combination of approaches selected will vary with the amenability of the child's disturbance; the personality, training, and philosophy of the particular mental-health specialist; the facilities available, and so forth. Since there are as yet no surefire treatment approaches, a diversity of approaches ranging from the physiological to the psychological might well be regarded as a healthy sign.

SUMMARY

Childhood psychoses, though relatively rare, have been a topic of great interest and concern to mental-health professionals. Despite the vast literature on this condition, there is considerable controversy as to definition, etiology, and treatment. The fundamental impairment in these disorders centers around the child's lack of contact with reality. Disturbances in language and speech, impaired interpersonal associations, inappropriate emotion, and retardation in educational performance are among the secondary symptoms. Rimland, who regards infantile autism as a separate disorder rather than as a variation of childhood schizophrenia, notes some fifteen points on which the two disorders purportedly differ. It is frequently necessary to differentiate childhood schizophrenia from such disorders as mental retardation, brain damage, and other severe personality and language disturbances.

Theories of etiology can be divided into the psychogenic and the somatogenic. Psychogenic explanations focus on faulty child-parent relationships, family interaction patterns, and reinforcement conditions in the home. Somatogenic explanations focus on a possible biological basis as reflected in the genetic or biochemical makeup of the individual. There may well be different types of childhood schizophrenia, each of which has a different weighting of constitutional and environmental forces.

In the light of the divergent etiological positions, it is not surprising to find a multitude of treatment stances. Followup studies of schizophrenic youngsters who have received psychotherapeutic treatment indicate that, at best, only 1 in 4 achieves a reasonably adequate adjustment. Behavioristic therapies seemingly increase the response repertoire of these children, but do not successfully alter the basic disturbance. Examples of psychoanalytic and learning-theory approaches to educational therapy were presented in this chapter. Because of the severity of this condition, total environmental change in the form of a residential milieu is often a common mode of treatment. Electroshock treatment has been largely replaced by the use of psychoactive drugs. Hopefully, future research and practice will provide new insights into the causes and treatments of these baffling conditions.

SUGGESTED READINGS

Axline, V. *Dibs in search of self.* New York: Ballantine Books, 1964.

Bettelheim, B. *The empty fortress.* Glencoe, Ill.: Free Press, 1967.

Hewett, F. *The emotionally disturbed child in the classroom.* Boston: Allyn & Bacon, 1968.

Kety, S. Biochemical theories of schizophrenia: Part A. In T. Millon (Ed.), *Theories of psychopathology.* Philadelphia: Saunders, 1967. Pp. 118-138.

Millon, T. (Ed.) *Theories of psychopathology.* Philadelphia: Sanders, 1967.

REFERENCES

Ayllon, T., & Michael, J. The psychiatric nurse as a behavioral engineer. *J. exp. Anal. Behav.*, 1959, **2**, 323-334.

Bahn, A., Chandler, C., & Eisenberg, L. Diagnostic characteristics related to services in psychiatric clinics for children. *Milbank mem. Fund Quart.*, 1962, **15**, 289-318.

Bakwin, H., & Bakwin, R. *Clinical management of behavior disorders in children.* (3rd ed.) Philadelphia: Saunders, 1966.

Bender, L. Childhood schizophrenia: clinical study of one hundred schizophrenic children. *Amer. J. Orthopsychiat.*, 1947, **17**, 40-56.

Bender, L. Current research in childhood schizophrenia. *Amer. J. Psychiat.*, 1954, **110**, 855-856.

Bender, L. Treatment in early schizophrenia. *Progr. Psychother.*, 1960, **5**, 177-184.

Bender, L., & Freedman, A. M. A study of the first three years in the maturation of schizophrenic children. *Quart. J. Child Behav.*, 1952, **4**, 245.

Bender, L., & Grugett, A. E. A study of certain epidemiological factors in a group of children with childhood schizophrenia. *Amer. J. Orthopsychiat.*, 1956, **26**, 131-143.

Bender, L., & Guerevitz, S. Results of psychotherapy with young schizophrenic children. *Amer. J. Orthopsychiat.*, 1955, **25**, 162-170.

Bennett, S., & Klein, H. R. Childhood schizophrenia: 30 years later. *Amer. J. Psychiat.*, 1966, **122**, 1121-1124.

Berger, A. A test of the double-bind hypothesis of schizophrenia. *Fam. Process,* 1965, **4**, 198-205.

Bettelheim, B. *Love is not enough.* Glencoe, Ill.: Free Press, 1950.

Bettelheim, B. *The empty fortress.* Glencoe, Ill.: Free Press, 1967.

Bettelheim, B., & Sylvester, E. A therapeutic milieu. *Amer. J. Orthopsychiat.*, 1948, **18**, 191-206.

Blau, A. The nature of childhood schizophrenia. *J. Amer. Acad. Child Psychiat.*, 1962, **2**, 225-235.

Boatman, J. J., & Szurek, S. A. A clinical study of childhood schizophrenia. In D. Jackson (Ed.), *The etiology of schizophrenia.* New York: Basic Books, 1960. Pp. 388-440.

Brown, J. L. Follow-up study of preschool children of atypical development (infantile psychosis): later personality patterns in adaptation to maturational stress. *Amer. J. Orthopsychiat.*, 1963, **33**, 336-338.

Committee on Child Psychiatry. *Psychopathological disorders in childhood: theoretical considerations and a proposed classification.* New York: Group for the Advancement of Psychiatry, 1966.

Davidson, G. The training of undergraduates as social reinforcers for autistic children. In L. P. Ullmann & L. Krasner (Eds.), *Case studies in behavior modification.* New York: Holt, Rinehart & Winston, 1965. Pp. 146-148.

Des Lauriers, A., & Halpern, F. Psychological tests in childhood schizophrenia. *Amer. J. Orthopsychiat.*, 1947, **17**, 56-57.

Eisenberg, L. The autistic child in adolescence. *Amer. J. Psychiat.*, 1956, **112**, 607-112.

Eisenberg, L. Fathers of autistic children. *Amer. J. Orthopsychiat.*, 1957, **27**, 715-724.

Ekstein, R., Bryant, K., & Friedman, S. Childhood schizophrenia and allied conditions. In L. Bellak (Ed.), *Schizophrenia: a review of the syndrome.* New York: Logos Press, 1958. Pp. 555-693.

Ferster, C. B. Positive reinforcement and behavioral deficits of autistic children. *Child Develpm.*, 1961, **32**, 437-456.

Ferster, C. B., & DeMyer, M. K. A method for the experimental analysis of the behavior of autistic children. *Amer. J. Orthopsychiat.*, 1962, **32**, 89-98.

Frank, G. H. The role of the family in the development of psychopathology. *Psychol. Bull.*, 1965, **64**, 191-203.

Gianascol, A. Psychodynamic approaches to childhood schizophrenia: a review. *J. nerv. ment. Dis.*, 1963, **137**, 336-348.

Goldberg, I. Tutoring as a method of psychotherapy in schizophrenic children with reading disabilities. *Quart. J. Child Behav.*, 1952, **4**, 273-280.

Goldfarb, W. *Childhood schizophrenia.* Cambridge: Harvard Univer. Press, 1961.

Goldfarb, W., Braunstein, P., & Lorgo, I. A study of speech patterns in a group of schizophrenic children. *Amer. J. Orthopsychiat.*, 1956, **26**, 544-555.

Goldfarb, W., Goldfarb, N., & Pollack, R. Treatment of childhood schizophrenia: a three-year comparison of day and residential treatment. *Arch. gen. Psychiat.*, 1966, **14**, 119-128.

Goldfarb, W., Goldfarb, N., & Scholl, H. The speech of mothers of schizophrenic children. *Amer. J. Psychiat.*, 1966, **122**, 1220-1227.

Gottesman, I. I., & Shields, J. Schizophrenia in twins: 16 years' consecutive admissions to a psychiatric clinic. *Brit. J. Psychiat.*, 1966, **112**, 809-818.

Halpern, F. The Rorschach test with children. In A. Rabin & M. Haworth (Eds.), *Projective techniques with children.* New York: Grune & Stratton, 1960. Pp. 14-28.

Hewett, F. Teaching reading to an autistic boy through operant conditioning. *Reading Tchr,* 1964, **17**, 613-618.

Hewett, F. Teaching speech to an autistic child through operant conditioning. *Amer. J. Orthopsychiat.*, 1965, **35**, 927-936.

Hewett, F. Educational engineering with emotionally disturbed children. *Except. Child.*, 1967, **33**, 459-467. (a)

Hewett, F. A school in a psychiatric hospital. *Ment. Hyg.*, 1967, **51**, 75-83. (b)

Hewett, F., Taylor, F., & Artuso, A. The Santa Monica Project. *Except. Child.*, 1968, **34**, 387.

Hingtgen, J., Sanders, B., & DeMyer, M. Shaping cooperative responses in early childhood schizophrenics. Paper read at meeting of American Psychological Association, Philadelphia, August, 1963.

Hingtgen, J. N., & Trost, F. C., Jr. Shaping cooperative responses in early childhood schizophrenics: II. Reinforcement of mutual contact and vocal responses. In R. Ulrich, T. Stachnik, & J. Mabry (Eds.), *Control of human behavior.* Glenview, Ill.: Scott, Foresman, 1966. Pp. 110-113.

Hirschberg, C. The role of education in the treatment of emotionally disturbed children through planned ego development. *Amer. J. Orthopsychiat.,* 1953, **23**, 684-690.

Johnson, J., & Juul, K. Learning characteristics in a schizophrenic boy. *Except. Child.,* 1960, **26**, 135-138.

Kallmann, F. J. *The genetics of schizophrenia.* New York: Augustine, 1938.

Kallmann, F. J. The genetics of human behavior. *Amer. J. Psychiat.,* 1956, **113**, 496-501.

Kanner, L. Autistic disturbances of affective contact. *Nerv. Child,* 1943, **2**, 217-250.

Kanner, L. Early infantile autism. *J. Pediat.,* 1944, **25**, 211-217.

Kanner, L. Irrelevant and metaphorical language in early infantile autism. *Amer. J. Psychiat.,* 1946, **103**, 242-246.

Kanner, L. Problems of nosology and psychodynamics. *Amer. J. Orthopsychiat.,* 1949, **19**, 416-476.

Kanner, L. Emotionally disturbed children: a historical review. *Child Develpm.,* 1962, **33**, 97-102.

Kaufman, I., Herrick, J., Willer, L., Frank T., & Heims, L. Four types of defenses in mothers and fathers of schizophrenic children. *Amer. J. Orthopsychiat.,* 1959, **29**, 460-472.

Kessler, J. W. *Psychopathology of childhood.* Englewood Cliffs, N.J.: Prentice-Hall, 1966.

Klebanoff, L. Parental attitudes of mothers of schizophrenic, brain-injured and retarded and normal children. *Amer. J. Orthopsychiat.,* 1959, **29**, 445-454.

Leitch, M., & Schafer, S. A study of the TATs of psychotic children. *Amer. J. Orthopsychiat.,* 1947, **17**, 337-342.

Lidz, T., & Fleck, S. Schizophrenia, human interaction, and the role of the family. In D. Jackson (Ed.), *The etiology of schizophrenia.* New York: Basic Books, 1960. Pp. 323-345.

Lifton, N., & Smolen, E. Group psychotherapy with schizophrenic children. *Int. J. Psychother.,* 1966, **16**, 23-41.

Lovaas, O. I., Freitag, G., Gold, V., & Kassorla, I. Experimental studies in childhood schizophrenia. *J. exp. Psychol.,* 1963, **66**, 67-73.

Lovaas, O. I., Freitag, G., Gold, V., & Kassorla, I. Experimental studies in childhood schizophrenia: analysis of self-destructive behavior. *J. exp. Child Psychol.,* 1965, **2**, 67-84.

Lovaas, I., Berberich, J., Perloff, B., & Schaeffer, B. Acquisition of imitative speech by schizophrenic children. *Science,* 1966, **151**, 705-707.

Lucas, A. Psychopharmacologic treatment. In C. R. Shaw (Ed.), *The psychiatric disorders of childhood.* New York: Appleton-Century-Crofts, 1966. Pp. 387-402.

Mahler, M. S. On child psychosis and schizophrenia: autistic and symbiotic infantile psychoses. In R. S. Eissler, A. Freud, H. Hartmann, & E. Kris

(Eds.), *The psychoanalytic study of the child.* Vol. 7. New York: International Universities Press, 1952. Pp. 286-305.

Mahler, M. S. On early infantile psychosis. *J. Amer. Acad. Child Psychiat.,* 1965, 4, 554-568.

Mahler, M. S., Furer, M., & Settlage, C. F. Severe emotional disturbances in childhood: psychosis. In S. Arieti (Ed.), *American handbook of psychiatry.* New York: Basic Books, 1959, Pp. 816-839.

Mariner, A. A critical look at professional education in the mental health field. *Amer. Psychologist,* 1967, 22, 271-281.

Mischler, E., & Waxler, N. Family interaction processes and schizophrenia: a review of current theories. *Merrill-Palmer Quart.,* 1965, 11, 269-315.

Morse, W. C., Cutler, R. L., & Fink, A. H. *Public school classes for the emotionally handicapped: a research analysis.* Washington, D.C.: Council for Exceptional Children, 1964.

Piotrowski, Z. A comparison of congenitally defective children with schizophrenic children with respect to personality structure and intellectual type. *Proc. Amer. Assn ment. Defic.,* 1937, 42, 78-90.

Potter, H. W. Schizophrenia in children. *Amer. J. Psychiat.,* 1933, 12, 1253.

Rabinovitch, R. An evaluation of present trends in psychotherapy of children. *J. psychiat. soc. Wk,* 1954, 24, 11-19.

Rank, B. Adaptation of the psychoanalytic technique for the treatment of young children with atypical development. *Amer. J. Orthopsychiat.,* 1949, 19, 130-139.

Rimland, B. *Infantile autism: the syndrome and its implications for a neural theory of behavior.* New York: Appleton-Century-Crofts, 1964.

Risley, T., & Wolf, M. Experimental manipulation of autistic behaviors and generalization into the home. Paper read at meeting of American Psychological Association, Los Angeles, September, 1964.

Rosen, B. M., Bahn, A. K., & Kramer, M. Demographic and diagnostic characteristics of psychiatric clinic outpatients in the U.S.A., 1961. *Amer. J. Orthopsychiat.,* 1964, 34, 455-468.

Rosenblum, S. Practices and problems in the use of tranquilizers with exceptional children. In E. Trapp & P. Himelstein (Eds.), *Readings on the exceptional child.* New York: Appleton-Century-Crofts, 1962. Pp. 639-657.

Shaw, C. R. *The psychiatric disorders of childhood.* New York: Appleton-Century-Crofts, 1966.

Skinner, B. F. Some contributions of an experimental analysis of behavior to psychology as a whole. *Amer. Psychologist,* 1953, 8, 69-78.

Speers, R., & Lansing, C. Group psychotherapy with preschool children and collateral group therapy of their parents: a preliminary report of the first two years. *Amer. J. Orthopsychiat.,* 1964, 34, 659-666.

U.S. Department of Health, Education, and Welfare. *Patients in mental institutions, 1963.* Washington, D.C.: Government Printing Office, 1964.

Weakland, J. The double-bind hypothesis of schizophrenia and the three party interaction. In D. Jackson (Ed.), *The etiology of schizophrenia.* New York: Basic Books, 1960. Pp. 373-388.

White, R. W. *The abnormal personality.* New York: Ronald Press, 1964.
Wolf, M. M., Risley, T., & Mees, H. L. Application of operant conditioning procedures to the behavior problems of an autistic child. *Behav. Res. Ther.,* 1964, **1**, 305-312.
Wynne, L., & Singer, M. Thought disorder and the family relations of schizophrenics. I: a research strategy. *Arch. gen. Psychiat.,* 1963, **9**, 191-198.
Zimmerman, E., & Zimmerman, J. The alteration of behavior in a special classroom situation. *J. exp. Anal. Behav.,* 1962, **5**, 59-60.

Part III

Intervention and
Prevention
Strategies

Therapeutic Approaches

In contrast to the discussions of psychotherapy in the earlier chapters of this book, which dealt with the treatment of specific disorders, the discussion in this chapter will deal with the general problem of theoretical approaches to therapy with children. The plan is to consider first the differences between therapeutic approaches for children and those for adults. Then we will turn to certain of the better-known systematic approaches to child therapy, followed by a detailed consideration of those approaches which utilize play as a medium of expression. There follows an assessment of the effectiveness of various treatment approaches. Finally, the chapter concludes with a presentation of recent innovations in treatment approaches which are receiving favor among psychologists.

DIFFERENCES BETWEEN ADULT AND CHILD PSYCHOTHERAPY

The basic principles of psychotherapy with children are not essentially different from those of psychotherapy with adults, but the immaturity and dependent status of the child necessitate certain modifications in the emphasis and application of these principles (White, 1964). Hence it seems appropriate to examine certain differences that exist between children and adults so that we may better understand the bases for the widespread use of play techniques and for other changes in therapeutic methods with children.

MOTIVATION FOR TREATMENT

As Table 14 shows, one important difference occurs in the approach to the therapy situation. The adult typically comes to treatment recognizing that he has a personal problem. Although he may need the support of others to reach this decision, the ultimate responsibility for seeking help is his. Few children, however, request psychotherapeutic help. Rather, they are usually placed into therapy by an adult, with little or no explanation as to why. The child may be experiencing strong anxiety or suffering from emotional deprivation, but it is doubtful that these states can be utilized to motivate him to look forward to therapy. Not only do children lack motivation in the usual adult sense to work on their own problems, but they not uncommonly have fears regarding what the therapist will do to them. Some children readily adjust to the playroom without the assistance of the therapist. In these instances, therapy can proceed without specifically designed attempts to establish a therapeutic relationship.

But there are children who question their presence at the clinic, who are angry and defiant, who become passive, or who are indifferent. With these children, an explanation which reflects the therapist's respect for the child is indicated. Care must be exercised lest the child feel that the therapist is "taking sides" with the mother or the teacher. A reality-based explanation geared to the child's developmental level is recommended in such instances. In brief, the child's anxieties, suspicions, and low level of motivation frequently require demonstration to him that the therapist is an empathic, benign, and helpful companion as the first step in establishing a therapeutic relationship. Some therapists, like Anna Freud (1946) and Pearson (1949),

TABLE 14. A SUMMARY OF DIFFERENCES BETWEEN ADULTS AND CHILDREN WITH IMPLICATIONS FOR CHILD THERAPY

Factor	Adult	Child	Treatment Implication for Child
Motivation for treatment	Often self-referred; better motivated to work on his difficulties.	Referred by others; lacks motivation to work on own problems.	Some therapists feel the need for initial sessions to develop a therapeutic relationship upon which to base later, more intensive therapy.
Insight into treatment objectives	More likely to share common goals with therapist and to be aware of his own role in therapy.	More apt to lack common goals with therapist.	The child must find therapy intrinsically interesting; his needs for exploration and manipulation should be utilized.
Linguistic development	Satisfactory verbal facility.	Limited verbal facility; greater use of nonverbal communication.	Speech-mediated interactions are minimized, with more emphasis on nonverbal communication.
Dependence on environmental forces	More independent of environment.	Very dependent on environment and significant others.	Treatment must accord more attention to dealing with significant others in the child's life and to external reality pressures.
Plasticity of personality	More "set" in his ways; defenses are better established.	More pliable and open to therapeutic influence; less integration and internal consistency in personality.	Intervention procedures should be undertaken before personality becomes stabilized; less need for depth-therapy techniques, as the child is more susceptible to environmental influences.

advocate an initial orientation and "getting-acquainted" approach in the beginning sessions to prepare the child for more intensive treatment later.

INSIGHT INTO TREATMENT OBJECTIVES

A related barrier to therapy is centered about the fact that the therapist and child lack the commonality of purpose more characteristic of adult therapy. Whereas the adult client is likely to be cognizant of certain common goals of treatment that he shares with the therapist and is somewhat more accepting of the impending personality reorganization, the child (because of his more limited cognitive and experiential background) may well lack insight both as to the roles that he and the therapist are to assume and as to the purposes of treatment. He may appreciate neither the desirability nor the possibility of behavioral change. Given this lack of common goals, much of the child's desire to remain in treatment must come from satisfactions inherent in the treatment setting itself. Fortunately, play therapy seems suited to this end.

LINGUISTIC DEVELOPMENT

Another very fundamental difference is the child's relative lack of verbal development. True enough, he can communicate verbally with adults, but he is apt to find the formal sort of psychiatric interview too stilted to permit a comfortable feeling in the situation. The child's limited experience may be reflected in an uncertainty as to how or what to label his feelings, whereas the use of concrete materials of play renders the child more secure since he is able to manipulate and control these tangibles with more assurance than he can the abstractions of words. Evidence from developmental studies in cognition would also indicate, especially for children below junior-high-school age, the suitability of concrete materials as opposed to verbal abstractions as a means of expression (Piaget, 1960). Lippman (1962) observes that children often show greater anxiety in direct interviews than in play. Limited verbal facility may engender feelings of inadequacy and failure on the part of the child, thus adding to the difficulty in establishing a trusting relationship with the therapist. As Watson (1951) notes, suspicion and hostility are likely to be encountered particularly with young or intellectually dull children as well as with delinquents.

Many of these problems can be alleviated through the medium of play therapy because play is something these children can comprehend and use as a means of communication. Since play therapy entails substantially less speech-mediated interaction than does psychotherapy with adults, nonverbal aspects are accorded a more important position. According to Watson (1951), this is a two-way proposition. The therapist must be especially alert to the child's facial expressions, postural adjustments, and expressive movements, realizing that these may well be the child's primary means of expression. In turn, the child reacts to similar nonverbal behavior on the therapist's part. Many therapists believe that how the therapist feels is more important than what he says and does.

The above remarks are not intended to deny the fact that some prepubescents communicate very well through langauge. In such instances the necessity of nonverbal forms of communication might well be markedly reduced.

DEPENDENCE ON ENVIRONMENTAL FORCES

The child's dependency on the adults in his life also has implications for treatment. Whereas the adult is relatively independent of the significant others in his environment, the child is still very much at their mercy. The adult can quit his job, change his residence, and replace companions much more readily than the child can quit school, change homes, and substitute peer groups. As a consequence of his immature and dependent status, the young child is more subject to environmental stresses and strains. Since the child in treatment is typically still living in the situation which caused or contributed to his difficulties, emphasis must be devoted to the child's current reality conditions.

Since it is commonly accepted that the child's disturbance is often inextricably bound up with problems of the significant others in his surroundings, many therapists do not advocate psychotherapy with children younger than 14 years of age unless the parents are also willing to become involved in the treatment process (White, 1964). Parental involvement necessitated by the child's dependency status poses challenges, however, which demand skillful management in the therapy program; for example, there may be parental rivalry with the therapist for the child's affection. More will be said about working with parents in the chapter on environmental intervention.

PLASTICITY OF PERSONALITY

Another difference centers around the lack of crystallization in the child's personality. Because the child's personality is relatively unde-veloped, unformed, and changing rapidly, it tends to be more pliable than the enduring adult personality. Hence, the potentiality for change should be greater prior to the establishment of a more consistent and more stable personality structure. Defense mechanisms are apt to be less deeply rooted and therefore more amenable to the types of relearning experiences offered in the therapy setting. Because of the greater fluidity and more elastic nature of the personality, greater lability and inconsistency of behavior as well as an intermingling of reality and fantasy in the child can be anticipated (Slavson, 1952; Watson, 1951). Consequently, the course of child therapy is likely to be characterized by greater discontinuity than is adult therapy, as exemplified by shifts from one activity to another, from reality to fantasy, and from deeper to more surface aspects of the difficulty. The greater fluidity and inconsistency which characterize the child's personality might also imply that less effort be directed toward the "uncovering" aspects of therapy and more toward the "covering-up" aspects. Further, these characteristics of child personality underscore the need for the therapist's ability to distinguish between more permanent or repetitive problems and those of a transitory character.

DIFFERENCES RELATED TO PLAY THERAPY

Slavson (1947) has cited other differences which further highlight the potential value of play techniques. Illustratively, the child is considerably more impulsive than the adult; he is less subject to repressive forces and more willing to act out and speak about matters that are embarrassing to an older person; his fantasy life is closer to the surface; his attention span is shorter; he is more concerned with locomotion and expression, so that physical activity is of greater importance to him. The implications of these differences are reflected in Slavson's group-therapy approach, which is discussed later in the chapter.

PLAY THERAPY

The child has a rich fantasy life which in early years he can express in a spontaneous and vivid manner, and unless strong repressive forces are at work, his fantasies can be utilized for uncovering and alleviating conflicts. Daily observation reveals that small children have a remarkable facility for switching back and forth between reality and fantasy —from their own subjective inner world to the objective outside world of reality. They also use toys and play to express externally their inner fantasies. In doing so, they build up a world which is just as important and meaningful to them as reality. It is this expressive capacity and fascination on the child's part which is utilized by the therapist during treatment. Thus, play therapy is based upon the fact that play is the child's natural medium of self-expression. The therapeutic use of play provides an opportunity for the child to formulate his feelings and problems, in much the same manner that the more linguistically facile adult talks out his difficulties in certain types of adult therapy.

Play, like adult conversation, is not therapeutic in itself; it is but an avenue for understanding the inner conflicts of the child. The more verbally oriented adult can often translate his troubles into words, whereas the child uses the language of play. All proponents of expressive or evocative play therapy view the establishment of a therapeutic relationship as a prerequisite for successful treatment. If this relationship is lacking, there may be play but not play therapy in any genuine sense. As Watson notes (1951),

Psychotherapy with children requires that the child be given an opportunity to interact with an adult (the therapist) who takes a different attitude toward his problem from that he has previously experienced. This the therapeutic attitude supplies, no matter how it is expressed. Of course, merely making it available is not enough; the child must experience it. Although play may share in the development of this interaction, the attitude may be maintained in its absence. Play is merely one way of allowing the therapist to interact with a child patient.

Thus, play becomes a medium of therapy, and as such it must occur within the framework of a relationship that is established through the participation of two people. It is the uniqueness of this relationship and of the circumstances that produces the special meaning to what the child does, whether it be playing or talking or just sitting. Froebel (quoted in Jackson & Todd, 1950) commented several decades ago:

Child's play is not mere sport. It is full of meaning and serious impact. Cherish it and encourage it. For to one who has insight into human nature, the trend of the whole future life of the child is revealed in his freely chosen play.

HISTORICAL BACKGROUND

The study of the treatment of emotional disturbance in children is a relatively recent development compared to the attention given emotional disturbance in adults. Contributions to child treatment have come from psychoanalysis, psychology, genetic psychology, and social work, among other sources. All have increased our knowledge of the child, but the greatest contributions to the treatment of problem behavior in children have come from those directly concerned with psychopathology. Outstanding is the work by Freud and his students.

One of Freud's major concerns was the development of a treatment for adults having neurotic symptoms. In his investigations he concluded that the problems of the neurotic adult derived from sexual conflicts in early childhood. From his clinical experience with adult patients, he inferred that young children have an active sexual life and vivid fantasies. In 1906 he presented a case entitled "Analysis of a Phobia in a Five-Year-Old Boy"—the celebrated "Case of Little Hans"—to support his contentions (1909). Freud did not conduct the analysis; it was carried out by the boy's father, himself an analyst. Although the interpretations of some of the findings might be questioned, this report did, nevertheless, represent the first application of psychoanalysis to the problems of children and hence gave impetus to a lively interest in child analysis.

About 1920 Hermine Hug-Hellmuth, a psychoanalytically oriented educator, began to treat maladjusted children within the framework of Freudian theory. She used play as a basic part of her procedures with children under 7 years of age and as an aid to communication at later ages. When dealing with children aged 7 or 8, she believed that the analyst could often facilitate the therapeutic process by sharing in the play activities. In essence, her approach, which combined Freudian theory and educational methods, consisted in observing the child at play and in translating each pattern of behavior into the analyst's set of symbols.

It was not until some ten years later, however, when Anna Freud and Melanie Klein reported their observations and theoretical discussions of the therapeutic process with children that child psychoanalysis began to be practiced on a sizable scale. Although both adhered to general psychoanalytic theories of child therapy, each formulated treatment procedures which differed in many significant respects, as will be discussed later in this chapter.

The pioneer efforts of these women greatly influenced the thinking of mental-health specialists in this country. Perhaps of more direct consequence was the establishment of the child-guidance movement. While many individuals figured in this movement, it was Lightner Witmer who in 1896 founded the first child-guidance clinic as a consequence of his interest in the school-aged child with problems. Shortly thereafter, other clinics were founded, with practices based on an integration of psychoanalytic and psychobiological principles as exemplified by Sigmund Freud and Adolf Meyer. By 1921, a large number of clinics attached to mental hospitals, schools, courts, colleges, and social agencies were employing a case-study and team approach to the disorders of children. The National Committee for Mental Hygiene and the Commonwealth Fund supported the developments of these clinics, and as they expanded, advances were made in the techniques of child therapy. By 1930, there were more than 500 such clinics.

Characteristically, child psychoanalysis and child therapy have differed in that the latter represents a less intense approach and is more apt to use environmental interventions. Accordingly, in child therapy the child is seen less frequently, and work with the parents might be undertaken. As Wattenberg (1966) notes, therapists today are realizing that the child's reality conditions are as important as how the child feels.

THE PLAYROOM AND SUGGESTED MATERIALS

Since play provides such an important medium of expression in therapeutic work, the arrangement of the office and the choice of play materials deserve careful consideration. In terms of general characteristics, the playroom should afford privacy of location and be durable, that is, constructed to withstand wear and tear and consisting of washable walls and floors, protected glass, and so forth. Soundproofing is also desirable. If possible, the same room should be used each time so as to maximize the child's sense of security and comfort in the setting. Play materials should be simple in construction and easy to handle in order to give the child a feeling of satisfaction and a sense of accomplishment.

The selection of toys warrants thoughtful judgment because the kind of toys used can either facilitate or hinder the expression of the child's impulses. Stated another way, some toys lend themselves more readily to the eliciting of certain types of themes or behaviors. Toy soldiers, military equipment, and pegboards to be hammered are frequently made available to elicit aggressive behavior, thus allowing negative and repressed youngsters to externalize and objectify their hostile feelings. Nursing bottles, nipples, baby carriages, and rattles are often used to elicit the regressive behaviors so common in the inadequate-immature child. Doll play facilities—a dollhouse fully furnished, wetting dolls, rag dolls, amputation dolls, and dolls representing various family members—have been used to permit the expression of feelings and attitudes regarding the family setting. Running water, sand boxes, crayons, watercolors and finger paints, clay, scissors and paper for cutting, and a chalkboard have been found to encourage expressive play.

Although not the most productive types of material for expressive play, checker games have also been utilized with some success especially in handling certain resistances in child analysis (Loomis, 1957). Similarly, mechanical toys are not recommended since the mechanics often interfere with creative play. Water play, on the other hand, seems to offer a versatile medium and is particularly appropriate for cases involving overactivity or constriction of behavior or interest in the environment (Hartley, Frank, & Goldenson, 1952). Although not all of these materials are essential to successful therapy, their presence in variety tends to encourage the freer expression of a greater diversity of problems.

Ultimately, the selection of materials is an individual matter varying somewhat with the individual therapist or the specific problems. Some therapists find that only a few toys in the playroom are advisable, since a wealth of toys often proves too distracting. As a rule, however, it has been found that once a child starts working with a particular type of material, he pays no attention to the rest of the material in the playroom. As the therapist becomes acquainted with the child's problems, he can make up a box of specific play materials that are suited to the child's needs, interests, and problems. The child will not uncommonly request more toys than are available, but the skillful therapist will not always accede to the child's demands, for the continued removal of frustrating circumstances not only deprives the child of opportunities to express feelings of anger and resentment but also delays his learning to cope with situations as they exist.

Major Varieties

Solomon's Activist Approach

Solomon (1951) advocates a directive and active role for the therapist. He asserts that many therapists are too passive and wait too long for something to happen in the treatment setting. There are three ways in which Solomon attempts to facilitate the therapeutic process:

1. By assuming a more active role and by keeping the play-session conversation in the third person, the therapist provides the child with greater anonymity and consequently reduces defensiveness.

2. Activity on the therapist's part, instead of frightening the child, presumably lowers resistances since both the therapist and the child are playing together on a level meaningful to the child.

3. Finally, the directive role played by the therapist in stimulating the child's fantasy through the use of suggested play activities leads to an uncovering of the child's inner life.

During the course of play therapy, much information regarding the home situation is obtained. Information revealed in the content of the child's play is considered important in that it allows the therapist to offer the parents more intelligent guidance, hopefully reducing operative reality stresses.

Over the years, Solomon has placed increasing emphasis on the emotional responses of the child rather than on dramatic aspects of his constructions, although he continued to use controlled play situations. There is some experimental evidence for his beliefs in the work of Pintler (1945) and Phillips (1945), whose research on the relative effectiveness of different variables in doll play revealed that when the variable was that of high experimenter-child activity versus low experimenter-child activity (passivity), abreactions of an aggressive nature began earlier and were more pronounced in the high-activity group. Also, the amount of nonstereotyped thematic play and the number of theme changes were greater under conditions of high interaction between experimenter and child.

Solomon is quick to stress the relationship between the therapist and child since he considers this the most important aspect of therapy. Anxiety generated by his more active approach is handled by the introduction of a "therapist doll" upon which the child can release his feelings. As Solomon (1951) asserts,

It has been the experience of the writer that a great deal of therapeutic movement can be released when the therapist actively introduces into the play situation the doll representing himself. Even when this is done, the anonymity is preserved for as long a period of time as the child desires, and emotions centering around the therapist-child situation proceed in effigy. Usually, after the therapist doll is introduced into play, it takes on a greater degree of importance in the configuration of the play than even the sibling doll or parent doll figures. Thus, the child uses a relationship much closer to the therapist to air some of the problems resulting from the disturbed inter-personal relationships within the home. As the child releases aggression, either oral or anal in character, or as he expresses tender sentiments, he comes to grips with his instinctive expressions. Guilt feelings or direct fear of punish-ment become living expressions in the transference situation. As the child survives his own instinctive expressions, he gains greater confidence in all of his human relationships.

As the child continues in therapy, several phenomena occur. There are expressions of the child's thinking, the release of anxiety and aggressive impulses, the working-through of dependency needs, the affording of alternatives to the feeling of impending danger, the provision of an atmosphere for the release of tender impulses, the lessening of guilt feelings, and the stabilizing of ego structure.

The age factor is thought to be of comparatively little significance once cortical development is sufficient to permit symbolization. Thus, Solomon has used play therapy with children of all ages, including adolescents. He does prefer, however, to relate treatment to the type of problem presented by the child. Accordingly, he differentiates therapeutic measures for the aggressive-impulsive child, the anxiety-phobic child, the regressive-reaction-formation group, and the schizoid-schizophrenic youngster.

Levy's Release Therapy

The role of emotional release as an ingredient common to all forms of child therapy has been widely recognized. Levy (1938, 1939) has developed a systematic approach using this therapeutic ingredient called *release therapy*. Through the use of the child's play, the therapist allows the child to act out his anxieties. Although the therapist's attitude during the session is one of permissiveness, the play situation has been carefully structured by the therapist prior to the session. The therapist, according to Levy, should make a judgment as to the cause of the child's problem on the basis of interviews with the parents. Levy, like Solomon, is not averse to assuming an active role in the therapy sessions. Thus, he will sometimes direct the play by selecting certain toys and inviting the child to play with him.

Levy has also experimented with dolls as a therapeutic medium with children. He has, in fact, developed an amputation doll which can be taken apart and reassembled. After the doll has been identified by the therapist as the child's mother, father, or sibling, the youngster is allowed to play with it as he desires, even destructively. Indeed, the therapist may sometimes actively encourage the child's expression of hostility. Levy feels that this technique is particularly suited to cases of sibling rivalry. Furthermore, he notes that children go through certain stages in resolving their sibling rivalries. Initially, there is apt to be an inhibition or "prevention of hostility" by the child. He is not yet sure how safe it is to express his genuine feelings. Gradually, in an atmosphere of permissiveness and encouragement, the child becomes more willing to reveal his hostility toward the sibling. Having expressed aggression toward the brother or sister, the child may attempt to rationalize his behavior by becoming extrapunitive, thus blaming the therapist or the sibling for his own actions. In some cases, the child engages in "undoing" and may try to reassemble the doll.

Levy has provided explicit criteria for the selection of cases deemed suitable for his release therapy:

1. The child should be under 10 years of age.
2. There should be a definite reaction pattern precipitated by a specific event, for example, a frightening experience, the birth of a sibling, the death of a parent, or some similar episode.
3. The problem should not be of long standing.
4. The traumatic experience should be in the past, that is, not continuing at the time of referral.
5. The child should be from a relatively normal family situation.

If these five conditions obtain, Levy feels little need to involve the parents beyond their role as informants in the case-history interviews. It should be noted that the majority of disturbed children would be excluded from treatment if Levy's criteria were stringently applied.

The expression of feeling is a necessary but not sufficient condition of therapeutic movement. The crucial variable for Levy is the relationship between child and therapist. The relationship, however, does not assume the status of a transference neurosis, as in Klein's psychoanalytic approach discussed below. What is achieved through the use of Levy's approach is the desensitization or counterconditioning of the child's fears. Some have charged that this desensitization technique is effective only with circumscribed fears having a specific and noninterpersonal basis. The cases described by Wolpe (1958) and Lazarus and Rachman (1957) suggest that even cases of generalized disturbances of an interpersonal nature might be effectively treated by this method. Thus, Levy's approach may have wider applicability than even he assumed.

Note that interpretation plays a minimal role in release therapy. Levy contends that children between the ages of 2 and 5 need not know the nature of their difficulties or of their relationship to the therapist in order to improve. Emotional release and a positive relationship with the therapist are the two basic elements making for successful treatment.

Klein's Psychoanalytic Approach

Melanie Klein, utilizing a psychoanalytic approach in the treatment of neurotic disorders, assumes that the free play of children is equivalent to the free association of adults. Her fashioning of play therapy after adult psychoanalysis is really not surprising, in that she likens the character of the child to that of the adult. As in adult psychoanalysis, the primary goal of child analysis is modification of the child's personality through the systematic exploration of the unconscious by means of the transference relationship (Klein, 1955). Klein assumes that a transference neurosis—the transfer of either strong positive or strong negative feelings toward the analyst—does occur in the treatment of disturbed children. The display of such intense emotion has no realistic basis in the therapeutic setting but instead presumably derives from earlier parent-child conflicts. Attention is directed to the development of a transference relationship before instinctual conflicts are brought into the child's awareness. The external life of the child is largely ignored. Klein also assumes that the superego even at this stage of development is severe and that the ego is undeveloped. Thus, there is a need to protect the emerging ego from the restrictive superego. The ego must be strengthened in relation to the superego. The parents' role in treatment is, therefore, minimal in that the parents represent external reinforcers of the child superego.

Klein substitutes free play for free association in order to uncover conflicts buried in the unconscious. Behind every playful action is a symbolic meaning which represents unconscious material. Basically, this approach consists of direct verbal interpretations to the child concerning the meaning of his play. The child is presumably able to attain greater insight than might be expected from his level of cognitive immaturity because infantile repressions are less powerful and because the connections between conscious and unconscious are closer than in the adult (Klein, 1955). Consistent with such views, Klein not uncommonly begins to interpret the meaning of the child's actions to him as succinctly and clearly as possible. To achieve the latter goal, she favors the use of the child's expressions in her analytic interpretation. Klein acknowledges that a single toy or play situation may have several meanings and that it is necessary to consider each child's use of symbols not only in relation to his own emotions and anxieties but also in relation to the entire treatment situation. Inspection of Klein's published interpretations suggests, however, that she has not always exercised such caution but instead reveals a leaping into direct interpretation based upon her previous experiences in play therapy. As might be expected, this approach has aroused substantial criticism and is little practiced in this country.

Anna Freud's Psychoanalytic Approach

Anna Freud (1946) also advocates a psychoanalytic orientation but maintains that the classical techniques of adult psychoanalysis require certain modification for applicability to children because the young are unable to develop a transference neurosis and because their ego ideal is still relatively weak. Although she has since modified her views regarding the possibility of a transference neurosis occurring in treatment, she continues to believe that it cannot equal that of the adult variety (A. Freud, 1965).

Whereas Klein (1955) expresses a definite preference for small, simple, nonmechanical toys, Freud (1965) discusses toys more for assessing the child's growth than for their use in therapy. She does find them useful in establishing a close relationship in the preanalytic phase of treatment which she regards as a necessary prerequisite to effective analytic interpretation. Free play, however, is not regarded as a substitute for free association. During the stage of analysis proper, various techniques are used as avenues to the unconscious. These include the taking of a case history from the child and the mother, the analyzing of drawings, and the interpreting of dreams. The technique of interpretation constitutes a cornerstone of psychoanalytic practice and is designed to promote insight on the child's part. Basically, interpretations center around connections between the past and the present, sometimes between a fantasy and a feeling, but most commonly between a defense and a feeling (Kessler, 1966).

Freud, again in contrast to Klein, highlights the need to work with parents, realizing that the initiation, continuance, and termination of treatment are contingent upon their insight and motivations. Moreover, Anna Freud is careful to note that psychoanalytic treatment is not indicated for all types of children. It may be contraindicated for the psychotic and for those who have a marked difficulty in establishing a relationship due to severe emotional deprivations in early life. The existence of severe infantile neurosis and the capacity for speech are regarded as two prerequisites for analytic treatment.

Allen's Relationship Therapy

It was Frederick Allen (1942), a psychiatrist, who provided leadership for the form of treatment termed *relationship therapy*. As the name implies, the therapeutic relationship is seen as the basic growth-inducing ingredient. Allen stresses the value of play in helping the child to relate to the therapist. The play materials are provided and the child is permitted freedom to use them as he likes. Though basically a permissive approach, certain rules pertaining to time limitations and property destruction are enforced.

The major focus is not on the content of the child's play, however, but on the way in which the child uses his play in relating himself to the therapist. Thus, through the medium of play, the child transfers to the therapist feelings and reactions which he has previously learned in his relations with significant others. The child, for example, may use the therapist to symbolize the good or bad parent or as one who possesses the power of magical cures. On other occasions, his relations with the therapist in the play setting may take the form of domination or exclusion. There is no delving into buried or original meanings of the play since the therapeutic relationship is used for the immediate experience that it is. The concern is with the situational present and not with unconscious forces. Whatever the child says or does reflects his attitudes about the immediate setting and relationship. Within the atmosphere of acceptance provided by relationship therapy, the child's self-healing process, which has heretofore lain dormant, is now activated by the interpretation of the child's relationship with the therapist. Such interpretations in the presence of an accepting person enable the child to achieve a redefinition of himself—an "affirmation of himself as an individual"—which is eventually translated into new forms of behavior outside the therapeutic setting.

Adherents of this approach view it as particularly suitable with difficulties originating in tensions reflecting disturbed interpersonal relationships and in cases where environmental intervention has failed. Children with severe personality disorders are also considered prime candidates for relationship therapy. Although Allen does not elaborate, he does reiterate the need for concomitant work with the parents.

Like nondirective therapy, relationship therapy takes an optimistic view with regard to the child's capacity for change; it assumes that the child has the capacity to solve his own difficulties. Interpretations of the therapeutic relationship in a safe climate serve to release those positive growth forces which enable the child to solve his difficulties. Accordingly, the therapist does not seek to impose his own standards on the child. The child is taken as he is, and the therapist does not attempt to take over responsibilities for him.

The following quotation from Allen (1942) conveys the flavor of his approach:

The child is taken at the point he is at in his own development and he will react with his own feelings to meet this experience. It may bring out the overt fear that emerges around each new experience which requires leaving behind the supports he has been able or willing to let go. He may enter this relation with a guarded, cautious attitude that allows little if any participation. He may attempt to assume complete control by an assertive, aggressive attitude which may be directed against the therapist or be a part of his activity which aggressively shuts him out. He may try to establish a side of himself that is completely adequate and then show he needs no help from anyone. He can do all his own changing, or even prove those changes have occurred before he came. But the important fact to be understood is that the child starts this experience with his own feeling, whatever form it may take, and in putting his own feeling into it, the experience immediately takes on a significance that links it with his growth problem. The therapist then has the opportunity to give meaning and direction to this new growth experience because he is a part of it. He is in the position to give immediacy to the child's turmoil and help him to a more livable balance as this relation is established, as it moves and, finally, as it ends. He begins to discover certain unique features of this new experience. Here he may be afraid without having efforts made immediately to remove his fear. He has met with a person who understands and accepts both his need and his right to be afraid without melting before it. He finds that he can be aggressive and hostile, and, at the same time, finds a person who can both accept the feeling and give limits to his expression. He finds a person who is interested in what he says, in what he is, and is not trying to squeeze him into a preconceived mold. He can have his own power without having it overwhelmed by the greater power of another. He comes expecting to be changed and finds a person interested and related to what he is now. Truly, this is a unique experience which is started with himself in the center of it.

Axline's Client-Centered Approach

Virginia Axline (1947), following closely the therapeutic approach of Carl Rogers, regards play as therapeutic because of the freedom of expression given the child within the atmosphere of a secure relationship with the therapist. As with relationship therapy, treatment begins in the first session. The child is taken as he is, accepted without censure from the therapist, given ample opportunity to express his feelings in as permissive a climate as the situation will permit, and helped to recognize and clarify his feelings. The notion of respect for the individual and his potential for self-determination is central to this viewpoint. Consistent with the idea of man as a self-autonomous individual, no attempt at interpretation or manipulation is consciously made. Rather, the therapist, sensitive to the feelings of the child, reflects attitudes back to him so the child may achieve a better understanding of himself. Responsibility for growth is placed with the child, as it is assumed that he possesses not only the ability to handle his problems successfully but also an inner drive toward self-actualization and maturity as well. Thus, there is a basic trust that the client will make the best decision. The function of therapy is to create an atmosphere conducive to the release of these internal growth forces.

Although the role of the client is stressed, the therapist is by no means a passive agent, for it is his sensitive participation that helps the child to clarify his feelings and revise his self-concept. The therapist establishes a relationship which enables the child to reveal his real self and thereby facilitates the development of his personality. Hence, the therapeutic relationship again is seen as a crucial ingredient.

Axline, who has worked mostly with children aged 4 to 8, believes that a favorable outcome in therapy can be expected even though the parents are not involved in treatment. Nevertheless, she feels that work with parents can expedite the therapeutic process, especially in cases involving handicapped children.[1]

---

[1]For an excellent description of Axline's approach to play therapy, see her exciting and informative book, *Dibs in Search of Self* (1964).

Axline has given a succinct statement of her position in the following basic principles which serve as guidelines for the nondirective therapist:

1. The therapist must develop a warm, friendly relationship with the child, in which good rapport is established as soon as possible.

2. The therapist accepts the child exactly as he is.

3. The therapist establishes a feeling of permissiveness in the relationship so that the child feels free to express his feelings completely.

4. The therapist is alert to recognize the feelings the child is expressing and reflects those feelings back to him in such a manner that he gains insight into his behavior.

5. The therapist maintains a deep respect for the child's ability to solve his own problems if given an opportunity to do so. The responsibility to make choices and to institute change is the child's.

6. The therapist does not attempt to direct the child's actions or conversation in any manner. The child leads the way; the therapist follows.

7. The therapist does not attempt to hurry the therapy along. It is a gradual process and is recognized as such by the therapist.

8. The therapist establishes only those limitations that are necessary to anchor the therapy to the world of reality and to make the child aware of his responsibility in the relationship.

The similarities between relationship therapy, which developed earlier, and client-centered therapy are readily perceived. The two approaches do differ, however, in that Allen does make interpretations, is willing to use supportive techniques if indicated, and is more variable in his method (Watson, 1951).

Slavson's Activity Group Psychotherapy

Slavson is best known for his *activity group psychotherapy,* which represents an adaptation of group therapy to children. In this approach, the group is regarded as a substitute family, with the therapist assuming the role of an impartial and calm parent substitute. Activity (for example, a group project) is substituted for the usual verbal interaction characteristic of adult group psychotherapy. Conversations do occur in the weekly meetings but in conjunction with the activities in which the youngsters are participating. Permissiveness, while a basic element in this approach, is carried out in a specifically structured setting. Through "passive restraint," the therapist conveys to the child and the group that he does not approve of certain behavior and that he does want to be a part of them. Another therapeutic element is that of social imitation. Slavson, through personal example, displays socially acceptable behavior and by so doing offers the disturbed child modeling cues for more desirable behavior. For example, at the end of the session, the therapist begins to clean up the room and the children gradually do likewise. Such therapeutic factors as emotional release, relationship, and insight are also considered operative although insight is not accorded a role of importance. The use of interpretation is accordingly deemphasized.

The goals of Slavson's (1947) approach are presented in the following quotation:

Generally, activity group therapy provides spontaneous discharge of drives, diminution of tension and reduction of anxiety through physical and emotional activity in a group setting that permits unimpeded acting out within the boundaries of personal safety, and through free interaction with fellow members that leads to a variety of relationships. Interpersonal and social situations consistently arise through which each discharges tensions, expresses emotions, discovers limitations, builds ego strength, finds some status for himself, develops relationships in a limited degree of derivative insight. The total situation is designed to supply substitute gratification, give vent to aggression, reinforce the ego, particularly in regard to feelings of failure and inadequacy, counteract deflated self-evaluation, release blockings to expression in some, and build self-restraint in others.

With respect to age, activity group psychotherapy is seen as suitable for use with youngsters between ages 7 and 14. With respect to disturbance, it is indicated for a wide variety of disturbed children—the acting-out child, the child with character disorders, and the child with neurotic disturbances.

After a period of from six to eight months, the child's social adjustment to the group has progressed to the extent that a return to the neighborhood group is possible. The permissive atmosphere of the group setting does, however, contraindicate the presence of the extremely hostile and uncontrolled child. The psychotic child would also not be considered for this type of treatment.

Comparison of Major Varieties

Table 15 provides a summary comparison of the theorists discussed in this chapter, including the behavior therapists, who are discussed

TABLE 15. A COMPARISON AMONG THE PROPONENTS OF THE MAJOR
THERAPEUTIC APPROACHES ON SELECTED DIMENSIONS

Dimension	Solomon	Levy	Klein	A. Freud	Allen	Axline	Slavson	Behavior Therapists
Therapeutic relationship	H	H	H	H	H	H	H	L
Expression of feeling	H	H	H	H	H	H	H	L
Pointing out feeling Recognition of feeling	M	L	H	H	H	H	L	L
Interpretation	M	L	H	H	M	L	L	L
Transference	L	L	H	M	L	L	L	L
Past history of individual	H	H	H	H	L	L	L	L
Parental involvement	H	L	L	M	H	L	L	M
Age range	L	H	L	N	N	H	H	L
Control of child's activity	H	H	L	L	L	L	L	H
Type of disorder	L	H	H	H	L	L	M	L

H = Heavy emphasis; M = Moderate emphasis; L = Little emphasis; N = No specific discussion.

later in the chapter. Note that Therapeutic Relationship and Expression of Feeling are regarded as essential ingredients by all except the behavior therapists. Theorists are somewhat more variable in the importance attached to Pointing Out Feeling, with the client-centered therapists stressing Recognition of Feeling, the psychoanalytically oriented therapists stressing Interpretation, and the behavior therapists deemphasizing this total dimension. Use of the Transference relationship is restricted primarily to the psychoanalytic group, with Melanie Klein according it a more central role in treatment than Anna Freud. The psychoanalytic theorists, together with the structured play therapists, Solomon and Levy, attach considerable importance to the Past History of Individual, whereas the other theorists focus on the patient's situational present. Considerable variation is observed with respect to Parental Involvement among the theorists discussed. Levy, Slavson, and Axline have generally deemed their treatment as more suitable for a specific Age Range than have other theorists. The theorists are fairly well dichotomized with respect to Control of Child's Activity; the structured approaches (Levy, Solomon, and the behaviorists) are at one end of the continuum, and the "free" play therapists at the other. On the final dimension, Type of Disorder, certain theorists (Levy, Klein, and Freud) view their treatment approaches as appropriate for specific types of behavioral deviations, while other theorists are more willing to treat a greater variety of disorders.[2]

EVALUATION OF PSYCHOTHERAPY

EMPIRICAL STUDIES

Parents and educators often turn to mental-health specialists when attempting to resolve the problems their children or pupils present. Today there are approximately 2,000 outpatient clinics and more than 400 hospitals with psychiatric units offering mental-health services (Bower, 1970). The question naturally arises, How effective is the treatment provided by these facilities? The authors can recall numerous occasions when they sat in on case conferences with mental-health specialists and school personnel and heard a sigh of relief from the participants once the child was recommended for psychotherapy.

How realistic is it to feel such a sense of relief? Generally speaking, results at termination of treatment indicate that from two-thirds to three-fourths of children seen at child-guidance centers show improvement. Typical of such findings was a large-scale national investigation of outpatient psychiatric clinics in 1959, conducted by Norman, Rosen, and Bahn (1962), who discovered an improvement rate of 72 per cent. Followup studies, moreover, indicate that children treated on an outpatient basis maintain their improved status (Levitt, 1957). The results of psychotherapy with residential treatment cases yield similarly high improvement rates both at the time of termination of treatment (Reid & Hagen, 1952) and at the time of followup (Rubin, 1962). Hence, data obtained on outpatients and inpatients at the close of therapy and at the time of followup seemingly suggest that the grounds for the sigh of relief alluded to earlier are realistically based.

There are, however, two disquieting aspects regarding the outcomes of psychotherapeutic treatment of children. First, of approximately 200,000 children seen in outpatient psychiatric clinics in 1959, only

---

[2]For additional discussion of expressive therapies with children, see Hammer and Kaplan (1967) and Haworth (1964).

one-fourth were accepted for direct treatment of some kind, another fourth were clinic-terminated as unsuitable for treatment, and half were clinic-terminated with the majority of such cases being referred to the originating agency (Norman, Rosen, & Bahn, 1962). As Redl (1966) notes, the model of "the holy trinity" (psychiatrist, psychologist, and social worker) is obsolescent, and the need for new modes of treatment to cope with the new mixtures of childhood disturbances is apparent. Schofield (1964), in a somewhat similar vein, points out that psychotherapists have not been trained to deal with some of the more common types of problems being referred to them, namely, difficulties symptomatic of social distress and discomfort.

Second, professional rejoicing over the high improvement rates for those accepted for treatment would have to be predicated upon the proposition that untreated disturbed youngsters do not improve. But an examination of the base rates for improvement without psychotherapy yields little support for such a proposition. The best-known studies on psychotherapeutic outcomes with children have been conducted by Eugene Levitt, and these will be discussed in some detail because of their significance and the controversy which they have engendered.

In attempting to take an objective look at the outcomes of psychotherapy with children, Levitt (1957) reviewed 18 reports of evaluations at the close of treatment and 17 reports at the time of followup. The studies reviewed were conducted between 1929 and 1955 and involved more than 7,500 clients who might be crudely labeled as having neurotic disturbances. About two-thirds of these children were classified as either much improved or partly improved at termination of treatment, and more than three-fourths of these children were so classified upon followup some five years later on the average. However, using "defectors" from therapy as a control group, that is, children who had been accepted for treatment but who had withdrawn from the waiting list before treatment began, Levitt obtained comparable improvement rates (72.5 per cent).

In his latest review, Levitt (1963) reported on studies which appeared between 1957 and 1963, thus bringing his evidence up to date. Like his earlier findings, the more recent ones offer little comfort to the proponents of traditional therapeutic approaches in that they failed to offer any satisfactory evidence that psychotherapy increases the likelihood of relief accorded to emotionally disturbed children.

Levitt went one step further in his latest report by analyzing the results for various diagnostic groups. As shown in Table 16, the data tentatively suggest that the lowest therapeutic rates occurred for cases of delinquent and acting-out behaviors and that the highest improvement rates were for specific maladaptive symptoms like enuresis and school phobia.

TABLE 16. A SUMMARY OF STUDIES ON SELECTED PSYCHIATRIC DISORDERS OF CHILDREN [SUMMARY OF EVALUATION DATA FROM TWENTY-TWO STUDIES — LEVITT, 1963]

Type of Disorder	Number of Studies	Much Improved (N) (%)		Partly Improved (N) (%)		Unim- proved (N) (%)		Total (N)	Over-All (%) Improved
Neurosis	3	34	15	107	46	89	39	230	61
Acting-out	5	108	31	84	24	157	45	349	55
Special Symptoms	5	114	54	49	23	50	23	213	77
Psychosis	5	62	25	102	40	88	35	252	65
Mixed	6	138	20	337	48	222	32	697	68
Total	24*	456	26.2	679	39.0	606	34.8	1741	65.2

*The study of [P. Annesley. Psychiatric illness in adolescence: presentation and prognosis. J. ment. Sci., 1961, 107, 268-278.] contributed data to three classifications.
Source: E. Levitt. Psychotherapy with children: a further review. Behav. Res. Ther., 1963, 1, 45-61. Reprinted with permission of Pergamon Press.

In still another study, Levitt, Beiser, and Robertson (1959) reported on 192 clients who had had ten or more therapy sessions at the Institute for Juvenile Research in Chicago, one of the largest child-guidance centers in the country. The treated group and the defector controls were compared on 26 variables through psychological tests, objective facts about adjustment, parental ratings, self-ratings, and the clinical judgment of interviewers. There were no significant differences found between the two groups on any of these outcome variables. On the average, five years had elapsed since treatment, and the average age at the time of followup was 16. Thus, the findings of this long-range followup study support those of Levitt's other reviews which dealt a serious blow to the contention that therapy facilitates recovery from neurotic and emotional disturbances in children.

As might be expected, Levitt's findings have not gone unnoticed. The major objections to his studies have centered around the use of defectors as a control group and the use of inexperienced therapists.

Critics (Eisenberg & Gruenberg, 1961; Heinicke, 1960; Hood-Williams, 1960; Ross & Lacey, 1961) contend that defectors are inappropriate as control baselines, because they may be less seriously disturbed youngsters who are able to respond in a therapeutically favorable way to the diagnostic assessment alone. Levitt (1963) readily admits the possibility of a "therapeutic diagnosis" issue; yet his findings were that interim improvement between diagnostic assessment and the offer of therapy was the sole explanation for termination of treatment in only 12 per cent of the cases. Thus, it seems unlikely that the interim improvement in symptoms can adequately account for the over-all improvement rate. Besides, the interim-improvement phenomenon should also have presumably existed in the case of the treated group, thereby balancing this factor in the defector group. Despite having compared the defector group and treated cases on 61 factors, including two clinical estimates relative to severity of disturbance, Levitt found few differences. Hence, although it can be said that the use of those who had been accepted for treatment but who dropped off the waiting list prior to actual treatment may result in the selection of a biased group, Levitt's study does not show this to be the case. Nevertheless, the use of defectors as a control group of subjects remains a controversial issue.

As to the second major objection to Levitt's studies, Kessler (1966) noted that almost half the children in the 1959 study were seen by student therapists with less than one year's experience, and only one-third of the child patients were treated by therapists who had more than three years' experience. Granted that many inexperienced therapists use clinics to gain experience before entering private practice, it does not follow that the use of inexperienced therapists minimizes the prospect for a favorable therapeutic outcome. In fact, there is some evidence to suggest that inexperienced therapists achieve better results than do their more experienced colleagues, perhaps because of the greater enthusiasm of the former. Moreover, it may be that non-professional therapists can perform as well as professional therapists (Rioch et al., 1963; Poser, 1966; Truax and Carkhuff, 1967).

There is still another problem which must be considered in evaluating the results of psychotherapy: the placebo effect, which in medicine refers to the observation that patients respond favorably when administered either sugar pills or a saline solution instead of an appropriate medication. Since the placebo effect is of a psychological nature, its role cannot be ignored in evaluating the outcomes of psychotherapy. This effect is regarded by some authorities as a nonspecific result of psychotherapy and as playing a possible role in the consistently high rates of psychotherapeutic improvement (Rosenthal & Frank, 1956). It is interesting to note, in this connection, that the majority of disturbed children improve regardless of age, sex, treatment setting, affiliation of the therapist, length of time spent in treatment, and whether or not they complete the treatment.

Others would argue that the efficacy of psychotherapy with children is limited to the placebo effect since the two-thirds improvement rate in therapy is about the same as the improvement rate resulting from the placebo effect in illnesses with emotional components. Basically, the placebo effect can take two forms: the use of suggestion or authority by the therapist and/or the attention, interest, and concern shown the child (Patterson, 1959). A genuinely rigorous experiment, as Ginott (1961) notes, requires a comparison of three groups to which subjects have been randomly assigned: (1) a therapy group, (2) a no-therapy group, and (3) a placebo group who have play sessions at the clinic but without a therapist. As Ginott (1961) contends, "Thus far, there is no evidence to indicate the superiority of play therapy over dancing lessons in the treatment of shyness nor its superiority over boxing lessons in the treatment of aggressiveness."

SPONTANEOUS REMISSIONS

Granted that the issue is still a hotly debated one, the evidence bearing on psychotherapeutic outcomes indicates that the effectiveness of expressive treatment procedures has not lived up to expectations. Yet, it is comforting to note that the majority of neurotic-like children do achieve a reasonably adequate adjustment regardless of whether or not they receive professional treatment. Thus, despite the child's defenses having failed and his having reached a low ebb, the odds are that he will not stick at this low point (White, 1964).

What factors are responsible for the spontaneous reduction of deviant behavior? Certainly, one factor which cannot be discounted is the placebo effect, mentioned above, for the child's behavior, especially as it reaches a low ebb, is apt to elicit attention, concern, and authoritative reassurance that the behavior will improve.

Alternative explanations which employ learning-theory constructs— such as aversive stimulation, extinction, positive reinforcement, and so forth—also enable us to account for spontaneous remissions in children. Aversive stimulation is most likely operative in cases where the untreated neurosis becomes so painful that the child himself actively seeks to improve his lot in life. Secondary gains no doubt play a reinforcing role in certain cases of neurosis, but "secondary pains" are also operative. As White (1964) asserts, the neurotic adjustment is apt to be an unpleasant one which motivates the child to seek "a new balance of forces toward remission." The authors can readily recall school-phobic youngsters who, suffering from the unpleasant state of having nothing to do at home, willingly attempted a return to school despite their initial anxieties.

According to Eysenck (1963a, 1963b), spontaneous remissions can also be expected simply on the basis of extinction since the presentation in everyday life of the conditioned stimulus that produces the troublesome behavior without the presentation of the reinforcing stimuli is likely to eliminate the maladaptive responses. Positive reinforcement for adaptive behavior following extinction, discrimination learning based on expectations related to cultural conceptions regarding appropriate behavior for one's developmental level, and nonsystematic desensitization also probably account for the elimination of maladaptive behaviors in untreated cases.

In addition to explanations based on the placebo effect and learning theory, evidence bearing on this issue of spontaneous recovery is forthcoming from the study of personality development in children. Such study has indicated the child's substantial ability to withstand environmental insult. The notion of the child as a delicate individual who must be protected from stresses, strains, and traumas and who must have exceptional amounts of "tender, loving care" is obviously distorted. The child not only possesses a substantial capacity for compensation and adjustment but also a remarkable capability for self-repair when damage is inflicted (Anderson, 1948). Fortunately, the child is a durable creature. The authors, like many other teachers and clinicians recalling their experiences with children from seriously disturbed homes, have wondered why the children were as well adjusted as they were, in light of the environmental insult. This observation is not intended to deny the role of parental and social pathology in childhood disorders but is mentioned simply to illustrate the resiliency of the child's personality.

The findings presented on intervention efforts lend support to

Redl's (1966) contention that we need new modes of treatment to cope with the new types of disturbances which have arisen. In large measure, youngsters have been referred to the psychiatric clinic even though they did not fit the classical model provided by the trinity of psychiatrist, psychologist, and social worker. It is little wonder that half of the clients come back, like the proverbial bad penny, to the agency initiating the referral. As those in charge of the daily management of disturbed children stress, we need services that are closer to the real-life situation of the children than the clinic model permits. Furthermore, we need new team members—the educational therapist, the public-health nurse, the pediatrician, the teacher—in addition to the traditional mental-health specialists if we are to implement a more realistic approach to the problems presented by today's disturbed youth (Redl, 1966). At this point, we will explore two relatively recent innovations—behavior therapy and the community mental-health movement—which permit a more reality-based intervention approach.

RECENT INNOVATIONS

BEHAVIOR THERAPY

Since modern psychology has been largely dominated by theories of learning, it is understandable that the most distinctive contribution made by psychologists to treatment efforts has come in the area of learning theory. In large measure the application of learning-theory concepts to the modification of deviant behavior can be attributed to the increasing number of clinical psychologists since World War II, the emphasis on more sophisticated training in research methodology at the doctoral level, the questioning of the traditional methods of psychotherapy, and the growing dissatisfaction with the appropriateness of the medical model for extension to behavior disorders (Ullmann & Krasner, 1965). Through the efforts of Dollard and Miller (1950), Shoben (1949), and Mowrer (1950), psychodynamic views were recast in learning-theory terms but, as Ullmann and Krasner (1965) assert, a new approach to *doing* therapy was not forthcoming, simply a new way of *talking about* therapy. Of the various learning-theory approaches to therapy, behavior therapy is attracting the most attention today and is probably the most relevant to the treatment of childhood disorders.

Basically, behavior therapy refers to the systematic application of learning-theory principles to the rational modification of deviant behavior (Franks, 1965). The term *behavior therapy* embraces not a specific technique but a variety of methods stemming from learning theory and focusing on the modification of deviant behavior. As such, it represents a meeting point for experimental and clinical psychology, fields which traditionally had been apart from each other.

While the roots of modifying behavior date back to the early Greeks, systematic attempts to produce behavior changes as a consequence of manipulated environmental contingencies are a relatively recent phenomenon. Watson's classic study in 1920 on the development of a phobia in a very young child played a key role by demonstrating that the emotional response of the human infant can be conditioned to previously innocuous objects. Thus, although 11-month-old Albert originally showed no fear in response to the sight of a white rat, he displayed a conditioned fear response soon after the simultaneous pairing of a white rat and the striking of a steel bar. Moreover, this fear spread to other furry animals and to furry objects, such as beards and cottonwool. This conditioned fear response also tended to persist throughout the months that Albert was available for study (Watson & Raynor, 1920).

Four years later, another experiment demonstrated that it was possible to eliminate a child's phobia. Jones (1924), using 3-year-old Peter, showed that a fear response which had generalized could also be eliminated through the use of a conditioning process. After conducting research on several other preschoolers, Jones concluded that direct conditioning and social imitation were effective means for eliminating fears. In that same year, Burnham (1924) published *The Normal Mind,* a book which anticipated techniques to be used by later behavior therapists.

Additional work in the treatment of tics, nailbiting, and stuttering (Dunlap, 1932) and fears (Jersild & Holmes, 1935) also contributed to both theory and practice. Mowrer and Mowrer's (1938) work on the conditioning of enuretics also represented a significant advance in the application of learning theory to children's disorders. But it was not until twenty years later that the next important step was made, when Wolpe (1958), a psychiatrist, formulated a systematic theory of neurosis and psychotherapy based on the principle of reciprocal inhibition (techniques designed to inhibit anxiety responses). Finally, in 1963, the journal *Behavior Research and Therapy* was established for those interested in behavior modification (Rachman, 1963).

Contrasts with Expressive Therapies

One of the first areas of disagreement between expressive therapies and behavior therapies centers around the issue of symptomatic treatment versus treatment of the underlying pathology. Psychoanalytically oriented therapists have traditionally shied away from the treatment of symptoms in accordance with the "symptom-underlying-disease medical model" discussed in Chapter 2. Accordingly, the psychoanalytically oriented view the behavior therapist as naively pragmatic. Relying on a hydraulic-energy analogy, the Freudians view the symptom as an outlet for a highly charged pentup energy which must find relief in one form or another. Neurotic symptoms thus represent the manifestation of the central conflict. Hence, the Freudians maintain that if one simply removes the symptom and not the underlying motivational forces, substitute symptoms can be expected. Moreover, according to the Freudian exposition, the therapist, by his attempts at symptomatic treatment, actually runs the risk of doing some further psychological damage to the patient by blocking energy release. It is not surprising, in light of this model, that the expression of feeling is considered a basic therapeutic ingredient in traditional forms of psychotherapy for both children and adults. In both Freudian and Rogerian therapies, the therapist is permissive since the tendencies toward self-realization or the biological urges will out inevitably, once provided with an accepting atmosphere which permits expression.

The learning theorists, on the other hand, view symptoms very differently. For Eysenck (1960), there is no neurosis underlying the symptom; there is just the symptom. As he boldly asserts, "Get rid of the symptom and you have eliminated the neurosis." In a similar, but somewhat milder vein, Franks (1965) adds,

Even if we assume that the present symptom owes its origin to some past trauma, it need follow neither that the trauma is of direct concern to the subject in the present nor that focusing attention upon the original traumatic situation inevitably must bring about the elimination of the present symptom. There is thus justification for concentrating on what is of concern, namely the symptom. It may be that it is not the original and long-past trauma which is still causing the present persisting symptom which is bringing about the emotional disturbance.

It is interesting to note that psychoanalytically oriented therapists do not conjecture as to the psychic damage which might ensue as a consequence of not treating symptoms, for example, enuresis. In the behavior-therapy approach, there is thus no search for relatively autonomous internal agents and processes in the form of dammed-up energy, complexes, unconscious psychic forces, free-floating libidos, or other hypothetical entities (Bandura & Walters, 1963). The learning theorist objects that such hypothetical conflicts are not directly subject to manipulation and, therefore, cannot play a major role in behavior modification. According to learning theory, there is little justifiable basis for the notion of symptom substitution from either a theoretical or an experimental standpoint. The behaviorist views the symptom as a dominant response which has been learned in relation to a specific stimulus situation. If this response or symptom is removed, the next most dominant response in the hierarchy is apt to occur. The behaviorist admits that the response obtained after behavioristic treatment may on occasion be a maladaptive one, but he does not regard the production of another undesirable behavior as inevitable or as symptom substitution in the Freudian sense of the term.

What would the behavior therapist do in the event that another maladaptive behavior occurred after treatment? He would continue to eliminate such responses from the behavior repertoire until adaptive behaviors occur. Contrary to widespread opinion, there is little if any evidence to substantiate the notion of symptom substitution (Grossberg, 1964). It is evident from the above that the behavior therapist makes an explicit attempt to produce new behavior in his client. Indeed, the modification of behavior is the central target of treatment. The nondirective therapist, on the other hand, never explicitly encourages his client toward certain courses of new behavior; he assumes that the individual will choose the right behavior or make the best decision once his internal growth forces have been released. Psychoanalytically oriented therapists are likewise reluctant to steer the client toward new modes of behavior.

This brings us to another difference between the two approaches. Behavior therapy represents a directive and manipulative approach, in which the therapist imposes the solution on the client. Expressive therapies, conversely, seek to treat the client without influencing him, by merely relieving the disabling psychic impairment (such as anxiety) and allowing him to find his own solution. The first view controls the individual from the outside; the second view permits self-determination. Two points should be noted as being germane to the manipulation versus the understanding issue. First, all therapists, regardless of orientation, most likely exert some influence on the client and his future actions. Thus, differences in the degree of manipulation between these two approaches may not be as great as initially suspected. There is, indeed, sufficient evidence to document the subtle influence of therapist manipulation in dynamic treatment approaches (Bandura, 1961; Greenspoon, 1962). Hence, if objection is to be voiced, it must not be focused on the issue of manipulation per se, but on the type of manipulation. Moreover, it would seem that some control, especially as it is oriented toward the well-being of both the individual and society, is necessary and desirable. The use of manipulation, ironically enough, enables the client to assume more flexible behaviors and thereby achieve greater individual self-determination by freeing him from present rigid and maladaptive behaviors. Second, while the behavioristic approach may be designated as manipulative, it is basically in keeping with the American tradition of achieving results in the most direct way. Ruesch and Bateson (1951) note that things typically have to be done fast in America and that therapy is no exception to the rule.

A third point of disagreement involves the role of the therapeutic relationship and transference. The evocative therapies, which tend to sanctify the therapist-client relationship, customarily devote considerable attention to such factors as rapport, understanding, acceptance, permissiveness, insight, emphasis on feelings, and at times the transference relationship. The procedures and objectives of behavior therapy, on the other hand, are such that these factors are given less attention, primarily because they are not regarded as essential prerequisites for successful therapy (Franks, 1965). The induction of cognitive contingencies may well be beneficial in behavioristic treatment (Peterson & London, 1965), but insight per se is not seen as a basic ingredient. It may be, as Bandura and Walters (1963) suggest, that insight is an outcome of the therapeutic process rather than an essential cause of successful treatment. As a consequence of its deemphasis on insight as a therapeutic ingredient, behavior therapy may be better suited to a wider child clientele than are the more conventional therapies. As Franks (1965) writes,

Unlike much of psychoanalytically oriented therapy, a behavior therapy program need not be restricted to the more sophisticated members of the society. It usually can be adapted to those who are intellectually, emotionally, or culturally at a disadvantage or whose knowledge of the therapist's language is limited.

Other evocative therapies would likewise seem inappropriate to children of low intelligence and/or of lower cultural standing in that the emphasis on permissiveness and/or the achievement of insight are too sociologically foreign to the culturally disadvantaged and to those of less than normal intelligence. Whereas the expressive therapies, with their emphasis on insight and self-knowledge, appeal to a more privileged and educated population, they are not appealing to most deprived people (Riessman, 1962). The mechanical and gadgetry aspects, together with the more directive atmosphere of behavior treatment, may lead to a more substantial initial gratification and therefore to greater motivation for therapy on the deprived youngster's part.

Evaluation

To date, there has been little experimental validation of the use of behavior therapy with children. The case-study approach, in which each child serves as his own control, has constituted the main avenue of exploration and assessment. There is some evidence to suggest that the results of behavior therapy with adults cannot be reduced to the placebo effect (Grossberg, 1964), but such a claim can neither be affirmed nor denied with respect to behavior therapy with children because of the paucity of rigorous scientific experimentation. The authors suspect that behavior therapy will register its greatest success in disorders which are due primarily to faulty learning and in disorders which involve specific symptomatology to be overcome. Although conclusive judgments would be premature, the results to date have been sufficiently encouraging to warrant further investigations in this area. The absence of demonstrated effectiveness of the evocative therapies, coupled with the shortage of trained mental-health specialists, would seem to leave us little other choice. Indeed, we can ill afford to ignore what appears to be a promising intervention approach. The extension of this approach to groups and the development of a core of psychotechnicians could prove a productive means of tackling the nation's foremost health problem on a larger scale by providing reality-type treatment services which are in close proximity to the child's life setting.

Many mental-health workers are unwilling to substitute the modification of behavior for personality reorganization as a goal of treatment. Controversy regarding the goals of therapy will probably rage for some time to come. Behavior modification is a less ambitious objective than that of other therapy approaches, which seem to undertake a total rebuilding of the individual. Yet, as Lewis (1965) asserts,

If we cannot aspire to reconstruction of personality that will have long range beneficial effects, we can modify disturbing behavior in specific ways in present social contexts. This more modest aspiration may not only be more realistic, but it may be all that is required of the child-helping professions in a society that is relatively open and provides a variety of opportunity systems in which a child can reconcile his personal needs with society's expectations of him.[3]

COMMUNITY MENTAL HEALTH

There is much discussion of *community mental health* today, but there is little agreement as to the precise meaning of the term. It is different things to different people. The myriad of meanings is not surprising in light of the varied and sundry activities subsumed under this umbrella term. Basic to all definitions of this concept is the fact that it points to a declining role of the traditional state hospital and the rise of the community mental-health center with all of the attendant auxiliary services essential for the treatment of the mentally ill. According to Dunham (1965),

In its ideal form the community mental health center would provide psychiatric services, both diagnostic and treatment; for all age groups and for both inpatients and outpatients in a particular community. In addition, the center would have attached closely to it day and night hospitals, convalescent homes, rehabilitative programs or, for that matter, any service that helps toward the maximizing of treatment potential with respect to the characteristics of the population that it is designed to serve. Also attached to this center would be several kinds of research activities aimed at evaluating and experimenting with old and new therapeutic procedures.

Hume (1964) has delineated nine functions of community psychiatry:

(1) *Community organization work,* that is, assessment of community resources for psychiatric patients, evaluation of their use, measurement of unmet

---

[3]For further discussion on the issue of evaluation, see Franks (1968).

needs (i.e., community self-surveys) plus participation with other agency representatives and community leaders . . .

(2) *Program administration* (including planning, evaluation, management, staffing, and financing) of either direct or indirect, partial or comprehensive, community mental health services for the whole population . . .

(3) *Supervision,* not only as an administrative adjunct, but also as a method of improving the professional performance of all the staff of a community mental health service or program.

(4) *The training of lay leaders,* health educators, or specialists in the use of mass media, in order that they may disseminate information and general education to the public on mental health matters.

(5) *In-service training,* that is, organized programs of mental health education for the nonpsychiatric professions such as medicine, nursing or the law, and for the staffs of nonpsychiatric agencies such as schools, welfare, public health or probation departments.

(6) *Consultation* to nonpsychiatric agencies and professions in connection with a wide variety of mental health problems encountered within such agencies in their work with people.

(7) *Research* in community psychiatry, such as case studies, program evaluation, biostatistical and epidemiological studies, mental health surveys, and studies of psychiatric institutions as social systems.

(8) *Utilization* of the laws touching upon community psychiatry, for example, enabling acts and welfare, family, and commitment laws.

(9) *Development of leadership,* participation in committee work and other group endeavors, and promotion of communication.

Bower (1970) has succinctly listed five essentials of a community health center. It must provide (1) inpatient services; (2) outpatient services; (3) hospitalization services, including at least day care; (4) emergency services; and (5) consultation and educational services to community agencies and professional personnel. Bower notes that these centers are being established, not in the large, metropolitan areas (where mental-health professionals have already congregated), but in middle-size cities with a population of approximately 65,000. He views this trend as desirable in that the community-center idea is better suited to the needs of moderate-size communities than it is to the needs of large urban areas. Although psychiatrists and psychologists will be on the staff, they will be heavily outnumbered by social workers.

Problems to Be Solved

Since community mental-health programs are of relatively recent vintage and assume a diversity of functions, it would be premature to pass judgment on them. Nevertheless, some concerns have already been expressed. Foremost among these is the type of training being given community mental-health specialists. It is apparent that current training programs in psychology and psychiatry have to be radically revised if the many functions listed above are to be performed. Currently, there appear to be few commonly accepted standards with regard to training requirements for community mental-health consultants beyond clinical training and experience (Haylett & Rapoport, 1964). A second problem centers around the danger that the change may be merely of the *locus* of function and not the *type* of treatment rendered.

Other serious questions which must eventually be answered have been raised by Dunham (1965):

What are the possible techniques that can be developed to treat the "collectivity"? Why do psychiatrists think that it is possible to treat the "collectivity" when there still exists a marked uncertainty with respect to the treatment and cure of the individual case? What causes the psychiatrist to think that if he advances certain techniques for treating the "collectivity," they will have community acceptance? If he begins to "treat" a group through discussions in order to develop personal insights, what assurances does he have that the results will be psychologically beneficial to the persons? Does the psychiatrist know how to organize a community along mentally hygienic lines and if he does, what evidence does he have that such an organization will be an improvement over the existing organization? In what institutional setting or in what cultural milieu would the psychiatrist expect to begin in order to move toward more healthy social relationships in the community? These are serious questions and I raise them with reference to the notion that the community is the patient.

To this list of difficulties, we add Bower's (1970) belief that the major obstacle to the community mental-health approach centers in the danger of fragmentation of services stemming from the autonomy and isolation which exist in various community agencies.

In sum, the idea of mental-health professionals going into the life situations of people in a community at key points where adjustment difficulties are apt to arise, for example, the schools, is an intriguing one. Only evaluation over time will determine how viable this idea is.

SUMMARY

This chapter opened with a discussion of certain differences between children and adults that have import for child psychotherapy. Differences in motivation for treatment, insight into the goals of treatment, linguistic development, environmental dependency, and the modifiability of personality development highlight the need for such treatment changes as "getting-acquainted" sessions, utilization of the child's inclination to manipulate and explore, stress on nonverbal communication, and increased attention to external reality factors. As might be inferred from a consideration of these differences, play therapy is often well suited to children.

Therapeutic approaches vary with respect to the importance attached to such variables as the expression of feeling, the intensity of the therapeutic relationship, the degree of parental involvement, and so on. Evaluative studies indicate that the vast majority (as many as three-fourths) of youngsters given therapy do improve. It has not been clearly established that this rate of improvement surpasses that of untreated disturbed youngsters, however. Behavior therapy and community mental health, two of the more recent treatment approaches, seem to have appreciable potential as reality-based interventions.

SUGGESTED READINGS

Bandura, A. *Principles of behavior modification.* New York: Holt, Rinehart & Winston, 1969.

Bloomberg, G. (Ed.) *The existentialist approach to psychotherapy with adults and children.* New York: Grune & Stratton, 1965.

Franks, C. M. *Assessment and status of the behavior therapies.* New York: McGraw-Hill, 1968.

Hammer, M., & Kaplan, A. M. *The practice of psychotherapy with children.* Homewood, Ill.: Dorsey Press, 1967.

Ullmann, L. P., & Krasner, L. *Case studies in behavior modification.* New York: Holt, Rinehart & Winston, 1965.

REFERENCES

Allen, F. *Psychotherapy with children.* New York: Norton, 1942.

Anderson, J. Personality organization in children. *Amer. Psychologist,* 1948, 3, 409-416.

Axline, V. *Play therapy.* Boston: Houghton Mifflin, 1947.

Axline, V. *Dibs in search of self.* New York: Ballantine Books, 1964.

Bandura, A. Psychotherapy as a learning process. *Psychol. Bull.,* 1961, 58, 143-157.

Bandura, A., & Walters, R. H. *Social learning and personality development.* New York: Holt, Rinehart & Winston, 1963.

Bower, E. M. Mental health. In R. Ebel (Ed.), *Encyclopedia of educational research.* (4th ed.) New York: Macmillan, 1970. Pp. 811-828.

Burnham, W. H. *The normal mind.* New York: Appleton-Century-Crofts, 1924.

Dollard, J., & Miller, N. E. *Personality and psychotherapy.* New York: McGraw-Hill, 1950.

Dunham, H. W. Community psychiatry: the newest therapeutic bandwagon. *Arch. gen. Psychiat.,* 1965, **12**, 303-313.

Dunlap, K. *Habits: their making and unmaking.* New York: Liveright, 1932.

Eisenberg, L., & Gruenberg, E. The current status of secondary prevention in child psychiatry. *Amer. J. Orthopsychiat.,* 1961, **31**, 355-367.

Eysenck, H. Learning theory and behavior therapy. In H. Eysenck, *Behavior therapy and the neuroses.* London: Pergamon Press, 1960. Pp. 4-21.

Eysenck, H. Behavior therapy extinction and relapse in neurosis. *Brit. J. Psychiat.,* 1963, **109**, 12-18. (a)

Eysenck, H. Behavior therapy, spontaneous remission and transference in neurotics. *Amer. J. Psychiat.,* 1963, **119**, 867-871. (b)

Franks, C. Behavior therapy, psychology and the psychiatrist: contributions, evaluation and overview. *Amer. J. Orthopsychiat.,* 1965, **35**, 145-151.

Franks, C. M. *Assessment and status of the behavior therapies.* New York: McGraw-Hill, 1968.

Freud, A. *Psychoanalytic treatment of children.* London: Imago, 1946.

Freud, A. *Normality and pathology in childhood.* New York: International Universities Press, 1965.

Freud, S. Analysis of a phobia in a five-year-old boy. *Standard edition of the complete psychological works of Sigmund Freud,* 1909, **10**, 5-149.

Froebel, F. Quoted in L. Jackson & K. Todd, *Child treatment and the therapy of play.* (2nd ed.) New York: Ronald Press, 1950.

Ginott, H. *Group psychotherapy with children.* New York: McGraw-Hill, 1961.

Greenspoon, J. Verbal conditioning and clinical psychology. In A. J. Bachrach (Ed.), *Experimental foundations of clinical psychology.* New York: Basic Books, 1962. Pp. 510-553.

Grossberg, J. Behavior therapy: a review. *Psychol. Bull.,* 1964, **62**, 73-88.

Hammer, M., & Kaplan, A. M. *The practice of psychotherapy with children.* Homewood, Ill.: Dorsey Press, 1967.

Hartley, R., Frank, L., & Goldenson, R. *Understanding children's play.* New York: Columbia Univer. Press, 1952.

Haworth, M. *Child psychotherapy.* New York: Basic Books, 1964.

Haylett, C. H., & Rapoport, L. Mental health consultation. In L. Bellak (Ed.), *Handbook of community psychiatry and community mental health.* New York: Grune & Stratton, 1964. Pp. 319-339.

Heinicke, C. Research on psychotherapy with children: a review and suggestions for further study. *Amer. J. Orthopsychiat.,* 1960, **30**, 483-493.

Hood-Williams, J. The results of psychotherapy with children: a revolution. *J. consult. Psychol.,* 1960, **24**, 84-88.

Hume, P. B. Principles and practices of community psychiatry: the role and training of the specialist in community psychiatry. In L. Bellak (Ed.), *Handbook of community psychiatry and community mental health.* New York: Grune & Stratton, 1964. Pp. 65-81.

Jersild, F., & Holmes, F. Methods of overcoming children's fears. *J. Psychol.*, 1935, **1**, 75-104.

Jones, M. C. A laboratory study of fear: the case of Peter. *J. genet. Psychol.*, 1924, **31**, 308-315.

Kessler, J. W. *Psychopathology of childhood.* Englewood Cliffs, N.J.: Prentice-Hall, 1966.

Klein, M. The psychoanalytic play technique. *Amer. J. Orthopsychiat.*, 1955, **25**, 223-227.

Lazarus, A., & Rachman, S. The use of systematic desensitization in psychotherapy. *S. Afr. med. J.*, 1957, **31**, 934-937.

Levitt, E. Results of psychotherapy with children: an evaluation. *J. consult. Psychol.*, 1957, **21**, 189-196.

Levitt, E. Psychotherapy with children: a further review. *Behav. Res. Ther.*, 1963, **1**, 45-51.

Levitt, E., Beiser, H., & Robertson, R. A follow-up evaluation of cases treated at a community child guidance clinic. *Amer. J. Orthopsychiat.*, 1959, **29**, 337-347.

Levy, D. Relationship therapy. *Amer. J. Orthopsychiat.*, 1938, **8**, 64-69.

Levy, D. Trends in therapy: III. Release therapy. *Amer. J. Orthopsychiat.*, 1939, **9**, 713-736.

Lewis, W. Continuity and intervention in emotional disturbance: a review. *Except. Child.*, 1965, **32**, 465-475.

Lippman, H. S. *Treatment of the child in emotional conflict.* (2nd ed.) New York: McGraw-Hill, 1962.

Loomis, E. A. The use of checkers in handling certain resistance in child therapy and analysis. *J. Amer. psychoanal. Assn*, 1957, **5**, 130-135.

Mowrer, O. H. *Learning theory and personality dynamics.* New York: Ronald Press, 1950.

Mowrer, O., & Mowrer, W. Enuresis: a method for its study and treatment. *Amer. J. Orthopsychiat.*, 1938, **8**, 436-459.

Norman, V., Rosen, B., & Bahn, A. Psychiatric clinic out-patients in the United States, 1959. *Ment. Hyg.*, 1962, **46**, 321-343.

Patterson, C. *Counseling and psychotherapy: theory and practice.* New York: Harper, 1959.

Pearson, G. H. J. *Emotional disorders of children.* New York: Norton, 1949.

Peterson, D., & London, P. A role for cognition in the behavioral treatment of a child's eliminative disturbance. In L. P. Ullmann & L. Krasner (Eds.), *Case studies in behavior modification.* New York: Holt, Rinehart & Winston, 1965. Pp. 289-294.

Phillips, R. Doll play as a function of the realism of the materials and the length of the experimental session. *Child Develpm.*, 1945, **16**, 123-143.

Piaget, J. *Psychology of intelligence.* Paterson, N.J.: Littlefield, Adams, 1960.

Pintler, M. Doll play as a function of experimenter-child interaction and initial organization of materials. *Child Develpm.*, 1945, **16**, 145-166.

Poser, E. G. The effect of therapist training on group therapeutic outcome. *J. consult. Psychol.*, 1966, **30**, 283-289.

Rachman, S. Introduction to behavior therapy. *Behav. Res. Ther.*, 1963, **1**, 3-15.

Redl, F. *When we deal with children.* New York: Free Press, 1966.

Reid, J. H., & Hagen, H. *Residential treatment of emotionally disturbed children.* New York: Child Welfare League of America, 1952.

Riessman, F. *The culturally deprived child.* New York: Harper, 1962.

Rioch, M. J., Elkes, C., Flint, A. A., Udansky, B. S., Newman, R. G., & Silber, E. National Institute of Mental Health pilot study in training of mental health counselors. *Amer. J. Orthopsychiat.*, 1963, **33**, 678-689.

Rosenthal, D., & Frank, J. Psychotherapy and the placebo effect. *Psychol. Bull.*, 1956, **53**, 294-302.

Ross, A. O., & Lacey, H. M. Characteristics of terminators and remainers in child guidance treatment. *J. consult. Psychol.*, 1961, **25**, 420-424.

Rubin, E. Special education in a psychiatric hospital. *Except. Child.*, 1962, **29**, 184-190.

Ruesch, J., & Bateson, G. *Communication: the social matrix of psychiatry.* New York: Norton, 1951.

Schofield, W. *Psychotherapy: the purchase of friendship.* Englewood Cliffs, N.J.: Prentice-Hall, 1964.

Shoben, E. Psychotherapy as a problem in learning theory. *Psychol. Bull.*, 1949, **46**, 366-392.

Slavson, S. General principles and dynamics. In S. Slavson (Ed.), *The practice of group therapy.* New York: International Universities Press, 1947. Pp. 13-39.

Slavson, S. *Child psychotherapy.* New York: Columbia Univer. Press, 1952.

Solomon, J. Therapeutic use of play. In H. Anderson & G. Anderson (Eds.), *An introduction to projective techniques.* Englewood Cliffs, N.J.: Prentice-Hall, 1951. Pp. 639-661.

Truax, C. B., & Carkhuff, R. R. *Toward effective counseling and psychotherapy training and practice.* Chicago: Aldine, 1967.

Ullmann, L. P., & Krasner, L. *Case studies in behavior modification.* New York: Holt, Rinehart & Winston, 1965.

Watson, J., & Raynor, R. Conditioned emotional reactions. *J. exp. Psychol.*, 1920, **3**, 1-14.

Watson, R. I. *The clinical method in psychology.* New York: Harper, 1951.

Wattenberg, W. W. Review of trends. In W. W. Wattenberg (Ed.), Social deviancy among youth. *Yearb. nat. Soc. Stud. Educ.*, 1966, **65**, Part I. Pp. 4-27.

White, R. W. *The abnormal personality.* (3rd ed.) New York: Ronald Press, 1964.

Wolpe, J. *Psychotherapy by reciprocal inhibition.* Stanford, Calif.: Stanford Univer. Press, 1958.

10

Environmental Interventions

Despite the general recognition that behavior can be encouraged or hindered by situational factors, the possibility of correcting adjustment problems by environmental change is often overlooked. Several factors are related to this reluctance:

1. The prevailing revered status attached to the home and family as the irreplaceable center for human development.

2. The view that behavior disorders are the outcome of internal (intrapsychic) conflicts.

3. The contention that psychotherapy is the only method for the permanent correction of behavior disorders.

The weight of these influences can be observed in the rationalization than any home is better than no home, the "rule" many children's clinics have against classifying a sub-teen-age child as psychotic, and the frank puzzlement which gives rise to a "wait and see" attitude rather than one of active intervention.

Information as to what the child requires for optimal development and which experiential deficits can result in devastating handicaps is accumulating. The bulk of this information has come from the so-called deprivation studies, which have shown the marked limitations on developmental potentials exerted by reduced stimulation. Deficits in sensory, motor, or social-emotional experiences are later identifiable in consequent deficiencies of competency in these same skill areas. There is accruing evidence that supplying the child with a stimulating environment leads to positive changes.

OVERVIEW

THE DEVELOPMENT OF COMMUNITY SERVICES

The provision of services for children obviously follows the prevailing theories concerning the causes of behavior disorders and the proper treatment required to correct the disabilities. At first, it was believed that little could be done to correct a behavior disorder. Treatment consisted of diagnosis and custodial care. The influences of the home and family were regarded as having a primary role in forming the child's personality. This view implied correction of impaired interpersonal relationships by psychotherapy provided directly to the children and indirectly through the parents. It became increasingly evident that children left to fend for themselves—provided with inadequate supervision, stimulation, and care of all kinds—faced a future filled with grave risks to their physical health, safety, and emotional well-being.

The failure to produce the needed supply of specific professional persons (psychiatrists, psychologists, and social workers) and the admission of the improbability of meeting this demand forced the consideration of more practical and feasible procedures for the delivery of essential corrective services. For example, at the Mid-Decade Conference on Children and Youth in Washington, D.C., it was reported that there were only 14,000 pediatricians in the United States in 1966, and few of them had resourceful psychiatric backgrounds. Faced with the sobering realization of this manpower problem, attention was directed to a concerted reevaluation of possible methods of changing behavior and a redefinition of conditions conducive to behavioral change. Pursuing this line to only a slight degree leads to the consideration that an approach of inducing "change" in behavior by creating situations which will accommodate certain kinds of behavior has a potential equal to that of an approach of changing behavior to fit a particular situation.

PRELIMINARY DIAGNOSTIC EVALUATION

Recognition of the fact that behavior is the outcome of many factors, internal and external, makes it necessary to carry out a detailed appraisal of the adjustment problem as a preliminary step in correction. Not only are personal and situational variables interacting to produce behavior, but even when the same forces are interacting to give rise to behavior, the arrangement of these factors may be different. The child who kicks his parents' shins may do so either in an impulsive release of rage brought on by temporary thwarting, as a well-established habit for releasing his aggressive self-assertion tendencies, or as a way of seeking wanted attention. On the one hand, thwarting, habit patterns, and seeking attention can and do find expression in numerous responses other than that of kicking parents' shins.

All this is to say that behavior and adjustment are individual matters. They can be changed, but not until the child's capacity for coping with stress, the types of pressures impinging upon him, and the toleration limits and outlets available in his surroundings have been ascertained. Diagnostic appraisal is the process of carrying out this total assessment.

Assessment of the Problem

An adjustment problem is usually indicated by the child's failure to achieve some developmental standard. Children are everywhere grouped with others of the same chronological age: play groups, church schools, nursery schools, public schools. In a culture which already tends to be preoccupied with the welfare of its children, this grouping makes it easy to compare the performance of children. Persons charged with supervising these groups typically give parents "progress reports" which indicate how the child is doing. Acting on information from these sources, many parents seek additional assistance for the child. They may consult their friends, minister, or the child's teacher. Frequently, a physician is consulted about the problem.

In other instances, parents may be busily occuped in providing economic necessities or managing a large family with many children. Some parents may find all their abilities absorbed in trying to keep their own personal balance and sanity. In any event, the children in such homes receive minimal care, even though the parents may be well intentioned. Children experiencing adjustment problems in such situations are dependent upon outsiders—caseworkers from community agencies, probation officials, ministers, recreation workers, or interested neighbors—for spotting their adjustment problems.

Whoever becomes involved in dealing with the difficulty begins by making a study of the total situation. This may be carried out formally or informally, briefly or over an extended time. Although each professional person (caseworker, minister, teacher, psychologist, physician) may see the child from a slightly different perspective, the intent is to examine the stress and possible danger to the child. Even though severely incapacitating at the time, a temporary developmental lag is to be treated in a different way than is a moderately impairing chronic problem. The social acceptability of the problem must also be considered. For whatever reasons it may be manifest, behavior which is not easily tolerated by society (overt aggressive acts) becomes the object of urgent efforts for change.

Included in the assessment preliminary to applying corrective procedures is an approximation of the child's capacities for coping with his problem. Foremost is a consideration of the child's general physical health. Formal measures of intellectual ability, social development, and emotional maturity, though desirable, are not always available, and assessment proceeds in a kind of all-or-none fashion. A younger child is usually regarded as having very limited personal resources, so that he must be protected from being overwhelmed by pressures on him. An older child has comparably greater personal assets for coping with pressures, so that he may require support rather than shielding.

Parents as a Potential Resource

Sizing up the parents is an essential step in formulating corrective action. It is helpful to know the details of the parents' own personality makeup and adjustment. Parental hostility, dependency, persistence, or antisocial orientations exert an influence on children, directly or indirectly. Such specific information is seldom available, but effective planning can be implemented on the basis of more easily acquired information. The amount of time the parent has actually available to spend with the child is, after all, a more real problem than the parent's wish or ideal. A parent may have the best intentions, but be absent from the home 90 per cent of the time because of the nature of his work (for example, employment necessitating traveling). Even when home all of the time, a parent who has many children will have proportionately little time to give to any one individual child.

Parental capacity to be of assistance to the child must also be ascertained. If the parent is taxed in maintaining his own day-to-day living, there is not likely to be much resource left over to give to the child. If the parent is of limited ability, there is a concomitant limitation in the extent to which the parent can profit from training in how to be a more adequate parent. Even if the parent is of average ability and willing to involve himself actively in helping the child, it is well to keep in mind that changes in adult behavior are not easily effected. Some individuals, otherwise competent, may have deeply ingrained personality traits which render them ineffectual in fulfilling a total parental role. The adequacy of the parent may ultimately best be determined by extended observation of the parent's success in fulfilling his role in the correction program. The hateful, blocking, thwarting parent is undoubtedly the most likely to hinder any steps for alleviation of the problem. Nevertheless, recent programs for special groups of children of migrant workers and of the socially disadvantaged have reported considerable success in training parents formerly thought to be of questionable adequacy to help their children learn to read and have better attitudes about school or work.

Other Situational Resources

In addition to the parents, there are generally other important persons (adults or older children) within the child's circle. These persons represent an important influence as helpful or obstructive contributors to the changing of disordered behavior. Scoutmasters, church workers, recreational workers, and teachers are present in varying numbers in the community. Other relatives or older siblings in the home should not be omitted in the assessment of resource persons.

Besides the backing represented in the persons in contact with the child, there are important, sometimes even essential, supports to be found in facilities available in the community. One of the most important of these community resources is the recreational program available. Chances to develop new skills in crafts programs, to play ball, to swim, and the like hold opportunities to experience successes, earn status, learn rules of the game, and acquire responsibilities as part of a team. Community child-guidance and family-service clinics offer counseling and other kinds of psychotherapy to children and families. Sheltered workshops, job-training schools, day schools, residential schools, summer camps, church or YMCA-sponsored recreational programs all increase the number of chances for the child finding success.

Totaling-Up the Assessment

The greatest skill is required in integrating information as to the factors contributing to the child's adjustment difficulty. The putting-together of the pieces may lead to a picture which indicates the essential steps for alleviation. A child may be doing poorly at home and at school because of a chronic health problem which drains his vitality. The parents may emerge as a potent resource, welcoming and putting into practice newly offered advice about child care. Or the parent, for various reasons, may have to be omitted as a source of support and assistance for resolving the child's problem. There may be other persons—playground supervisors, caseworkers, or teachers—whose influence on the child can be marshaled. The community may be an isolated and impoverished one with no planned recreational outlets or program and only meager church, school, or interest-group offerings. In some communities a range of facilities offering medical, psychological, recreational, vocational, psychiatric, and remedial services may be available.

In any event, the treatment program must take into account the child's individual assets for meeting adjustment demands. In some instances, it will be apparent that the child is basically able to deal with his situation, if he can be provided with temporary reassurance, support, or specific training. Teaching the child to swim, play a musical instrument, control aggressive impulses, or read can then strengthen an already sound personality organization. Proceeding along this path is contingent upon the availability of the facilities and professional specialists for carrying out the particular training. In other instances, it may be all too apparent that the undeveloped personality organization of the child is beset by formidable pressures. A "repotting" is necessary before the child can blossom forth in his full potential. There are no fixed rules for making the decision, and there is frequently considerable urgency associated with the process of developing a corrective procedure. Where the child's personal resources permit, a treatment strategy which seeks to straighten the bent twig is preferable to the more drastic approach of transplantation.

THE IMPLEMENTATION OF DIAGNOSTIC FINDINGS

The appraisal of an adjustment problem can entail a lengthy and involved set of procedures, including examination of the child, study of the home and family, evaluation of the parents' capacity to cooperate, and determination of available community resources. The carrying-out of a treatment program is often infinitely more complex. There is no central supervisory person or agency in many instances. Coordinating a treatment program is more cumbersome when agencies and professionals are reluctant to impinge upon one another's domain.

The responsibility for implementing a program is usually given to the parents. Otherwise, the child's guardian becomes the responsible person. The guardian may be a caseworker, an institutional superintendent, or a court judge. In a hospital setting it is the physician. The followup is seldom without problems, and workers typically must distinguish the ideal from the practical treatment regimen.

The Role of Children's Courts

Special courts for handling legal proceedings involving children appeared with the turn of the century. Collectively referred to as juvenile courts, they are also known as children's courts and family courts. In addition to the presiding judge, the juvenile-court staff includes probation officers and caseworkers. In larger metropolitan centers, the staff may be augmented by psychologists and psychiatrists. Children's-court proceedings tend to be very informal, with the court operating from a broadly liberal orientation, and in an advisement capacity. The courts have been most effective when they have assumed the role of guardianship for children. Guardianship is continued for an indefinite period of time and can be an effective control measure. Although children's courts usually only see that recommendations or changes suggested by caseworkers or other agencies are carried out, the courts have considerable resources to implement corrective procedures. Courts may stipulate attendance in a vocational or trade school, treatment by psychotherapy, the assignment of a caseworker to work with parents, placement in a foster home or children's residential home, or commitment to a correctional institution. Parents may contest decisions, but the courts usually have the support of other legal agencies and often hold in abeyance more stringent consequences which may be invoked in any review of proceedings.

Recognizing that they are often forced to deal with problem behavior in the terminal stages, juvenile officials have pushed for and obtained in approximately 40 states an important set of responsibilities. These are referred to as "protective services" and pertain to cases involving the neglect and abuse of children. This is a controversial but undeniably necessary extension of the state's authority. The state has two concerns at stake. On the one hand, neglected and abused children frequently wind up as wards of the state in one or another way. From another point of view, the child has certain rights and privileges which the state must guarantee. To complicate the matter, protective services can entail the deprivation of the rights and liberties of parents. The parent has a right to live as he pleases within broad limits; that is, he doesn't have to have a job, be married to live with someone, or spend his money on his family. Courts have decreed the rights of each citizen to include the freedom to marry, establish a home, bring up children, and enjoy privacy. The implementation of protective services thus brings into the arena a three-way conflict between society's rights, the child's rights, and the parent's rights.

Protective services can do much to correct the past trend of too little, too late. They offer a clear and direct procedure for intervention on behalf of children. Requests for protective services are made to a designated social agency working in close cooperation with juvenile courts. Referrals come from schools, police, neighbors, physicians, other social agencies, and other courts. Upon receipt of the referral, a caseworker makes a call to the home, where the parents are advised of the complaint, and explains the routine of relevant legal procedures (which vary slightly from state to state). The caseworker carries out an investigation and offers assistance (counseling, day care, or the like) to the parents. He reports his findings to the court. If the parent accepts the plan outlined by the caseworker, no court action is taken. If the parent refuses to cooperate, the court pursues a sequence of actions. A probation officer or caseworker may be assigned to work with the parents and supervise the child. Continued lack of cooperation can result in the child being removed from the home and legal proceedings being initiated against the parent. The entire plan places much dependence upon the wisdom of the judge in interpreting such vague conditions as "proper care" and situations "prejudicial to the child's well-being." Protective services represent a significant intervention step and will undoubtedly be greatly extended in future applications. Recent decisions to the effect that a child must be represented by legal counsel in any court action may intensify the entire issue of "protection" vs. "rights" of children.

MODIFICATION APPROACHES

The discussion of environmental modification will deal with procedures designed to assist the child by varying some aspect or component of the surroundings. Environmental modification techniques are the most frequently used intervention procedures. The child is not removed from his home, and the emphasis is on reducing the press of forces which impinge upon the child or on strengthening the child's capacity for dealing with the elements making up his environment. In a sense, the environment is changed, but the change is in the nature of a rearrangement of the situation. The relationships among the various parts of the child's situation are redefined and readjusted. For example, the child's contacts with well-intentioned but interfering grandparents may be stopped. Parents may be advised of the importance for assigning jobs as a way of instilling a sense of responsibility in the child. Physical health may be improved by specific medical or surgical procedures. The child's ability to meet successfully demands from his surroundings may be bolstered by specific training such as remedial instruction or the teaching of particular skills.

Environmental modification can be viewed as a kind of psychological first aid administered after it has been ascertained what capacity the child has for responding and what response is expected of him. The decision must indicate that the adjustment balance can be restored by modifying specific disturbing influences or by adding new experiences. The focus is on the control of external forces so as to promote the continuation of optimal development of the child. The assumption is made that the child has skills and abilities sufficient for profiting from the new opportunities. The general objectives are those of providing structured socialization contacts, training in specific skills, retraining of specific habitual outlets for aggressive or destructive behaviors, encouraging socially acceptable outlets for fantasies, bringing new opportunities for status and identification, or continuing supervisory care on a temporary basis.

Briefly summarized, the goals of environmental modification are:

1. Guiding mental attitudes into socially acceptable channels.
2. Restoration of self-confidence and personal security.
3. Replacement of discouragement with encouragement.
4. Establishment and promotion of good work habits.
5. Increasing opportunities for socialization.
6. Learning of specific skills needed for work or school.

In the course of achieving these goals, the entire environment is searched and advantage is taken of all opportunities. The community resources are usually to be found in some one of the following groupings of services. It must be pointed out that the availability of facilities is a function of the size of the community. Large communities tend to have more of a variety of all resources. The discussion presented at this point also makes only brief reference to educational resources and programs for the maladjusted child since educational intervention facilities were treated in conjunction with the specific disabilities discussed in Chapters 3 through 8.

RECREATIONAL COMMUNITY PROGRAMS

Park and Playground Facilities

Most cities of any size offer organized recreational activities on some type of regular schedule. These include playground equipment; areas for playing baseball, football, basketball, volleyball, and tennis; swimming pools; and other sports activities. In some communities there are regular special classes with instruction available in arts and crafts, dancing, tumbling, trampoline, or baton twirling. There is usually some supervision, and the instructional staff is augmented during school vacation periods. In the summer, daycamping activities and nature study may be offered. Fees are usually minimal, but transportation can be a problem in some instances. Organized recreational programs can offer a wholesome use of leisure time, new friendships, chances for success in athletics, and opportunities in learning how to function as a member of a socially approved group.

Summer Camps

Summer camps are sometimes a part of community recreation programs but are more likely to be sponsored by churches, the YMCA, or the YWCA. There are numerous private camps, but the fees for private camps limit their availability. Fees and transportation are less costly for the semiprivate camps. Summer-camp experiences emphasize the fostering of independence and self-reliance. There are also excellent opportunities for contacts and training in the give and take of group social relationships. Training in arts and crafts, archery, fishing, canoeing, or horseback riding can be a unique experience and give the child a sense of being "expert" in a prestigious skill area. This "expertise" can be a solid contribution to self-ideas of competence or positive ego building.

After-School Programs

Schools in large cities have had recreational programs or after-school "study" centers for many years. These programs are usually offered in areas where other recreational opportunities are limited and where there is a high percentage of homes without parental supervision during the working day. An example is New York City's All-Day Neighborhood School, when an extra teacher is assigned for each grade level from kindergarten through grade 6. These teachers work from 11:00 A.M. to 5:00 P.M. From 11:00 A.M. to 3:00 P.M., the teachers are engaged in remedial work with individuals and small groups. From 3:00 to 5:00 P.M., they conduct an "activity" program composed of homework study, interest clubs, individual hobbies, field trips, organized games, and individualized recreational reading. Initiated in 1936, the New York City program appears to be an exemplary model which merits general emulation. It would be difficult to provide such a comprehensive and pertinent set of opportunities, ranging from remediation through planned use of leisure time, in any other single program.

Other Recreational Centers

Other recreational activities are made available by churches, the YMCA-YWCA, scouting organizations, businessmen's organizations (Kiwanis, Rotary, Optimists), and civic groups. Included are a variety of youth centers, where dancing and informal get-togethers are scheduled under supervision. The YMCA-YWCA and scouting organizations offer individual and group activities from weight lifting to team sports. They also have instruction in hobbies and crafts. Churches are increasingly entering the field of providing recreational programs, usually directed toward the adolescent. These community programs can be excellent opportunities for social contacts. They are able to supply both male and female identification models. The hobby and craft programs may develop long-standing recreational interests along socially approved lines.

SPECIALIZED COMMUNITY PROGRAMS

General Hospitals, Medical Clinics, and Crippled-Children's Clinics

Despite the tremendous advances made in the field of medicine, these services remain difficult to obtain for many children. Part of the problem may be that knowledge has been discovered at a much faster rate than trained persons have become available for applying the information. Adequate medical and surgical treatment is basic to insuring that the child will be maximally prepared to cope with life's demands. Physical health can make the difference in all-important initial success or failure experiences. Repeated failures or the inability to participate fully in play activities may foster a nucleus of self-doubt and a diminished zest for persistence. The chances for obtaining specialized medical care are greater in populous urban centers than in small or medium-sized communities, mainly because medical specialists gravitate to metropolitan areas.

Large general hospitals are organizing children's clinics modeled after those until recently seen only in association with medical schools. The cost of medical services is a formidable barrier for children from less economically advantaged families. Public facilities, such as crippled-children's services, are frequently limited as to the kinds of conditions or children they can accept. Privately sponsored facilities, such as

Shriners Hospitals for Crippled Children, have limited capacities. Nevertheless, adequate medical care is paramount in the prevention of later adjustment problems, so that physicians, clinics, or hospitals providing these services must be searched out.

Mental-Health, Guidance, and Counseling Clinics

The support of federal financing has made it possible for community mental-health or child-guidance clinics to become established in most cities of more than 50,000 population. Typically, these mental-health clinics are staffed by psychiatrists, social workers, and psychologists. These specialists carry out diagnostic evaluations and provide various types of psychotherapy. A major part of the treatment offered by mental-health clinics consists of counseling for parents and play therapy for children. Costs are generally minimal, but the demands for services are great. Most mental-health clinics have extensive waiting lists, even though treatment is on a voluntary basis. Clients are selected on the basis of being able to participate as outpatients, that is, persons who are not so incapacitated as to require hospitalization (inpatients). The parent must contact the clinic, but suggestions as to the advisability of this self-referral may come from schools, courts, physicians, ministers, or other social agencies. Unfortunately, it is difficult for many persons to find immediate rewards in psychotherapy, as attested by the large number of clients—estimated as high as 50 per cent— who are seen for only one or two contacts.

Family-service agencies, which closely resemble the organization and staff complement of the mental-health clinic, have had rapid national growth. These agencies are found in most large urban centers, although they are more numerous in the northeastern quarter of the United States. Historically, family-service agencies were a practical answer to the predicament expressed as "I need money, not counseling." These agencies are distinguished by their organization around the function of providing practical, on-the-spot casework, rather than psychiatric service. Consistent with this orientation, they perform a minimum of diagnostic functions. The staff consists mostly of trained caseworkers who make use of many techniques in dealing with families in crises. Counseling services are available, often in the form of patching up and improving relationships between parents, but the caseworker is willing and expects actively to assist the family in finding a more suitable house or better jobs or in living on a planned budget. The caseworker frequently contacts the family in home visitations rather than waiting for the family to come to the agency's offices. Family-service agencies work with clients on a voluntary basis. They can usually be counted upon to provide rapid service, but they may elect to refer to other facilities "difficult" cases, such as those requiring hospitalization or regarding a psychotic disorder. Their practical approach often brings quick results, and they are likely to be in close working contact with all other community agencies.

Vocational Counseling and Training Agencies

Vocational training and job preparation are based on the recognized necessity of employment as an economic essential for adult life and on the alarming number of youths who are unprepared for gainful employment. For a number of years, the Division of Vocational Rehabilitation (DVR) has marshaled powerful resources in preparing and assisting handicapped persons to find employment. The DVR is possibly the most important single resource which can be brought to bear in assisting qualified persons. Medical and surgical treatment, educational or specific vocational instruction, and psychotherapy are among the major areas for which the DVR will pay the costs of rendering the individual able to work. Because of the success which the DVR has demonstrated in work with the handicapped, similar services are being extended to other youths through such recently activated programs for job training as the Office of Economic Services and the Office of Economic Opportunity (OEO).

Representing an ultimate development in dealing with adjustment problems, "sheltered workshops" offer a daywork situation which is arranged to accommodate the individual. The workshop can be viewed as a permanent employment situation for persons with very limited resources, such as the severely mentally retarded, or as a temporary training experience for assisting individuals to overcome a specific disability, such as the impulsive emotionally disturbed. Sheltered workshops have a small staff complement and emphasize vocational activities. They may be associated with other community agencies, such as churches, schools, or parent groups. As yet, sheltered workshops are not widespread, but they are increasing in number and community support. They accept clients on referral from other community agencies, from public schools, and from residential schools. Clients are often paid a small wage, money left over after defraying the operating expenses of the workshop.

Special day schools which give training in specific marketable skills, such as welding, automobile repair, building maintenance, or packing products, have become a part of most large school systems. These facilities are limited to older youth, but they are an essential resource. Adolescents who have dropped out of school or who are not academically oriented often distinguish themselves in trade schools. The success of these training schools is so generally recognized in contributing to youth adjustment that they have been incorporated as central components in recent programs initiated by the President's Commission on Juvenile Delinquency.

PROGRAMS OF TEMPORARY SHELTER

Nursery Schools

These are predominately privately operated centers for children who are close to the usual school-entrance age. Nursery schools originally appeared on the scene as a kind of supplement to the home experiences of children of working parents, the mother often working only part-time. Since most nursery schools are privately operated, they may vary widely as to physical facilities, staff competency, and quality of program. In some, the emphasis is on educational rather than mothering activities, and the program often closely resembles that of the public-school kindergarten. Children generally attend for a relatively short period of time. Unfortunately, there have been occasional reports of glaring inadequacies, bordering on neglect, which have resulted in many states instituting licensing standards for approved nursery schools. Nursery schools can provide programs excellent in every respect, but the cost is generally prohibitive for those children who may be most in need of this help.

Day-Care Centers

Day-care centers are publically supported facilities designed to provide substitute maternal care for the child during a major part of the day. The emphasis is on meeting basic physical, emotional, intellectual, and social needs of the child during his school attendance. Day-care centers are usually conveniently located in neighborhoods carefully selected on the basis of anticipated need; that is, where both parents are likely to be working, where family incomes are low, and where recreational facilities are minimal. Most of the publically financed day-care centers have a well-trained staff of specialists who work with children. They have well-planned programs, including appropriate motor- and language-stimulating activities, and there is attention to needs for rest and proper diet. In some instances, transporation may be provided. The interest in preschool education has resulted in an increase in these day-care centers. Some are expanding the services they offer, to include temporary residential care.

THE ROLE OF THE PARENT

It should be apparent that environmental modification relies heavily upon working with the parent. The child is regarded as having the capacity to cope with his environment with only slight rearrangements or temporary supporting measures. Environmental-modification approaches focus upon elimination, replacement, addition, or improvement of the existing surroundings. To accomplish those objectives, use is made of community resources, medical clinics, clubs, social groups, children's agencies, recreational programs, and vocational-training centers. It is essential to know what experiences, opportunities, or services each such facility will present. Ideally, the referring person is acquainted with the caliber of the caseworker, group leader, or supervisor of each facility.

Generally, the parent must make the request for service, so that he remains a key aspect of the treatment program. Whenever possible, work with the parent should center on help for the child and should avoid the parent's personal problems. Until other evidence is accumulated, it must be assumed that the parent has made an honest request for assistance and is able and willing to follow through with suggestions. Diagnostic-evaluative impressions must be shared with the parent in meaningful terms, and the parent apprised of the treatment objectives and plan. The following steps outline a guide for working with parents:

1. Allow for parental participation in the problem.
2. Involve the parent to the extent of his capacity and willingness.
3. Do not waver or become lost in a search for specific causes.
4. Be reassuring by taking charge of the problem and making specific recommendations which can be carried out.

ALTERATION APPROACHES

The procedures to be used in alleviating an adjustment problem are dependent upon the findings gained in diagnostic appraisal. As a general rule, the less the total life organization can be disrupted, the better the possibilities of the child being able to profit from the treatment. (A poor home is better than no home.) When there are indications that moderate rearrangements of the existing environment will not be adequate for correcting the problem, more drastic measures must be considered. Less frequently used than environmental modification, environmental alteration has the objective of bringing about a total change in the child's surroundings. Alteration is dictated by the assumption that the child, for one reason or another, cannot continue in his present situation.

Because such a rearrangement of the child's life has incumbent implications of far-reaching consequences, it must be embarked upon only after the most careful appraisal. It is essential to ascertain that the child will be able to profit from, rather than merely to tolerate, the new situation. To place a severely mentally retarded child in a highly stimulating, enriched, and achievement-demanding home may be the beginning of a change for the worse. Not only the potential for adjustment but the plasticity of the child must be considered. Age, then, becomes an important variable. Havighurst (1960) has found that foster homes are of limited value in effecting personality changes in children after they reach preadolescence. The implication for treatment is that correction of the difficulty need not demand the remaking of the total personality. Changes directed to the consideration of those parts of the personality which are most impaired may be adequate for rendering the child socially competent.

A total incapacitation of personality development is seldom encountered, and partial changes may render the child socially competent. In such instances, a new family with a different set of parents may be sufficient for the continuation of normal development. This setup is especially true for the child who is young and possesses at least average physical and psychological resources. In other cases, it is apparent that the child has only the most tenuous relationship with his present surroundings and has no choice but to develop highly maladjustive strategies for maintaining himself in that situation. Psychotherapy may be futile in alleviating the pressures upon such a disabled child; he must have the protection of a completely controlled environment. Institutional placement becomes a necessity for the preservation of the child and the only hope for eventually building his capacity for tolerating a noninstitutional situation.

There are no hard-and-fast rules which can be followed in every case. Watson (1951) has suggested a list of criteria which may be helpful in deciding whether or not to transplant a child to a new environment:

1. The parents reject the child and are inaccessible for change by existing resources.

2. The parents' own needs cause them to be so deeply involved with the child as to prevent the child profiting from any environmental modifications and yet the parents are unable to accept treatment for themselves.

3. The child is delinquent and lives in a family group which contributes to his delinquency.

4. The mother is absent from the home, and there is no adequate mother substitute.

5. The care of the child places a disproportionate drain on the resources of the parental home (parents or child are extremely limited, severely retarded, and the like).

6. The child has not been able to profit from help supplied by other procedures and facilities.

7. Diagnostic study indicates that a totally new environment is the only likely way to help the child.

Facilities available for placement of the child vary from a completely new family to a controlled and structured residential institution.

FOSTER-HOME PLACEMENT

Finding a new family for the child is a procedure which has long been made use of in providing for children's needs. It is in many ways a "natural" approach which attempts to continue the customary developmental situation found in our society, the family unit. The human neonate is totally unable to provide for himself. The dependency upon adults tapers off as the child's maturing capacities permit him to assume more self-reliance, but full independence is not achieved until late in the adolescent period. Foster-home placement is a necessity for the infant even when there are no indications of adjustment problems. Sudden loss of both parents, for example, requires some provision for replacing the parents. In other instances, the parent may decide to give up a child, as, for example, a young unmarried mother. These placements are generally made through a process of adoption, a legal procedure usually arranged by a caseworker and entailing court action.

Of greater relevance to intervention as a way of correcting a child's adjustment problems is action which takes him from his parents. This is a drastic step in which the recognized rights of the parent are superseded in the interest of protecting the rights of the child and/or society. Removal of the child from his original home is carried out by some interested agency acting with court sanction. The actual process is generally supervised by a caseworker. Removal of the child is undertaken only after detailed diagnostic study which establishes the child's basic potential for an adequate adjustment and the inadequacy of the current home situation.

Upon being taken from his parents by court action, a child may be deemed suitable for adoption and placed in a permanent new home. It is difficult to obtain the evidence demanded by legal requirements in establishing proof of abuse, neglect, or conditions detrimental to the child's psychological well-being. Therefore, many children, especially older ones, are more likely to be adjudicated to the custody of the court rather than being taken outright from parents. This motion gives the court and cooperating social agency necessary legal authority for controlling the child's placement. It has the advantage of permitting the court to act quickly and makes it more likely that the child will be placed in another home when the foster parents do not have to legally adopt the child. Prospective adoptive parents frequently are reluctant to commit themselves to the binding responsibility of formal adoption. The placement of the child in a home by the court, with the court retaining custody of the child, may also permit the court to allocate money for the support of the child, thus lessening the financial obligation of the foster parents. The court has legitimate reasons for maintaining an evaluative relationship with the child in the foster home. Court control can be an effective bargaining device for insisting upon certain minimal conditions and standards within the home. If the child and the foster-home parents do not hit it off well, it is a relatively easy matter to place the child in another home.

Child candidates for foster-home placement are referred by social agencies, probation and juvenile officials, and children's institutions. As can be gathered from the preceding discussion, there are many advantages to the courts' retaining custody of the child and purchasing the necessary services of a family and home for the child. Many children are able to profit from the new home and family, extinguishing old and maladjustive behavior patterns and acquiring new and socially acceptable responses. Other children, particularly young ones, are not able to profit from a new home or family; such children require a more structured and controlled environment.

INSTITUTIONAL PLACEMENT

For those children who have limited capacity for dealing with life adjustment demands, a situation is required in which there is scheduling, regulation, control of demands, and the supplying of highly particular training and procedures. These services are usually available in the continual-care programs of an institutional setting. For children having the most limited potentials for life adjustment, such as the severely mentally retarded, permanent institutional placement may be necessary. Other children can benefit from the services provided by an institution to the extent that they will be able to move out into a regular place in society and function adequately.

Specific Treatment: Short- or Long-Term

Included in this group are institutions which offer specific services. The service may be surgical or medical care to correct a physical defect (deformed leg or foot) or to diagnose and treat a medical problem, such as epilepsy or a metabolic dysfunction (diabetes). During the time the child is hospitalized, as for a lengthy series of surgical operations, he will require other services, such as psychotherapy or educational tutoring. Other problems which necessitate residential facilities for treatment are those requiring specific and prolonged therapy and special education and training. The deaf, blind, language-disabled, socially deviant, and emotionally disturbed are examples. Residential schools for the cerebral-palsied, blind, or deaf are to be found in most states. The emphasis is on providing particular training, and the staff is made up largely of teachers trained in the special educational problems of these exceptional children. Children are in these schools only for the usual school year, going home in the summers. After a few years, a majority have had enough special help to be able to keep up in regular schools.

Another type of residential school where children may be admitted for up to several years for special service is the institution dealing with social and emotional problems. Schools concerned with social deviants are more numerous, and several may be found in even less populous states. More popularly known as "training schools," "reformatories," or "detention homes," these institutions were originally designed to take the place of jails and adult reformatories. The emphasis was on control and supervision of the children committed to the institution by court decree. Gradually, improvements have been made to include education and casework-counseling services to the children. Institutions for the socially deviant are among the most overcrowded facilities to be found. They have all too often served more as crime schools for the children committed, so that most workers are reluctant to make this type of placement.

Residential facilities for emotionally disturbed children have always been in critically short supply. Privately operated institutions, generally bearing the title of "school," are so costly as to be prohibitive for all but a few children. In some states, schools for the emotionally disturbed are being opened under state auspices. These are frequently in association with existing state mental hospitals. Those in conjunction with medical schools tend to have the most complete staff complement and a favorably low staff-patient ratio. Residential institutions for the emotionally disturbed have as their special service various types of treatment for emotional disorders. Psychotherapy, chemotherapy, education, and an emphasis on family living units are typical. The Sonja Heinkman Orthogenic School, associated with the University of Chicago, is an excellent example of the milieu approach to treatment. Some larger cities have semiprivate residential schools for the emotionally disturbed. In general, there is a long waiting list even for the expensive private schools. Admission to state-operated schools is usually by court-ordered commitment. Parents or guardians must arrange the admission for either a public or a private institution.

Complete Home: Long-Term or Permanent

A second major group of residential institutions is organized to provide a home for children on a permanent basis. These institutions, sometimes referred to as "orphanages" or simply as "homes," are also designated as "group homes" in the current technical literature. They are frequently privately operated, especially by church groups, but most counties and large cities also have such facilities for dependent or abandoned children. A number of children are adopted or placed in regular homes from these institutions. But, for a significant number of children, the institution becomes their permanent home and they reside there until they are "graduated" or reach the release age, often about 18 or 19 years of age. The emphasis is on providing the routine as well as the physical and emotional needs of family home life. There are institutional "parent" persons and frequently casework service. Larger institutions (more than 30 children) are often organized on the "cottage" plan. Children are assigned to small groups for living in one of several residence buildings, like a large house, on the institution's grounds. Necessary special services—medical, dental, or educational—are generally purchased or arranged for the children from sources in the surrounding community. Developmental institutions have the advantages of stability and consistency, but children in residence can fall into a pattern of isolation unless frequent contacts with the community are included in the total program.

PLACEMENT OBJECTIVES AND OUTCOMES

Objectives

The removal of a child from his home is likely to arouse a number of controversial feelings. In some ways, such a step seems to threaten the very existence of society by breaking up the basic societal unit, the family. Nevertheless, some form of placement is vital for some children; for example, there is obvious justification in hospitalizing a child for a series of bone-graft operations that will require months to complete. The child whose parents are suddenly removed or absent from the home must have a continuation of care and supervision. But there are other reasons for which placements are made. The practice is to remove the child from a home environment judged to be one in which the child can never learn to adjust or to attain stability. If the decision is that the child must have a neutral, highly structured environment which makes minimal demands on him in order to protect and then strengthen his capacity for adjustment, then placement in an institution is made.

Demands and Conditions of Placement

The intention of placement as a method for permitting the child to continue the pattern of normal development is not debatable. There are many successful outcomes which provide tangible evidence as to the effectiveness of placement. Placement as a technique for intervention has, in fact, become widespread and gives every indication of gaining even more general use and acceptance.

Workers dealing with children have often been intrigued with a technique which looks good on paper, but in practice proves disappointing. Some techniques for changing behavior, including some which require the greatest skill in diagnostic evaluation or training and time from the worker, appear to have little observable benefit for the child or may even make him worse. For example, a carefully made diagnostic study may indicate that a severely rejected child should be placed in an orphanage. As a consequence, the child may interpret the action as tangible evidence that he is rejected. To add to the problem, he may view his being taken from his home as severe punishment. In discussing this possibility, Fine (1966) cautioned,

Anyone who undertakes to move a child from residential treatment to a foster home, even one especially selected to meet the anticipated needs of the disturbed youngsters, is taking a calculated risk, though the decision is made out of the best clinical judgment that the patient is ready to move.

Fine goes on to discuss how children can react to the suddenness of the change and the associated new pressures. It is a shock for some children to find that having another person interested in them demands interpersonal responsibilities they have not acquired. The child may resist intensively and actively these new responsibilities, negating any possible benefit from the change. Fine concludes by suggesting that placements be made only reluctantly and with generous support for the new parents and for the child.

A study carried out by Jenkins and Sauber (1964) listed the reasons given for placement of children in New York City from May through August of 1963. A total of 891 children (all over 6 months old) from 425 families were placed, for these reasons:

29%—physical illness of an adult in the family
11%—mother had mental illness
17%—child had severe emotional problems
10%—severe parental neglect or abuse
33%—miscellaneous, including parental incompatibility, parental

incompetence, drug addiction, alcoholism, arrest, child abandonment, and unwillingness of caretakers other than parents
to continue care in the home.

It was found that the majority of the families from which these children were removed lived in conditions of poverty and lacked supportive
community services. The problems confronting the families seem to
be directly related to pressures associated with limited finances. Of
the 425 families, 44 per cent were one-parent families, mostly headed
by the mother. Only 38 per cent of the families were receiving public
assistance at the time of the placement. Followup study of the children placed revealed the surprising information that 49 per cent
spent no more than 3 months in placement; 16 per cent were in
placement for less than one week. Emotionally disturbed children
were in foster care for the longest period of time.

The findings obtained by Jenkins and Sauber imply that greater
use of existing community resources, such as casework services,
mental-health clinics, and day-care centers, could assist these families
under stress. Financial supports also seem to have the same potential
for the alleviation of pressures. The most surprising data concern
the followup on the length of time spent in placement. It seems
obvious that homemaker service, purchase of a caretaker, or temporary shelters could easily avoid the necessity of making from
one-fourth to one-half of the placements reported in this study.

Outcomes as Gauged by Children's Reactions

Intervention approaches have the objective of improving the child's
chances for realizing his potential for adjustment. However, the pressures for action have often been so great that there has been limited
opportunity to follow the outcomes of intervention. Yet the question
must be raised: How effective are such intervention approaches as
placement in another home or in an institution? The question may
best be answered by the children themselves.

A study conducted by DeFries, Jenkins, and Williams (1964)
compared the responses of two groups of children matched on sex,
age, IQ, and socioeconomic background. At the start of the study, all
of the children were emotionally disturbed wards of the New York
Department of Public Welfare. One group remained under treatment
in a residential institution. Children in the other group were placed
in foster homes where they and the foster parents were also supplied
psychotherapy. Surprisingly, children in the foster-home placement did

less well than did those who continued to live in the institution. Foster-home placement seemed to have the adverse effect of accentuating the children's feelings of being different. Most unexpected were these children's reports that their needs for satisfying affectional relationships were not fulfilled in the foster homes. Older children seemed to encounter somewhat more adjustment stress in foster-home placement than did younger children. In a review which questioned the adequacy of "the good old foster home" for dealing with disturbed children, Redl (1966) came to this conclusion:

As an institution for the safeguarding of the mental health of vulnerable children, the foster home of yesterday is either extinct or not sufficient any more. It is an obsolete answer to a current problem of huge proportions.

Redl made a strong plea for well-implemented residential treatment centers to care for disturbed children.

Recounting his experiences in dealing with long-term institutionally placed children, Moss (1966) reported that most institutionalized children have little idea of how and why they came into placement and of what is planned for their future. They may harbor bitter feelings of having been victimized or experience chronic pain in being rejected by parents or society in general. An orientation of inadequacy, helplessness, and accompanying hopelessness may easily develop if the child's predicament is not realized and dealt with. Moss recommends including the child in discussions about his future as a way of instilling a more healthy outlook.

It is apparent that intervention can be highly effective by way of making it possible for children to overcome adjustment difficulties. While many children who are given selected assistance will be able to continue patterns of normal development, the same procedures may compound and prolong adjustment problems for other children. Placement is most likely to aggravate adjustment and must be sparingly used and closely observed for signs of unfavorable consequences. The objectives of intervention involving placement must be made explicit to the child and to the parents. Foster-home placement appears to be especially hazardous for older children.

PROBLEMS IN INTEGRATING SERVICES

OVERLAP

Even when services to children are well defined and services to dependent families are clear-cut, there remains a large gray area in which the services overlap. The problem is made more difficult by the fact that these services are seldom defined or definable with specificity and by the fact that the children usually are in some type of placement. Jenkins and Sauber (1964) found that the families of children given placement services typically were living on the edges of poverty and lacked the support of existing community services. Parents were sometimes bogged down by more demands for being parents than they could muster, but family problems were also frequently related to inadequate economic resources.

Buell (1952) found that 6 per cent of the families in one area were receiving 68 per cent of the available community services. He describes the "multiple agency contacting" family, which often adds to the pressures impinging on it by being involved with four or five agencies. Each agency must make a diagnostic intake study preparatory to assisting the family. These diagnostic studies are often remarkably similar. The recommendations may depend on the agency's area or particular service. One worker tells the family to clean up the living quarters, another wants the children taken to school immediately, another tells a parent to enter the hospital tomorrow, yet another wants the parent to take the job the worker has found or financial aid will be terminated, and a juvenile officer comes by to take a child for questioning. Such an array of demands is enough to disrupt even the most stable of families. Puzzled as to which "boss" should be heeded, the parents may believe the safest course of action is to do nothing. A smoldering resentment at all the pressure may find expression in passive, uncooperative attitudes which are exceedingly difficult to deal with.

THE NEED FOR CENTRALIZATION

It becomes apparent that some organization and coordination of services is essential, for multiple agency contacts obviously increase the pressures on an already disabled family unit. There is also the matter of tying up the services of personnel already in short supply in duplications of intake interviews, home visits, and related diagnostic study. Not only is there misuse of specialist personnel, but the actual delivery of available services is impaired when there is no central coordination. Any one community agency should be able to deliver services directly (casework, financial aid) or indirectly (surgical care, temporary placement). Ways are being found to circumvent artificially drawn but real barriers based on professional areas of competence. But these must presently be approached indirectly and thus are time-consuming. A direct approach would be more efficient and possibly more effective.

The gray areas in the delivery of children's services are in parent-child relationships, protective services, and supervisory care. It is here that the details of planning and coordination must be carefully worked out. One of many possibilities is for the school to be designated as the center of coordination, in recognition of the major influence of the school upon the child. The entire matter is a complex one, demanding the integration of parents' rights with children's rights. In view of the many legal aspects, the solution may eventually be worked out through court actions. New York and Idaho have made significant advances in facilitating court action on behalf of children. Physicians, who are frequently the first to be consulted regarding the need for services, are likely to be the least knowledgeable about community resources unless they are among the rare few who have had specific training in community services (Olshansky and Sternfeld, 1962).

EMERGING TRENDS

A continuing expansion in intervention services is to be expected. Despite the admitted limitations, some type of intervention stands as the most effective procedure for influencing the welfare of maladjusted children. Information collected by the Children's Bureau (1965) indicated that only one-fourth to one-half of those children known or estimated to be in need of services were receiving them in 1964. In a discussion of children's problems, Witmer (1964) reported that one-fourth of the children then living were in homes where the family income was inadequate to provide basic needs. Out of the practice of providing services, ideas and beliefs initially having only theoretical existence become solid and effective intervention techniques. Foster-home placement is currently the major child service, but there has been a reappraisal of institutional placement. Formerly regarded as punitive and ineffectual, institutions can contribute far more than mere custodial care for the child if they are provided with adequate staffs. The capacity for positive contribution is greatly strengthened when education is recognized as an important kind of therapy and when it is realized that many parents cannot be changed so that treatment directed to them may be wasted. The following sections review some of the major new developments in children's services.

PROJECT RE-ED

A grant from the federal government in 1961 launched a promising special study project to investigate facilities for the emotionally disturbed child of school age. The state mental-health departments of Tennessee and South Carolina are cooperatively involved in administering two residential schools which form the nucleus of the project. Each school enrolls 40 children aged 6 to 12 years. The children are subdivided into 5 working groups of 8 children each. For each of these groups a team of staff members is continuously assigned; the team includes teacher-counselors, teacher-counselor trainees, teacher aides, and resource persons from the special areas of art, music, and physical education. The staff team is assisted by volunteer workers. The schools have psychiatric, educational, social-work, and psychological-consultative services, but these are mostly given to diagnostic evaluation of the child and consultation for the staff members.

Treatment centers about the educational program as provided by or under the supervision of the teacher-counselor. Children are referred by local area schools and are informed that they will return there. From Sunday evening through Friday afternoon the children are in residence at the project school. Weekends are spent at home with the family, thus enforcing the parents' rights vis-à-vis the child. Outstanding innovations are the teacher-counselor as a mental-health specialist and the concept of coordination and control remaining with the local community school, along with reduced costs, intensive short-term intervention, mobilization of community resources, and a focus on behavioral and personal competence.

Project Re-ed has had a promising debut and seems to have much to commend it as a facility for the emotionally disturbed. It is not intended to take the place of psychiatric institutions for severely disturbed children, but it appears to have the capacity to prevent such severe personality disorganization.

ILLINOIS ZONE CENTERS

The need for some type of residential facility for emotionally disturbed children remains the most critical deficit of all services for children. The Illinois Department of Mental Health has put into operation a model plan for speeding up services to children. The state is divided into eight geographic regions, termed "zones." Centrally located in each zone is a center staffed and equipped to carry out extensive diagnostic evaluations. Added to the usual diagnostic team of psychiatrist, social worker, and psychologist is an educational specialist. The center has a limited number of residential spaces, which can be assigned either on an extended diagnostic-observation basis or on a temporary (or emergency) treatment basis. The staff of the center maintains contacts with all other possible treatment agencies in the zone area, and referrals may be made back to these agencies, as well as being received from them. A service most recently inaugurated sends staff members skilled in behavior-modification techniques into the homes of children having severe adjustment problems. The staff member remains to do on-the-spot training of parents in procedures appropriate for the disturbed child.

The zone centers have the advantages of being part of the community, being easily accessible, holding accommodations for short-term intensive care, and having a representative staff complement. They concentrate treatment by focusing on a specific symptom or disability which is preventing the child from getting along in school or in the community. At this time they have been in operation only a few months, so that there is no hard data regarding the effectiveness of what seems to be a much needed service organization.

HALFWAY HOUSES

The necessity for some type of mediating step to bridge the suddenly incurred changes from institutional life to community life has long been recognized. Very few institutions make a provision for this transition. The Division of Vocational Rehabilitation (DVR) is keenly aware of the problem and frequently has purchased this type of service for its clients. The problem is most severe for older adolescents and youths who have lived in an institution for several years. The Illinois Department of Mental Health has established a halfway-house unit made up of several residences in a large city. Youths released from state institutions may live in the halfway house for as long as two years while locating work, completing training, or simply getting used to "the grind." Counseling, financial assistance, and technical advice are available.

DAY-CARE CENTERS AS DIAGNOSTIC-OBSERVATION STATIONS

Data from the Children's Bureau (1965) reveal that only 2.6 per cent of federal funds for children's services in fiscal 1965 went to day-care centers. The demand for this type of service is growing rapidly. Professional workers have become aware of the potential of this service which is given primarily to preschool children. A pattern is evolving in which the staff of day-care centers is greatly strengthened and the centers become continuous observation stations. In this way potential behavior problems can be detected early, and prompt treatment can prevent more serious or chronic problems.

NEW PERSONNEL CATEGORIES

It is generally recognized that needed professional workers may never be trained in sufficient quantity. Some of the most imaginative developments have been concerned with solving the manpower shortage. Leaders in the field have urged trying out what are sometimes referred to as "auxiliary" or "subprofessional" personnel. In describing the effectiveness of such persons, Brieland (1965) lists three possible types of subprofessional workers who can make important contributions in children's services:

1. Case aide—a caseworker trained at the bachelor's-degree level.
2. Preprofessional—a college graduate trained in a field related to casework.
3. Volunteer—an assistant who may or may not have had college training, but who enjoys working with children and is willing to tutor, take children on trips, supervise games, and so on.

There are enthusiastic reports of the successful use of such subprofessional workers. In Chicago, college students organized and manned a volunteer program called Helping Hands, in which tutoring, recreational, and enrichment activities were provided after school for disadvantaged children. In New York City, Philadelphia, and Los Angeles there has been success in using "the poor to help the poor." Persons are employed as aides to work in subprofessional activities with the disadvantaged. This arrangement can provide needed employment in addition to speeding up the acceptance of services offered by an agency when these persons man neighborhood "information" centers.

It has been suggested that the only way to attack the vexing problem of getting services to migrant-worker families may be that of employing individuals from these same migrant groups to carry out activities of tutoring, counseling, and supervisory care for children. The success of such an effort remains to be verified, but the idea is illustrative of the innovative approaches which are evolving in a sincere effort to make it feasible for each child to have a maximum opportunity for realizing his potential.

DELIVERY OF SERVICES TO SPARSELY POPULATED AREAS

At several points, this chapter has mentioned the fact that large communities have more of the resources customarily utilized in intervention approaches. The intention has been to describe, rather than to sanction. Acute shortages in trained mental-health manpower are perhaps nowhere more evident than in sparsely populated areas. The provision of mental-health and welfare services to communities of less than 50,000 persons is indeed an urgent and challenging problem.

That there is no shortage in these areas of what is perhaps the most important of all resources—human ingenuity—is attested to by the number of communities which have met the problem. In some instances, counties are banding together to form a single service unit. In a centrally located center, mental-health clinics, vocational-rehabilitation offices, general hospitals, and other welfare-service facilities are situated. In another plan, a group of specialists may have a regular schedule of working in several medium-size towns for one or two days a week. Mental-health specialists have sometimes worked out schedules which allow them to work in a regular consultative capacity with local-community paraprofessionals (ministers, teachers, public-health nurses, physicians) who are apt to have the most direct day-to-day contacts with persons needing help.

The involvement of interested citizens of the community in planning programs for the delivery of services to the populace is in its own right an essential service. Persons who may be participants in such community-action projects may find helpful the recommendations for improving services to children compiled by Jenkins and Sauber (1964):

1. Round-the-clock intake services.
2. Greater interagency coordination.

3. Provision of funds to pay relatives and family friends to care for the children.

4. Expansion of family and group day-care facilities.

5. More shelter-care resources.

6. Increased supply of long-term placement resources for emotionally disturbed children.

7. Expansion of and more flexibility in homemaker services.

8. Expansion of community psychiatric services.

9. Improved means for reporting child abuse and neglect.

10. Increased service aimed at strengthening family life.

SUMMARY

There is an appreciable concern on the part of mental-health specialists as to the role of environment in shaping personality. Despite the relative affluence of our society, many youngsters are exposed to potentially harmful environmental conditions which are in need of change. Basically, environmental-intervention approaches follow two major trends. Environmental-modification procedures are those in which the child remains with his family, but pressures in his surroundings are reduced or strengthening supportive assistance is given. In environmental-alteration procedures, the child is removed from an intolerable environmental situation and placed in a new situation, generally a foster home or residential institution. Both approaches have the common objective of doing everything possible to enable the child to continue normal growth processes. Each approach may have correlated services of psychotherapy, recreational outlets, medical services, socialization experiences, ego-building activities, or special educational services.

Intervention approaches demand the effective collaboration of all child-welfare specialists. One of the major problems in the delivery of services has been the chronic shortage of trained professionals. Attempts to resolve this manpower shortage have resulted in many innovations, including subprofessional workers, "big brother" programs, homemaker services, and community-located residential schools.

SUGGESTED READINGS

Bower, E. M., & Hollister, W. G. (Eds.) *Behavioral science frontiers in education*. New York: Wiley, 1967.

Caplan, G. (Ed.) *Prevention of mental disorders in children*. New York: Basic Books, 1961.

Cowen, E. L., Gardner, E. A., & Zax, M. (Eds.) *Emergent approaches to mental health problems.* New York: Appleton-Century-Crofts, 1967.

Gildea, M. C. L. *Community mental health.* Springfield, Ill.: Thomas, 1959.

Shore, M. F., & Mannino, F. V. (Eds.) *Mental health and the community: problems, programs, and strategies.* New York: Behavioral Publications, 1969.

REFERENCES

Brieland, D. The efficient use of child welfare personnel. *Children,* 1965, **12**, 91-96.

Buell, B. *Community planning for human services.* New York: Columbia Univer. Press, 1952.

DeFries, Z., Jenkins, S., & Williams, E. C. Treatment of disturbed children in foster care. *Amer. J. Orthopsychiat.,* 1964, **34**, 126-139.

Fine, R. Moving emotionally disturbed children from institution to foster families. *Children,* 1966, **13**, 221-226.

Havighurst, R. J. *Education in metropolitan areas.* Boston: Allyn & Bacon, 1960.

Jenkins, S., & Sauber, M. *Paths to child placement: family situations prior to foster care.* New York: Community Council of Greater New York, 1964.

Mid-Decade Conference on Children and Youth. *Report.* Washington, D.C.: National Committee for Children and Youth, 1966.

Moss, S. Z. How children feel about being placed away from home. *Children,* 1966, **13**, 153-157.

Olshansky, S., & Sternfeld, L. Attitudes of some pediatricians toward the institutionalization of mentally retarded children. *Train. Sch. Bull.,* 1962, **59**, 67-73.

Redl, F. *When we deal with children.* New York: Free Press, 1966.

U.S. Children's Bureau. *Child welfare statistics—1964.* Washington, D.C.: Government Printing Office, 1965.

Watson, R. I. *The clinical method in psychology.* New York: Harper, 1951.

Witmer, H. L. Children and poverty. *Children,* 1964, **11**, 207-213.

11

Classroom Management of Behavior Problems

STATEMENT OF THE PROBLEM
THE PSYCHIATRIC VERSUS THE EDUCATIONAL MODEL
REDL'S PSYCHODYNAMIC APPROACH
  • GROUP MANAGEMENT [Common Group Malfunctions / Three Issues
  concerning Discipline] • INFLUENCE TECHNIQUES [Support of Self-
  Control / Situational Assistance / Reality and Value Appraisal / The
  Pleasure-Pain Principle] • LIFE-SPACE INTERVIEWING [Objectives /
  Guidelines for the Interview / Limitations]
BEHAVIORAL APPROACHES
  • RATIONALE • INTERVENTION TECHNIQUES [Positive Reinforcement /
  Extinction / Modeling / Punishment / Desensitization / Discrimination
  Learning] • ADVANTAGES

In keeping with the new outlook in school mental hygiene, teachers
have been assigned a central role in promoting the mental health of
their pupils. By and large, however, while teachers have been given
this added responsibility, they have not been adequately equipped
with the tools needed to fulfill their new role. One important aspect
of classroom mental health of substantial concern to teachers centers
around the problem of classroom discipline, and it is to this topic
that this chapter addresses itself. There are times in every teacher's
day when he must interfere with the pupils' behavior in order to
safeguard the classroom program of instruction as well as the psychological and physical safety of the pupils.

After a discussion of the inadequacy of professional technical assistance offered teachers in the past, attention will be focused on two
current approaches which have much to offer regarding daily classroom management. The basic concern will be with the control of
surface behavior rather than with the underlying attitudes, although

some consideration will also be given to the latter. The specific thesis of this chapter is that teachers *can* cope with problem behavior and do this as well as psychiatrists, psychologists, and social workers. While a "hands-off" policy prevailed in the past, it is becoming increasingly evident that teachers who are successful in managing the behavior of nondisturbed children are also relatively successful with emotionally disturbed children (Kounin, Friesen, & Norton, 1966).

STATEMENT OF THE PROBLEM

It is well known that many beginning school teachers, males as well as females, are concerned about matters of classroom discipline. Flesher (1945), for example, noted that discipline was the most frequently reported problem among beginning teachers. This same study also revealed that school administrators regarded the maintenance of discipline as the greatest problem of inexperienced teachers. Even experienced teachers, in coping with deviant behavior, are often at a loss on how best to proceed. That many teachers still use outdated and psychologically unsound disciplinary measures is shown in a study of 290 elementary teachers from 86 counties in a midwestern state (Slobetz, 1950). While it is heartening to report the use of positive disciplinary measures in an appreciable number of instances, it also appears that physical force, censure, and punishment of various sorts were used more than the situation warranted.

Teachers seem especially concerned about the child with disorderly conduct, although less so than their counterparts did forty years ago. Back in 1928, Wickman (1928) asked teachers and mental-hygiene specialists to rate the severity of various behavior problems and discovered that the two groups rated the problems quite differently. Teachers, in general, were more concerned about acting-out behaviors, such as stealing and disobedience; whereas the clinicians were most concerned about the withdrawn child.

In keeping with the mental-hygiene spirit of the times, the conclusion was that teachers should be taught more about the nature of problem behavior so that their value judgments would be more in line with those of clinicians. More recent replication of Wickman's research (Stouffer, 1959) indicates that teachers' judgments as to the seriousness of withdrawn behavior are, by and large, more consistent with those of professional clinicians. As shown in Table 17, however, normalCLASSROOM MANAGEMENT OF BEHAVIOR PROBLEMS

TABLE 17. THE TWENTY MOST SERIOUS BEHAVIOR PROBLEMS OF SCHOOL-AGED CHILDREN, TAKEN FROM WICKMAN'S ORIGINAL LIST OF 50 AND RANKED ACCORDING TO THEIR SERIOUSNESS BY MENTAL HYGIENISTS, TEACHERS, AND PARENTS

Mental Hygienists	Teachers	Parents
1. Unsocial, withdrawing	1. Unreliableness	1. Stealing
2. Unhappy, depressed	2. Stealing	2. Untruthfulness
3. Fearfulness	3. Unhappy, depressed	3. Heterosexual activity
4. Suspiciousness	4. Cruelty, bullying	4. Destroying school
5. Cruelty, bullying	5. Untruthfulness	materials
6. Shyness	6. Unsocial, withdrawing	5. Cheating
7. Enuresis (bedwetting)	7. Truancy	6. Cruelty, bullying
8. Resentfulness	8. Impertinence, defiance	7. Unreliableness
9. Stealing	9. Cheating	8. Truancy
10. Sensitiveness	10. Easily discouraged	9. Disobedience
11. Dreaminess	11. Resentfulness	10. Impertinence, defiance
12. Nervousness	12. Destroying school	11. Obscene notes, talk
13. Suggestible	materials	12. Impudence
14. Overcritical of others	13. Suggestible	13. Selfishness
15. Easily discouraged	14. Heterosexual activity	14. Unhappy, depressed
16. Temper tantrums	15. Domineering	15. Masturbation
17. Dominating	16. Temper tantrums	16. Suggestible
18. Truancy	17. Selfishness	17. Domineering
19. Physical coward	18. Nervousness	18. Easily discouraged
20. Untruthfulness	19. Disobedience	19. Profanity
	20. Laziness	20. Lack of interest in work

Source: Adapted by permission of the author and publisher from two tables in G. A. W. Stouffer, Jr., The attitudes of parents toward certain behavior problems of children. *Tchrs Coll. Bull.*, 1959, 5, 173-174.

teachers and parents are most concerned with behavior that defies authority and moral dictates. Over-all, the parents tended to have attitudes similar to those of teachers in the late 1920's.

Are teachers mistaken in their greater concern with antisocial behavior than with introverted behavior? Perhaps not. As was mentioned in the earlier discussion on the stability of deviant behavior, it is the shy child whose behavior tends to be nonpersistent over time, whereas the behavior of the seriously aggressive child signifies the more serious psychological implications for later adjustment. Curiously, despite longitudinal data on the stability of aberrant behavior in children, it still seems today that many clinicians and educators accept the implications of the Wickman-type studies, which chastise teachers in varying degrees for their emphasis on the acting-out child.

Some teachers, feeling that it is not their responsibility to deal with emotionally disturbed children, wash their hands of the whole disciplinary affair. Realistically, however, it appears that they have little choice in this matter, at least for the foreseeable future. For example, despite a doubling of special-class provisions for behaviorally disordered children in the public schools between 1948 and 1958, only 2-5 per cent of youngsters so identified are placed in special classes. This means that approximately 95 to 98 per cent of emotionally handicapped pupils are in the regular classes. Bower (1961) contends that, in the average classroom, there are 3 youngsters who warrant the emotionally handicapped label. Hence, even though some teachers would prefer not to concern themselves with the management of problem behavior, this is not likely to be their fate. While it is true that schools refer more youngsters than does any other agency to professionally trained workers, it is equally evident that the teacher, nonetheless, remains the person who has primary responsibility for the classroom management of the disturbed child. One hour of therapy per week often does little to lessen the need for coping with the child's disturbing behavior during the remaining hours that he is in school.

Rather than decreasing the role of the teacher as it relates to the mental health of children, there is a definite movement in the direction of greater teacher involvement in such matters. Expansion of the teacher's role has stemmed largely from the following factors:

1. The shortage of mental-health workers has served to force expansion of mental-health forces to include school personnel, even though the role the latter are to play in this respect has not been clearly conceptualized or delineated. Authorities like Fritz Redl point to a need for additional mental-health professionals to supplement the traditional clinical team. Some speak of the need for "invisible" therapists.

2. The inadequacy of the clinic model to deal with the varieties of disturbed children that our society is producing is another factor. In one large urban area, almost 3 out of every 5 patients in child psychiatric clinics did not complete treatment (Frumkin, 1955). The abrupt termination of clinic treatment has been ascribed by some authors (Overall and Aronson, 1963) to a discrepancy between the expectations of the lower-socioeconomic patients and their middle-class therapists. Nationally, the fact that only 1 in 4 child psychiatric patients receive direct treatment of some kind also highlights the obsolescence of the psychiatric model (Norman, Rosen, & Bahn,

1962). While we have traditionally modeled intervention after the clinic concept of treatment, the need for a more reality-type mental-health approach is becoming increasingly recognized. Just as the mounting dissatisfaction with the clinic concept of treatment has led to the development of community psychiatry, so has it led to a new look in school mental hygiene. The current realization that the child's life conditions, for example, the school, are as important as his feelings must obviously involve teachers to a greater extent than in the past.

3. Evaluations of therapy with children have also forced us to try other methods. Even with cases for whom the clinic model is supposedly appropriate, for example, middle-class neurotic youngsters, the effectiveness of treatment remains to be demonstrated (Bahn, Chandler, & Eisenberg, 1962).

4. The rising popularity of behavior therapy has also resulted in a more central role for teachers in the quest for better mental health for our children. When the psychodynamic model was the preferred method, the teacher was accorded at best a second-string status on the clinical team. Today it may well be the mental-health specialist who will assume a supportive role (Gallagher & Chalfant, 1966).

THE PSYCHIATRIC VERSUS THE EDUCATIONAL MODEL

The values advocated by educators and those favoring a psychiatric model often clash, and the clash has led to a role conflict on the part of teachers. The divergence in values espoused by these two groups has been summarized by White (1965):

It would be fair to say that the mental health movement has revered warmth of feeling; spontaneity; insight; a high interest in others, particularly peers; the ability to communicate, especially one's feelings; warm parents; freedom to exercise judgment; warm teachers, and democratic classrooms. The same movement has been against: being compulsive; competitive striving; intellectualism; being either thing- or achievement-oriented; being emotionally unresponsive, as well as being angry or passionate; being a loner; not confiding in others; teachers who are curriculum-oriented; the regimentation of school life; group tests; red tape; and vice-principals in charge of discipline. Many of these are precisely the values revered by educators committed to the "cognitive" cause.

Because mental-hygiene specialists have not fully understood the teacher's role, they have made little available to teachers by way of specific and concrete practical suggestions pertaining to the management of the child's daily behavior. It is the sad truth that mental-health concepts advanced by psychodynamically oriented clinicians have proved of little value to teachers on the front lines. Teachers have asked for practical and concrete suggestions, says Morse (1961), only to be given general platitudes. Teachers have, therefore, been forced to rely on their own common sense and ingenuity. Admonitions to be accepting, nonthreatening, and understanding of the child's needs have not helped teachers very much in coping with aberrant behavior. Ausubel (1961) opines that permissiveness was perhaps overdone between 1935 and 1955 and that there has been a shift away from permissiveness in recent years. In giving advice to educators, mental-health professionals seem to forget about the following aspects of the teacher's role which makes it difficult for him to heed the advice given:

1. The teacher is a group worker; therefore he cannot usually work with just one child.

2. The teacher's primary goal is not to increase the child's personal insights but to achieve certain academic objectives.

3. The teacher must reflect cultural values; therefore, he cannot be permissively accepting.

4. The teacher deals primarily with conscious or preconscious processes; he is not prepared to handle unconscious processes and materials.

5. The teacher must focus on the reality problems as they exist in the situational present.

Because of these basic differences in outlook, the folklore of mental-hygiene concepts disseminated in teacher-training courses has most likely promoted the mental health neither of children nor of their teachers. In fact, personal adjustment and academic achievement were seen as incompatible objectives. Teachers, being asked to do what they cannot, have consequently been made to feel anxious, inadequate, helpless, and guilty. The result has been that they are less well prepared to fulfill their mental-health roles.

There are certain theoretical models, we believe, which yield more specific and practical aids for classroom management than the psychiatric model permits. Furthermore, these intervention models, namely, Redl's psychodynamic approach and the behavioral approach, are more consistent with the teacher's role than is the traditional psychiatric model.

REDL'S PSYCHODYNAMIC APPROACH

In this section we will consider management techniques stemming from a psychodynamic model developed by Redl for use with severely antisocial children. Unlike other psychodynamic management models, Redl's approach offers specific and practical techniques which are consistent with the teacher's role. The methods he advocates can be useful not only in the immediate control of classroom discipline problems but also in the long-range working-through of mental-health goals for the child. Moreover, the techniques are useful for group as well as individual management.

GROUP MANAGEMENT

Cognizant that no pattern of teacher-pupil interaction alone is sufficient to establish and maintain discipline, Redl (1966) underscores the importance of group psychological factors in the production of classroom difficulties. Rather than viewing discipline cases as a consequence of a given child's particular disturbance, he argues that the large majority of such cases involve a mixture of individual disturbances and factors peculiar to the group atmosphere surrounding the incident in question. It is necessary, therefore, to conduct an analysis of the individual and group factors together with their respective importance in the production of misbehavior in a given situation. The teacher, who is first and foremost a group leader, consequently needs skills not only in child-study techniques but also in group analysis, for the one-to-one teacher-pupil relationship is an ideal rarely obtained in reality. Even in special-education classes for emotionally handicapped children, where class size averages from 8 to 10 pupils, the teacher must be well versed in group-management skills.

Common Group Malfunctions

In analyzing some of the more typical things that go wrong in group settings, Redl cites the following six categories:

1. *Dissatisfaction in Work Process.* Basic dissatisfaction sometimes stems from curricula and teaching approaches which are inconsistent with the children's needs. Assignments which are too easy or too difficult for the pupil, verbal instruction which is too abstract or distant

from the child's social background, tasks which are unfairly assessed, and faulty scheduling or sequencing of classroom activities are just some of the problems found in this category. Some educators would go so far as to attribute most discipline problems to this complex factor, but Redl warns that to do so is as mistaken as assuming that all disciplinary cases are produced solely by personality factors. That frustrations do result from a discrepancy between situational demands and the child's ability to cope with them is well established, but to state this as the primary cause of disciplinary issues is an overstatement.

2. *Emotional Unrest in Interpersonal Relations.* Tensions stemming from strained interpersonal relations can also produce classroom discipline problems. Though the teacher is usually not the intended recipient of such outcropping tensions, he must nonetheless cope with the forthcoming disturbances. Typical of such difficulties are conflicts between cliques, between personal friendships and academic interests, and over the distribution of roles within the group. Such tensions can pose substantial trouble for the teacher, especially if the unrest becomes widespread and disrupts group harmony.

3. *Disturbances in Group Climate.* The punitive classroom climate is one of the most common causes of group disorders. Predicated upon a lack of respect for the individual and characterized by an atmosphere of fear, this climate has particularly deleterious effects on group order and morale. Resistance to teacher standards might well be, in this case, a sign of a healthy personality rather than an unhealthy one. The emotional-blackmail climate is based upon the teacher's withdrawal of love resulting in guilt feelings on the pupil's part if he violates the teacher's code. Climates characterized by vicious competition among students or a snobbish sense of group pride also represent unhealthy group tones.

4. *Mistakes in Organization and Group Leadership.* Though a teacher may be knowledgeable in terms of his subject-matter area and equitable in terms of his relationship with the class, he may encounter difficulties when it comes to the mechanics of group leadership. Being ill-prepared for group leadership, teachers are prone to problems arising from too much or too little group structure, a lack of sensitivity to student feelings, and a nonjudicious imposition of their own values on the pupils.

5. *Emotional Strain and Sudden Change.* Chronic anxiety, boredom, and resistance to classroom change on the pupil's part are well known, but often overlooked, enemies of classroom order.

6. *Composition of the Group.* No one has the solution to the problem of achieving the most effective grouping, although any teacher will readily admit that the makeup of his class is a factor of vital importance in the establishment and maintenance of discipline. Since variability in group composition is always present and can sometimes be very healthy, the issue, says Redl, is not one of heterogeneity versus homogeneity, but one of grouping on relevant variables. It is of prime importance that, though grouped according to relevant criteria, the extremes be avoided on criteria nonessential to the group's *raison d'être.* When analyzing the sources of misbehavior, the teacher would do well to consider such criteria as the socioeconomic level of his pupils, their independence-dependence level, their approach-withdrawal tendencies, as well as their self-governing abilities and interest levels.

Three Issues concerning Discipline

There are three basic problems regarding group discipline with which the teacher must come to grips, according to Redl. First, he must consider the effects of a given disciplinary action upon the individual and upon the group. Since discipline affects both the individual and the group, difficulty sometimes arises. For example, being very harsh and threatening may be good for a particular group at a particular time, but this technique may be harmful to the shy children in the group who do not respond therapeutically to this kind of atmosphere. Redl offers a guideline for individual-group decisions, namely, the law of "marginal antisepsis." This law states that a given technique that is appropriate for the individual must be at least harmless to the growth of the group and vice versa. Redl stresses the need for a "double-orientation" if teachers are to have hygienic discipline.

A second consideration hinges around the objective of group discipline. Does the teacher want to modify surface behavior or to seek a more deep-rooted change in attitude? Usually, both types of changes are sought, but complications arise since some techniques are more appropriate to one objective than the other. Again the law of marginal antisepsis applies. Any technique devised to alter disruptive momentary behavior should be at least harmless to the accomplishment of longer-range objectives of a basic attitudinal change and vice versa.

Third, the teacher must ask whether or not his disciplinary techniques are effective. Unfortunately, the yardsticks used are often misleading. For example, the teacher may, through a show of force, suppress certain aggressive behaviors in the classroom and feel that this technique works; yet he may not realize that his pupils are now more aggressive in the bus on the way home from school. Anyone who has ever sat in the teachers' lounge of a school is aware of how freely advice is given about disciplinary techniques that work. To determine whether they really work or not, Redl argues that one must consider the disciplinary techniques in light of the individuals in question, the effects on the group as well as on the individual, the influence on surface behavior versus attitudinal change, and, finally, the subsurface effects. Only after examination of these circumstances will one be prepared to answer the question of whether a technique works or not.

INFLUENCE TECHNIQUES

The influence techniques can be divided for purposes of discussion into four basic categories: (1) techniques supporting self-control; (2) techniques involving task assistance; (3) techniques of reality and value appraisals; and (4) techniques working the pleasure-pain principle (Redl and Wattenberg, 1959). We will confine our discussion to those methods of Redl's which have most relevance to the classroom. It should be borne in mind that these techniques are regarded by Redl and his associates as tools for helping the teachers through difficult or rough moments. They are not intended to replace a well-thought-out classroom program, in the broadest sense of the term.[1]

Support of Self-Control

The first group of techniques yields most effective dividends when used with children whose behavioral controls, though generally adequate, need strengthening at times. Basically these children are reasonably well motivated to do what is expected of them, but they have momentary lapses because of overexcitement, forgetfulness, and so forth. Once assisted by the teacher, these children are able to get back on the right track without much ado. The following techniques seem to work well with such youngsters.

---

[1]While we have not discussed educational programing in any detail, we heartily recommend Redl and Wineman's (1952) discussion of programing for ego support for a fuller treatment of this neglected topic.

1. *Signal Interference.* Most teachers realize the value of preventing misbehavior before it spreads. Cues from the teacher, such as giving a cool stare, pointing a finger, tapping the chalk, quietly mentioning the child's name, and so forth, are often sufficient to help many children regain control.

2. *Planned Ignoring.* Behaviors will sometimes disappear or diminish in frequency if not rewarded. A given misbehavior may thus cease of its own accord once the teacher intentionally ignores it. As is true of all techniques to be discussed, the teacher must decide when it is appropriate to use this approach. Although the technique works well with certain pupils and certain behaviors, it is subject to many of the same limitations that extinction has (see pp. 450-451).

3. *Interest Boosting.* A technique long used by teachers in drawing a pupil's wandering attention back to the work at hand is to convey interest in the child's work. This procedure serves to renew the child's interest in the task; the underlying assumption is that he has the skills necessary for successful completion.

4. *Humor.* Humor can also be used in handling behavior problems, that is, the friendly use of humor which elicits responses incompatible with anxiety and aggression. Sarcasm predicated upon teacher hostility is likely to elicit great covert or overt aggression and hostility. The use of humor shows a pupil that the teacher is human and that he is secure enough in his role to be able to joke. The authors recall one bright lower-class pupil who habitually defied direct orders. Through good-natured kidding and interest boosting on the teacher's part, the pupil was able to complete assignments. The fact that he was quite aware of the teacher's strategy did not seem to limit the effectiveness of the "humorous" approach.

5. *Diversion.* Another technique widely employed by both teachers and parents is that of diversion. It consists in distracting the child from his objectionable pursuits by directing his attention toward more desirable activities. Frequently, the asking of a simple question may suffice. The question serves to interrupt the undesirable activity and simultaneously to channel energies along more acceptable lines.

One of the main advantages of these techniques is that they prevent small incidents from blossoming into more difficult situations. Such incidents nipped in the bud are less painful to both the teacher and the pupil. Another advantage of these techniques centers around the cardinal rule for discipline: never intervene any further than is necessary to handle the situation. Stated otherwise, the use of intervention procedures should be parsimonious. While these techniques are based on common sense, many beginning teachers overreact to mild forms of student misbehavior, with the consequence that they use drastic forms of intervention when subtle interventions would do. It is imprudent to use physical restraint when a quiet glance in the offender's direction will suffice. Since the supportive techniques entail minimal interference, they are less apt to arouse counterhostility on the student's part. Moreover, once applied, the supportive techniques enable the student to regulate his own behavior in an acceptable manner once again.

It should be mentioned, however, that these techniques are less effective with children whose control systems are not intact. Further, these low-pressure methods are of limited value once misbehavior has advanced beyond the beginning stage and emotional contagion has spread. The teacher must know when to intervene, for the timing of disciplinary actions often determines their outcomes.

Situational Assistance

Some youngsters misbehave because the situational demands, social as well as academic, exceed the students' skills and abilities. Though students may have reasonably adequate behavior controls, misbehavior can sometimes be expected when goals are blocked and frustration ensues. The teacher can assist in such situations by manipulating the outside barriers which thwart the pupil. Such assistance may not solve long-range problems, but it does permit the energies of both the student and the teacher to be directed to the task at hand. The following list is not exhaustive.

1. *Hurdle Help.* The child sometimes misbehaves because he cannot understand or execute the required assignment. Rather than losing face in the eyes of his peers, he prefers not to ask for help. His sense of frustration and anxiety, resulting from his inability in this situation, is further heightened by his seeing that his classmates are working diligently on the task. Thus, he is prone to pester others. In such situations, a wise teacher offers the child the help needed to grasp the concept or skills involved rather than focusing on misbehavior.

2. *Restructuring the Class Setting.* Students, like most other human beings, become bored or overly excited on occasions. In certain

instances, it may be more profitable to alter the situation than to call attention to the restlessness. For example, instead of oral book reports in the traditional manner, tension due to restlessness could be relieved by having the students role-play the reports. If the teacher feels that restructuring classroom activities will benefit the learning process, he should feel flexible enough to make the necessary changes. In their study of certain dimensions of teacher behaviors as they relate to the behavior of emotionally disturbed children in regular classrooms, Kounin, Friesen, and Norton (1966) noted that programing to reduce pupil satiation was one concrete teaching technique which influenced the amount of classroom deviancy. It is easy to become a slave to a standardized program which no doubt affords a sense of security for both teacher and pupil. However, at some point, this security can lead to stagnation and inhibit further development of one's capacities for development and change. Some persons, teachers and pupils alike, may be able to tolerate less change than others, but probably all persons should have training in coping with change and variety.

3. *Routines.* Although some classrooms are too regimented and, therefore, subject to trouble, other classroom programs lead to trouble for exactly the opposite reason. Both acting-out and withdrawn students need and benefit from structure. The environmental predictability stemming from routine offers students guidelines for their actions and a sense of security. Routinizing classroom activities, such as the start of the school day, pencil sharpening, trips to the lavatory, and so forth, should help to minimize classroom behavior problems.

4. *Removing Seductive Objects.* Almost every parent recalls removing from the scene objects which result in his child's misbehaving. Beginning teachers soon realize that some objects hold an irresistible appeal to pupils, especially to those with inadequate behavioral controls. Some objects and children just do not mix well. Leaving science equipment, shop tools, athletic gear, and valuables about only invites trouble. Once a teacher becomes aware of what triggers certain students, he is wise to avoid these situations or objects. It serves no constructive purpose to expose youngsters with inadequate personal controls to temptations which they cannot resist.

5. *Antiseptic Bouncing.* Times arise when it is necessary to remove or restrain a child. The possibilities of physical danger and emotional contagion offer two examples when such action is necessary. Unfortunately, there are few places in the typical school building to

which a pupil may be nonpunitively exiled. In one well-staffed school system, a buzzer system was installed in the classroom so that the teacher could signal the social worker or school counselor when a child had to be ousted. Sending the child on errands to the office with a sealed note explaining the situation is also a technique permitting hygienic removal in cases of emergency. The authors know of cases in which volatile children had been taught to signal the teacher once they felt an outburst coming on so that he could head off the trouble by sending them out of the room to cool off and regain self-control before returning to class. Antiseptic bouncing not only enables the child to save face with his classmates but spares his teacher the problem of having to cope with temper flareups.

6. *Physical Restraint.* Sometimes a child erupts aggressively in the classroom and physical restraint is the only course of action open to the teacher. The authors remember one occasion during which a fifth-grade pupil felled his teacher, cursing and kicking her as she lay on the floor. Another teacher, quickly summoned, held the boy until he had calmed down. In such situations, it is important that the teacher's approach be protective and not counteraggressive. It is well to tell the explosive youngster gently that he is not going to be hurt, but simply that he is going to be restrained until he gets over his attack.

Reality and Value Appraisal

Another set of devices involves various kinds of appeals to values held by the youngsters. Illustrative of the variety of appeals that can be made are:

1. An appeal to a personal relationship between the teacher and the child; for example, "Jim, that noise bothers me."
2. An appeal to reality implications; for example, "You can get hurt by doing that."
3. An appeal to conscience; for example, "You're not that kind of child."

To use these appeals effectively, the teacher must be well aware of the child's value system. This technique requires sensitivity and empathy on the teacher's part.

Research by Kounin, Gump, and Ryan (1961) found that *task* appeals (for example, "We can't get the job done if you're going to make all that noise") elicited more favorable student reactions than did *personal* appeals (for example, "I don't like boys who make that kind of noise"). Students witnessing task-appeal techniques also rated their teachers as more skillful in handling children and expressed greater interest in the subject matter being taught than did students experiencing personal appeals. Centering on the immediate task thus seems to result in less classroom deviancy than does reliance on teacher relationship.

As with any other influence technique, the use of appeals can be overworked. If used sparingly, the seriousness of the incident or situation is impressed on the class. On the other hand, if it is overused, and there is a tendency to misuse this approach since the use of appeals makes teachers feel good, the technique loses much of its effectiveness. Another limitation arises when the teacher encounters a child who is markedly deficient in the values to which teachers commonly address their appeals. On the positive side, this technique can help to develop or strengthen the very values that will permit self-control.

The Pleasure-Pain Principle

Much of Redl's discussion of these topics might be subsumed under the learning-theory concepts of positive reinforcement and punishment. The basic rationale underlying the use of the pleasure-pain technique is that behavior which leads to unpleasant experiences for the child will be avoided. While acknowledging that such techniques as rewards, promises, threats, praise, blame, and punishment can have a constructive effect in modifying undesirable behavior, Redl is apparently more impressed with their limitations or misuses. For example, he considers that rewards and promises work well in the achievement of long-range goals with children whose egos are intact, but that these techniques are limited to the achievement of short-term goals with youngsters whose egos are impaired.

Let us examine Redl's discussion of punishment since there is current controversy surrounding the use of this technique. Redl and Wattenberg (1959) specify exact prerequisite conditions for the constructive use of this method:

1. There should be some concern by the child over his misdeed; that is, there should be a conflict between his control system and his impulses.

2. The child must know that the teacher basically likes and accepts him even though he has to punish him on this occasion.

3. The punishment meted out should, in the child's eyes, be a reasonable and preferably a natural consequence of his action.

Though, at first glance, these criteria do not seem too stringent, Redl believes that in reality these conditions are less commonly met than might be presumed. For example, some youngsters may not be upset by their behavior. Then again, teachers are probably more inclined to punish youngsters with whom they have a poor relationship.

In addition, to the cautions cited in our earlier discussion of punishment, Redl notes:

1. The timing of the punishment is highly crucial. If it occurs too soon, when the child is still in an irrational state, or too long after the incident, he is less able to see the relationship between his actions and the imposed consequences.

2. The teacher can be easily led to believe that he has achieved results which he has not. For example, the child may overtly conform to his teacher's demands, but he may be even more aggressive with his peers on the playgound.

3. The length or nature of the punishment should fit the offense and the child's developmental level. If the primary-school child is deprived of pleasant activities for prolonged periods of time, he comes to see the teacher as mean and the desired educational benefit intended is consequently nullified.

LIFE-SPACE INTERVIEWING

A most important skill for teachers is the ability to talk effectively with children, especially for purposes of managing problem behavior. To this end, life-space interviewing (LSI), or reality-interviewing as it is sometimes called, was developed. The main goal of this technique is to achieve some degree of behavioral conformity on the child's part. It can be used apart from or in conjunction with the influence techniques discussed earlier. It is not a moralistic approach but a dynamic one based in large measure on the teacher's empathic relationship with the child.[2]

---

[2]Extended treatment of this method is beyond the scope of this chapter, but we will attempt to present a general description of this type of interviewing. The student who wants to learn more is referred to Redl and Wineman (1952) and Newman (1963).

In contrast to counseling and psychotherapy, which generally take place in the interview room, LSI occurs in the more natural context of the child's daily environment. As far as teachers are concerned, what are most often needed are on-the-scene impromptu talks about specific troublesome incidents. To have a child discuss an incident with his counselor or therapist next week is of little assistance to the teacher who must somehow cope with the child's behavior here and now. Reality-interviewing thus affords a kind of needed instant therapy. The potency of LSI accrues from the fact that since the child's disequilibrium is greatest during times of crisis, the teacher is especially able through minimal assistance to influence adjustment outcomes which are hanging in a state of delicate balance. Stated otherwise, in crisis situations, people are better motivated to seek and use the help afforded them. It would, therefore, seem that critical incidents afford an excellent teaching opportunity for teachers.

Objectives

In essence, there are two broad goals of LSI: (1) clinical exploitation of life events, and (2) emotional first aid (Redl, 1959). At times, the purpose of the interview may be to help the youngster over momentary difficulties and back to his normal self. On other occasions, the teacher may attempt to work through some long-range goals with the child. A given incident may offer the teacher a long-awaited or golden opportunity to attack an issue which needs further explanation. In everyday practice, it is often difficult to know in advance of the interview which of the two broad objectives one will seek. Many times, both processes may be combined in a single interview.

Clinical Exploitation of Life Events. Attempts at clinical exploitation aimed at long-range clinical goals may involve:

1. Giving a reality "rub-in" to youngsters who habitually misinterpret interpersonal situations (for example, youngsters who think the teacher is "against" them) or who fail to derive meaning from social situations.

2. Demonstrating that the maladaptive style of life really involves more secondary pains than secondary gains.

3. Stimulating numb value areas by appealing to potential or dormant values of the child or his peer group.

4. Convincing the child through word and action that there are other ways of behaving (defenses) which are satisfying.

5. Expanding the child's own psychological boundaries to include other adults and teachers or to permit acceptance of formerly unacceptable aspects of himself.

Emotional First Aid. Like the clinical exploitation of life events, emotional first aid is accomplished through the process of empathic communication between the child and the teacher. The following goals are illustrative:

1. To drain off hostilities of daily frustrations so as to prevent an intolerable accumulation.

2. To provide emotional support when children are overwhelmed by feelings of panic or guilt.

3. To maintain a relationship with the child so that he does not retreat into his own world as a consequence of emotional upheaval.

4. To govern social traffic so as to remind wayward pupils of "house" policies and regulations.

5. To serve as an umpire in disputes, fights, and other "loaded transactions."

Guidelines for the Interview

Bernstein (1963) offers the following guidelines as being useful and supportive in school-oriented reality-interviewing:

1. Be polite. Offer the child a chair. Produce a tissue if it is needed. While teachers and other adults demand good manners from children, they are occasionally guilty of excessive rudeness toward the children.

2. Don't tower over a little child. Kneel or bend down to him. Have a small chair or stool in the office for really little children and another one for you to sit on. Be wary about lifting a kindergartner or first-grader onto a desk or table. Although a well-meant action, it may push a frightened child into a screaming panic because he feels trapped in midair and can't get down.

3. When you are sure of your ground, it can be a good approach to confront a child with your knowledge of his misdeed, and not give an inch. This can be a tremendous relief to the child who otherwise would have to clam up or spend twenty minutes denying the facts. Confrontation, however, is not likely to be successful with the child who feels that everybody is his enemy.

4. Be sparing with your use of "Why?" It is very difficult to explore reasons and all but impossible for a child to lay his motivations out

on the principal's desk for dissection. It is much better to say, "We can't have this art on the lavatory walls. I'm not going to let you continue. We have to talk about this a little."

5. Get conversation going about the actual situation. Obtain a description of what happened. *Listen* to what the child says.

6. If you think a child is overwhelmed with guilt or shame, begin by minimizing the weightiness of the problem at hand, for example, by saying, "This action doesn't bother me too much, but we had better look into it, for it can cause *you* trouble."

7. Say what you know the child wants to say but can't put into words. "You were very disappointed, weren't you? You had been counting on this talk for a long time and couldn't stand to have to wait any longer."

8. Be aware of the kinds of thinking demanded by the particular situation. Bright children frequently become involved in relationships which are beyond their grasp in terms of emotional and personality maturity.

9. Help the child with plans for specific steps to improve the situation.

10. At some point in the interview, give the child an opportunity to ask *you* questions, or say, "Is there anything you want to tell me?" or, "Is there something you would like me to try to do for you?" Be prepared for some remarkable questions and disclosures, but after you've done this a few times you'll be convinced of how helpless and frightened the misbehavers are and you'll be moved by the depth and intensity of their desire to be "in" and to be good.

Limitations

There is no question but that LSI can be a powerful tool for the hygienic management of classroom behavior problems. Like other approaches, LSI is subject to limitations, three of which are particularly prominent:

1. LSI is a highly complex and sophisticated clinical technique which requires more extensive supervised training in the form of seminars and practicum experiences (for example, the Fresh Air Camp at the University of Michigan) than most teacher-training institutions are willing or able to muster. The method requires considerable teacher sensitivity as well as an awareness of individual and group dynamics. The teacher must know what issues to select for clinical exploitation, which materials to interpret and which to leave untouched,

what the influences of the setting imply, and so forth. Moreover, since reality-interviewing is more art than science, it is difficult to communicate to others.

2. Teachers with 25-30 pupils often do not have time to conduct individual interviews. Advocates of this approach are well aware of this limitation and advise the use of a "crisis teacher" to circumvent this difficulty (Morse, 1962).

3. Since LSI is most effectively implemented in a totally hygienic milieu, it demands satisfactory cooperation among all members of the school staff, especially between the teacher and the principal, as well as an awareness of the psychosocial totality of the school setting. Initially, it might seem that securing the necessary cooperation would not be difficult among professional people, but a study by Long (1963) suggests otherwise. In his followup study of teachers trained in life-space interviewing, Long reported that many of the teachers stated that their fellow teachers were critical of and unsympathetic toward this approach. Consequently, most of the teachers gradually gave up on this approach. Long concludes that if universities are to teach LSI methods, then they should maintain contact with or train psychologists and counselors already in the public schools so that the necessary support for this approach can be provided. These findings also highlight the need for in-service training of administrators as well as teachers.

BEHAVIORAL APPROACHES

RATIONALE[3]

The behavioral approach is essentially interested in the modification of behavior. Little attention is devoted to the etiology of the troublesome behavior. The inner dynamics or the underlying phenomena are definitely relegated to a secondary status.

Before an exploration of the techniques emanating from this approach, it is appropriate to ask why teachers should focus primarily on maladaptive *symptoms* or behaviors rather than on *causes* of the maladaptive behavior. There are several reasons for this emphasis on symptoms:

---

[3]The material in this section has been reprinted, with minor editorial changes, from Harvey Clarizio and S. Yelon, "Learning Theory Approaches to Classroom Management: Rationale and Intervention Techniques," *Journal of Special Education,* 1967, 1, 267-274, by permission of the publisher.

1. Teachers, by virtue of their orientation, are not trained to probe the inner dynamics of behavior. They cannot deal with transference neuroses, interpret free associations, or explore dammed-up psychic processes. Indeed, mental-hygiene specialists themselves have large gaps in their knowledge relative to the causes of behavior even after extensive diagnostic workups have been made. The search for non-observable causes is further complicated by the fact that, typically, behavior is multiply caused; rarely is the etiology singular in nature. Not only are there multiple causes, but the causes interact, so that specific delineation of the causative factors becomes even more difficult. In certain cases, any one of the component etiological factors may not be sufficient, in and of itself, to produce deviant behavior. Yet, taken together, these factors are capable of producing such behavior. The difficulties associated with diagnosis in cases of multiple causes are illustrated in a study by Lambert and Grossman (1964), in which two teams of psychologists, neurologists, pediatricians, and educators were to determine independently if the learning and behavior difficulties of a given group of students had an organic basis. The results indicated that there was little agreement between the two teams as to the cause of the difficulty for individual students.

2. Even when teachers are able to identify or infer the underlying causes of deviant behavior, they are rarely in a position where they can directly manipulate the causes so as to modify their influences on the child's classroom adjustment. For example, if the problem lies in the parent-child relationship or in a brain lesion, there are seldom few, if any, constructive intervention techniques which a teacher can employ. Yet, the child's troublesome behavior persists and must be handled as hygienically as possible.

3. Even in those select cases in which the causes can be identified and manipulated directly, the maladaptive behaviors may persist. Consider the pupil whose reading disability is caused by a combination of faulty child-rearing practices and poor vision. If and when these etiological factors are identified and cleared up, attention still must be focused on this inadequate reading behavior in order for the child to be successful in reality. Until such efforts are undertaken, his mental health will most likely continue to suffer.

4. In certain cases, the behaviors or symptoms may, in and of themselves, become quite incapacitating and therefore warrant atten-

tion. This point is most dramatically illustrated in certain cases of reading disability where the relationships between education and emotional maladjustment are closely intertwined.

5. There is no reason to believe that when the teacher assists the child in modifying a given behavior, another undesirable behavior will inevitably take its place. The available evidence indicates that there is little support for this Freudian theory of symptom substitution (Grossberg, 1964). Symptom treatment can permit the breaking of a vicious circle of maladaptive behavior in which disabling symptoms either intensify the primary problem or become causes of other maladaptive behaviors. This latter possibility is illustrated in cases of learning disabilities which, though originally symptomatic of a more basic disturbance, came to produce additional anxiety, discomfort, and failure. By modification of the behavior, however, it is sometimes possible to reverse this downward spiral. For example, as the symptomatic behavior (for example, a reading disability) begins to clear up, the child is perceived and treated by others in a more favorable light. The parents view him as more worthwhile, as do his peers. Consequently, the child comes to view himself differently and to set new expectations for his own behavior.

6. Finally, as already implied, it is important to note that the teacher most commonly has no recourse other than to deal with behavior directly. However, if he can do this effectively, he will have gone far in meeting his mental-health responsibilities to his pupils. He should by no means disparage his accomplishments since he has restricted his assistance to a behavioral level. The science of psychology has not yet advanced to the stage that permits complete personality reorganization.

INTERVENTION TECHNIQUES

Having argued that the teacher should be primarily concerned with behavior per se rather than with its causes, let us turn to techniques stemming from behavior therapy which have relevance to the modification of deviant behavior in the classroom. Although the techniques to be presented are discussed separately for the sake of clarity, it should be recognized that more than one of them may be operative at the same time. Further, the teacher, to be most effective, often will combine several techniques.

Positive Reinforcement

The dispensation of rewards constitutes one of the main tools of the behavioral approach. In this technique, emphasis is placed on reinforcing the response made by the individual, and only minimal attention is given to the stimuli eliciting the response. Accordingly, the teacher presents the reward when the individual performs the desired response. Thus, the teacher who says, "I see that Johnny is ready to begin work, now that recess is over" is rewarding him for his attention and studiousness. Teachers have long recognized the value of making certain behaviors worthwhile to the learner.

One of the merits of this technique stems from its applicability to antisocial youngsters as well as to withdrawn children (Bandura & Walters, 1963). As mental-health workers know, there has been a regrettable dearth of psychotherapeutic approaches designed for the child with a conduct problem, despite the fact that such pupils typically are most disruptive to classroom procedures and societal order. Basically, the application of this method to seriously aggressive children involves the manipulation of three variables: (1) the schedules of reinforcement, (2) the interval factor, and (3) the type of reward.

1. With respect to the concept of reinforcement schedules, a distinction must be enforced between the acquisition of a specific behavior and its maintenance. There has been an unfortunate tendency to blur the distinction between the building of behavior and the maintaining of behavior (Lindsley, 1964). For the former, continuous or full-schedule reinforcement is most effective; whereas for the latter, partial or intermittent reinforcement is most parsimonious and effective. In other words, if the desired response is not yet an established part of the child's behavior, the youngster should be positively reinforced each time that he makes the desired response. Once the response has become ingrained in his behavior, however, partial reinforcement schedules should be used since behavior is more readily maintained and less subject to extinction under this pattern of reward. Thus, for example, the habitually hostile child who makes a friendly or non-aggressive response toward a classmate should be rewarded every time he does so. Once the more socially acceptable behavior toward others has been securely acquired, it would be best that the teacher reinforce such behavior every now and then rather than 100 per cent of the time. Similarly, the basically shy child should be reinforced for greater

assertiveness 100 per cent of the time until assertiveness becomes an established response for him. Once this point has been reached, a schedule of partial reinforcement should be adopted.

2. The interval variable merely refers to the passage of time between the production of the response and the presentation of the reward. The delay factor may be quite short initially for acting-out youngsters because typically these children have difficulty in postponing gratification. Step by step, however, the interval can be lengthened as the child acquires more adequate behavioral controls. Hence, initially the teacher may have to reward the conduct-disordered child immediately after his good behavior at recess time or in the laboratory. Eventually, if all proceeds well, he may have to reward the child once a day for his compliant behavior. The delay interval may also have to be short with youngsters whose self-esteem and self-confidence are severely impaired. A seriously disabled reader may, for example, need a reward, such as the teacher's praise or encouragement, immediately after he has sounded out a single word. Later, as he gains in reading skill and personal confidence, he may not need to be rewarded until he has completed a whole page or story.

3. The nature of the reward for some pupils may, at the start, have to be tangible and physical in nature. Though concrete in nature, the reward should always be paired with verbal social reinforcers; for example, "Lisa, you handled yourself well in that situation today" (Quay, 1963). By the pairing of verbal rewards with tangible rewards, the teacher's words—through association with the concrete satisfactions —gradually take on a reinforcement value of their own. Eventually, the reinforcers become less and less concrete (for example, a gold star on a chart) until a child can respond satisfactorily to verbal and abstract kinds of reinforcements, such as teacher approval. In the determination of the most suitable reinforcers for the children in question, consideration should be given to such factors as developmental level and social-cultural background. What is reinforcing for a lower-class child may be quite different from what is reinforcing for a middle-class child. Similarly, certain rewards may work better with 12-year-olds than with 7-year-olds. The need for caution in this regard is exemplified in research demonstrating that verbal praise is actually aversive for certain emotionally disturbed children (Levin & Simmons, 1962a, 1962b). For some youngsters, praise had a dramatic decelerating influence on the frequency of desirable responses.

In brief, through the use of positive reinforcement, the child is taught three characteristics needed for his ultimate return to a regular class: (1) to work on an intermittent reinforcement schedule, (2) to delay gratification, and (3) to work for symbolic rewards (Quay et al., 1966).

The main unresolved question with this technique centers around the issue of how to elicit the response from the child in the first place so that it can be rewarded. The technique of social modeling, which will be discussed below, may well provide at least a partial answer to this problem.

Extinction

While there is a substantial body of research demonstrating that the presentation of rewards facilitates the acquisition and maintenance of given behaviors, there is also a growing body of literature attesting that the simple withdrawal of reinforcers can reduce or eliminate troublesome behaviors. This procedure has been found effective with such varied problems as excessive talking, tantrum behavior, and academic errors (Williams, 1959; Zimmerman & Zimmerman, 1962; Warren, 1965).

Extinction is not always the most economical and effective means of bringing about behavioral change. Certain cautions should be recognized:

1. Deviant behavior may recur following the extinction trials. In other words, extinction does not always permanently abolish the misbehavior. If spontaneous recovery of the undesirable behaviors does occur, additional extinction trials will be needed.

2. As noted in the discussion of partial reinforcement, behaviors —troublesome or commendable—can be maintained even though they are only infrequently reinforced. What sometimes happens, since the teacher cannot always completely control circumstances in a classroom, is that many deviant behaviors (for example, talking out loud in class) are occasionally reinforced and thereby set up on a partial reinforcement schedule. Thus, instead of the abolition of the behavior via extinction, there is a rise in the frequency and intensity of deviant responses via partial reinforcement. It is sometimes extremely difficult *not* to reinforce maladaptive behaviors in the classroom setting. For example, the aggressive pupil who kicks the teacher or a classmate cannot help but be reinforced by the look of pain on the victim's

face. In the same regard, the inability to obtain cooperation needed from other teachers and pupils in the school to secure more complete control over the school environment also poses problems to the most effective use of extinction as an intervention technique.

3. Clinical observation suggests that some behaviors do not become extinct simply by the withdrawal of the reinforcer. Moreover, the teacher sometimes cannot or will not wait long enough for the extinction process to take place. This latter limitation is particularly acute in situations where the dangers of emotional contagion or self-inflicted injury are distinct possibilities.

Modeling

Bandura (1965) contends that modeling procedures represent a more effective means for the acquisition of new behavior patterns than does an operant-conditioning paradigm based on positive reinforcement. Moreover, once a behavior is acquired through imitation, it can often be maintained without external reinforcement since humans learn to reinforce themselves for behaving in certain ways.

As an intervention technique, modeling is based on the premise that a child will imitate the behaviors of others. It is an important technique, in that the learning of social skills in children is commonly acquired through examples of socially approved behavior presented by suitable models. Therapists and school teachers, as models, thus have considerable opportunity to influence the behavior of children. Despite having distinct utilitarian value, this technique has unfortunately been neglected in the management and modification of deviant behavior. Training institutions have long recognized the importance of modeling procedures in the preparation of future therapists and teachers, and therefore have attempted to provide adequate models in the form of critic therapists or teachers. However, less attention has been devoted by training institutions to the use of modeling procedures as a means of influencing the behavior of the clients or pupils with whom the teachers and therapists will have to work.

There are three main effects of exposure to models: (1) the modeling effect, (2) the inhibitory or disinhibitory effect, and (3) the eliciting effect (Bandura, 1965):

1. Through the modeling effect, children come to acquire responses which were not previously a part of their behavior. As noted earlier, modeling procedures are considerably more economical in trans-

mitting new responses than is the method of operant conditioning based on positive reinforcement, especially when a combination of verbalizing models and demonstration procedures is used.

2. The strengthening or weakening of inhibitory responses already existing in the observer can also be accomplished through modeling procedures. For example, children who see an agemate punished or rewarded for aggressive behavior tend to decrease or increase their aggressive behavior accordingly.

3. The eliciting or response-facilitation effect refers to responses that precisely or approximately match those exhibited by the model. Thus, observation of the teacher's response provides discriminative clues which trigger similar responses already in the pupil's behavior repertoire. This eliciting effect is distinguished from the modeling effect and the disinhibiting effect in that the imitated behavior is neither new nor previously punished.

The probability that a child will imitate a model is a function of more than sensory contiguity. Mere exposure to models is no guarantee that the child will imitate the desired behaviors. Attention-directing variables—such as motivational factors, previous experiences in discriminative observation, the distinctiveness of the modeling stimuli, and the expectation of reward or punishment—all contribute to the extent that the child will observe the behavior exhibited by the model. The rate, amount, and complexity of the modeling stimuli also influence the amount of the child's imitation (Bandura, 1965).

Punishment

Aversive conditioning, as punishment is sometimes called, is an intervention technique which has been used primarily to discourage undesirable behavior. This technique consists in the presentation of either physically or psychologically painful stimuli or the withdrawal of pleasant stimuli when the undesirable behavior occurs. Traditionally, the use of punishment as a technique for behavioral modification has not been advocated for the following reasons:

1. Punishment does not eliminate the response; it merely slows down the rate at which the troublesome behaviors are emitted.

2. This technique simply serves notice to stop inappropriate behaviors; it does not indicate what behaviors are appropriate to the situation.

3. Aggressive behaviors on the teacher's part serve as an undesirable model for the pupil.

4. The emotional side effects of punishment, such as fear, tenseness, and withdrawal, are maladaptive.

5. Punishment serves as a source of frustration which is apt to elicit additional maladaptive behaviors.

Acknowledging these cautions, some psychologists who are currently reevaluating the concept of punishment nonetheless contend that it does have a beneficial effect if applied to specific responses rather than to the general situation (Marshall, 1965). Indeed, teachers and parents—whatever their motivations—use verbal reprimands and other forms of corrections in their approach to classroom or home management. The judicious use of punishment as an intervention technique is most likely necessary because it is impossible to guide children effectively only through positive reinforcement and extinction. Ausubel (1961) rejects the idea that only positive forms of discipline are beneficial. He notes that a child does not come to regard rudeness as an undesirable form of behavior simply by the reinforcement of respect for others. In Ausubel's words:

It is impossible for children to learn what is *not* approved and tolerated simply by generalizing in reverse from the approval they receive for the behavior that *is* acceptable.

Punishment of specific responses can thus have an informative and beneficial effect.

Another positive value accruing from the use of punishment is that by holding undesirable behaviors in abeyance, it permits the teaching of desired behaviors through such intervention techniques as social imitation or positive reinforcement. Although punishment as an intervention technique has been used primarily with acting-out pupils, its use may be extended to certain cases of withdrawn behavior (Lovaas, 1965). Punishment, though controversial in nature, seems to be gaining in respectability as a tool in the behavior therapist's armamentarium.

Desensitization

Desensitization as an intervention technique has been used primarily with the phobic child. The basic objective is to have the child achieve a relaxed response in the presence of what were previously anxiety-producing stimuli. To accomplish this relaxed response, the subject is encouraged to perform a series of graduated approximations of the previously punished acts within a nonpunishing or actually rewarding situation. Through gradual exposure to the feared object or act, he comes to approach the once frightening situation in a calmer and more adjustive manner. The child thereby overcomes his specific phobia and is able to respond in a more constructive way when confronted with previously feared objects or situations.

One perfectionistic child who always earned "A" grades in order to ward off feelings of inadequacy and guilt was helped through use of this technique. The feared object in this case was a grade lower than "A." At the start, the teacher occasionally structured the classroom assignment so that this boy would earn an "A" grade. Once he was able to accept a slightly less than perfect grade, he was given a grade of "B+" and so on until he was able to set less perfectionistic standards for his behavior. This youngster, over a period of time, seemed to feel under less pressure and strain without appreciable sacrifice in the quality and quantity of his school work.

Another example involves the integration of a withdrawn child into group settings. In this case, the first-grade boy was too shy to sing in front of the class. He did not seem to mind singing, however, when he was with the entire group. The strategy was to get him to sing in progressively smaller groups until he would not be afraid to sing alone. Thus, the teacher initially had him sing with about half the class, the boys. She then had him sing in quartets and in trios, until by the end of the year he was able to sing a duet comfortably. Through use of this technique in other areas of socialization, the boy showed considerable gains in becoming more gregarious and outgoing.

Many remedial-skills teachers have also used this technique with severely disabled readers whose attitudes toward books were characterized by fear and hate, two emotions which are often very closely related. One teacher began with typewritten reading materials prepared from the child's own dictation of stories about incidents he enjoyed. Later in the year, comic books of an educational nature were used to develop reading skills. By the end of the year, the child was finally ready to return to books, the objects he feared so strongly just five months earlier.

Discrimination Learning

Children sometimes engage in maladaptive behaviors because they have transferred behaviors acceptable in one setting to a second setting where these behaviors are considered inappropriate and maladaptive. Thus, for example, the child who is overly dependent upon his mother may behave in a very dependent way toward his teacher. Such cases of inappropriate generalization sometimes can be handled through the use of discrimination learning.

Essentially, this process consists of labeling given behaviors as appropriate or inappropriate in a specific environmental context. Thus, for example, the teacher may inform the child in a nonpunitive way that she is not his mother and that she expects him to become more self-reliant as the year goes on. This labeling by the teacher serves to make the child more aware of both inappropriate and appropriate behaviors. Interestingly, children do not always have to be able to express such discriminations verbally in order to achieve the insight. To ensure effective results, the appropriate responses should be rewarded, and undesirable responses discouraged. Discrimination learning thus may be of service in conjunction with other techniques in managing conduct and personality problems in the classroom.

ADVANTAGES

As evidenced by the discussion of the limitations of each technique, the authors do not envision management techniques emanating from learning theory as a panacea. We concur with Whelan and Haring's (1966) observation that

a skeptical, cautious acceptance and application of behavioral procedures and tools is most appropriately warranted at the time. The crucial validation of these techniques must take place in regular classrooms.

While such validation has not yet been demonstrated, we believe that these intervention techniques possess certain advantages:

1. The fruitfulness of these techniques in modifying human behavior has been demonstrated in laboratory settings as well as natural settings. Grounded in research, these techniques permit the development of systematically trainable competencies among those individuals responsible for the building, modifying, and maintaining of behavior patterns in children.

2. They are consistent with that aspect of the teacher's role which requires that he reflect cultural expectations to the pupils and set standards for their academic and social behavior. Traditionally, it has been the teacher's job to change the behavior of those entrusted to him.

3. A behavioral approach offers specific and practical techniques for use in day-to-day classroom problems. While teachers already use some or all of these techniques, they frequently do so in an intuitive and/or inconsistent way, thereby reducing the efficacy of such intervention tools.

4. These techniques enable the teacher to strive toward more realistic and obtainable goals relative to their pupils' mental health. Troublesome target behaviors can be selected and then modified through appropriate intervention techniques. One of the major advantages of these techniques is the easy accessibility to observable behaviors which can be readily identified and treated (Ulrich, Stachnik, & Mabry, 1966).

5. One of the most important attributes of these techniques is their communicability; that is, they can be taught to teachers. While there are few if any teacher-training institutions currently offering systematic didactics and practicum training in such techniques, there will be a time when teachers in training will receive such skills in laboratory courses taken in conjunction with their formal course work. In the meantime, teachers in the field may be able to acquire this training through in-service meetings or through workshops. Theoretically, the school psychologist or clinical psychologist, by virtue of his clinical experience and background in learning theory, may well be in a position to conduct such training institutes. The development of a core of behavioral technicians could go far to alleviate the manpower shortage in the mental-health disciplines.

SUMMARY

While there remains a gap between the theoretical and the applied aspects of discipline, the principles and techniques discussed in this chapter should help to reduce the amount of deviant classroom behavior. The wise teacher will employ a number of these methods, thereby expanding his repertoire of management techniques and avoiding reliance on any given technique. He will also vary management techniques according to the situation and refrain from intervening any further than is warranted. Timing must also be carefully considered so that he does not wait until his own feelings as well as the child's get out of hand. Further, the experienced teacher patiently waits until circumstances are sufficiently in his favor before attempting to teach the child a lesson.

Despite the effective application of these techniques, it is unreasonable to expect that teachers will be able to handle every upset pupil. It must be remembered that teacher behavior and attitudes are but two of a complex of factors that influence pupil behavior. It should not be assumed, as Ausubel (1961) points out, that a pupil's misbehavior is solely the result of "aggressive, unsympathetic and punitive teachers." Further, regardless of the number of professional services available, teachers are going to encounter uncontrollable youngsters. What is most important in such instances is that teachers not feel guilty because of their inability to manage the aberrant behavior. Even in an ideal milieu setting, it is sometimes necessary to remove a seriously disturbed youngster. On the other hand, if a teacher is habitually having trouble with several pupils, many of whom are not ordinarily disorderly, he might well examine his classroom program and modes of handling children. He may find, for example, that the setting is overregimented and the curriculum boring.

Teachers sometimes frustrate themselves unnecessarily through unrealistic goal setting. In the present state of development in the mental-health disciplines, a teacher should not strive to convert a disturbed child into a fine, lovable all-American boy. A more realistic goal would be to seek the development of marginally acceptable behavior. Hence, instead of trying to produce a relatively rapid and total personality transformation, teachers might more realistically try to make him a more tolerable "so-and-so."

SUGGESTED READINGS

Clarizio, H. F. *Toward positive classroom discipline.* New York: Wiley, 1971, forthcoming.

Gnagey, W. *The psychology of discipline in the classroom.* New York: Macmillan, 1968.

Newman, R. G., & Keith, M. M. (Eds.) *The school-centered life space interview.* Washington, D.C.: Washington School of Psychiatry, 1963.

Webster, S. *Discipline in the classroom.* Scranton: Chandler, 1968.

REFERENCES

Ausubel, D. A new look at classroom discipline. *Phi Delta Kappan,* 1961, **43,** 25-30.

Bahn, A., Chandler, C., & Eisenberg, L. Diagnostic characteristics related to services in psychiatric clinics for children. *Milbank mem. Fund Quart.,* 1962, **40,** 289-318.

Bandura, A. Behavior modifications through modeling procedures. In L. Krasner & L. P. Ullmann (Eds.), *Research in behavior modification.* New York: Holt, Rinehart & Winston, 1965. Pp. 310-340.

Bandura, A., & Walters, R. H. *Social learning and personality development.* New York: Holt, Rinehart & Winston, 1963.

Bernstein, M. Life space interview in the school setting. In R. G. Newman & M. M. Keith (Eds.), *The school-centered life space interview.* Washington, D.C.: Washington School of Psychiatry, 1963. Pp. 35-44.

Bower, E. M. *The education of emotionally handicapped children.* Sacramento: California State Department of Education, 1961.

Flesher, W. R. The beginning teacher. *Educ. Res. Bull.,* 1945, **24,** 12-18.

Frumkin, R. M. Occupation and major mental disorders. In A. M. Rose (Ed.), *Mental health and mental disorder.* New York: Norton, 1955. Pp. 136-160.

Gallagher, J. J., & Chalfant, J. C. The training of educational specialists for emotionally disturbed and socially maladjusted children. In W. W. Wattenberg (Ed.), Social deviancy among youth. *Yearb. nat. Soc. Stud. Educ.,* 1966, **65,** Part I. Pp. 398-422.

Grossberg, J. Behavior therapy: a review. *Psychol. Bull.,* 1964, **62,** 73-88.

Kounin, J., Friesen, W., & Norton, A. Managing emotionally disturbed children in regular classrooms. *J. educ. Psychol.,* 1966, **57,** 1-13.

Kounin, J., Gump, P., & Ryan, J. Explorations in classroom management. *J. Tchr Educ.,* 1961, **12,** 235-246.

Lambert, N., & Grossman, H. *Problems in determining the etiology of learning and behavior problems.* Sacramento: California State Department of Education, 1964.

Levin, G., & Simmons, J. Response to praise by emotionally disturbed boys. *Psychol. Rep.,* 1962, **2,** 10. (a)

Levin, G., & Simmons, J. Response to food and praise by emotionally disturbed boys. *Psychol. Rep.,* 1962, **2,** 539-546. (b)

Lindsley, O. Direct measurement and prothesis of retarded behavior. *J. Educ.,* 1964, **147,** 62-81.

Long, N. Some problems in teaching life space interviewing techniques to graduate students in education in a large class at Indiana University. In R. G. Newman & M. M. Keith (Eds.), *The school-centered life space interview.* Washington, D.C.: Washington School of Psychiatry, 1963. Pp. 51-56.

Lovaas, I. Building social behavior in autistic children by use of electroshock. *J. exp. Res. Pers.,* 1965, **1,** 99-109.

Marshall, H. The effects of punishment on children: a review of the literature and a suggested hypothesis. *J. genet. Psychol.,* 1965, **108,** 23-33.

Morse, W. The mental hygiene dilemma in public education. *Amer. J. Orthopsychiat.,* 1961, **31,** 332-338.

Morse, W. The crisis teacher: public school provision for the disturbed pupil. *Univer. Mich. Sch. Educ. Bull.,* 1962, **37,** 101-104.

Newman, R. G. The school-centered life space interview. In R. G. Newman & M. M. Keith (Eds.), *The school-centered life space interview.* Washington, D.C.: Washington School of Psychiatry, 1963. Pp. 13-34.

Norman, V., Rosen, B., & Bahn, A. Psychiatric clinic out-patients in the United States, 1959. *Ment. Hyg.,* 1962, **46,** 321-343.

Overall, B., & Aronson, H. Expectations of psychotherapy in patients of lower socioeconomic class. *Amer. J. Orthopsychiat.,* 1963, **33,** 421-430.

Quay, H. Some basic considerations in the education of emotionally disordered children. *Except. Child.,* 1963, **30,** 27-31.

Quay, H., Werry, J., McQueen, M., & Sprague, R. Remediation of the conduct problem child in the special class setting. *Except. Child.,* 1966, **32,** 509-515.

Redl, F. The concept of the life space interview. *Amer. J. Orthopsychiat.,* 1959, **29,** 1-18.

Redl, F. *When we deal with children.* New York: Free Press, 1966.

Redl, F., & Wattenberg, W. *Mental hygiene in teaching.* New York: Harcourt, Brace & World, 1959.

Redl, F., & Wineman, D. *Controls from within.* New York: Free Press, 1952.

Slobetz, F. Elementary teachers' reactions to school situations. *J. educ. Res.,* 1950, **44,** 81-90.

Stouffer, G. A. W., Jr. The attitudes of parents toward certain behavior problems of children. *Tchrs Coll. Bull.,* 1959, **5,** 173-174.

Ulrich, R., Stachnik, T., & Mabry, J. (Eds.) *Control of human behavior.* Glenview, Ill.: Scott, Foresman, 1966.

Warren, A. All's quiet in the back of the room. Paper read at meeting of Council for Exceptional Children, Wichita, October, 1965.

Whelan, R. J., & Haring, N. G. Modification and maintenance of behavior through systematic application of consequences. *Except. Child.,* 1966, **32,** 281-289.

White, M. Little red schoolhouse and little white clinic. *Tchrs Coll. Rec.,* 1965, **67,** 188-200.

Wickman, E. *Children's behavior and teachers' attitudes.* New York: Commonwealth Fund, 1928.

Williams, C. The elimination of tantrum behavior by extinction procedures. *J. abnorm. soc. Psychol.,* 1959, **59,** 269.

Zimmerman, E., & Zimmerman, J. The alteration of behavior in a special classroom situation. *J. exp. Anal. Behav.,* 1962, **5,** 59-60.

12

The Prevention of Behavior Disorders

THE NEED FOR PREVENTIVE STRATEGIES
● *THE SCOPE OF THE PROBLEM* ● *THE SHORTAGE OF MANPOWER* ● *THE EXPENSE AND INADEQUACY OF TREATMENT*
DETERRENTS TO IMPLEMENTATION
THE FOCI OF ATTACK
● *BIOLOGICAL APPROACHES [General Physical Robustness / Genetic Aspects]* ● *SOCIOLOGICAL APPROACHES [Social Engineering / Deterrents]* ● *PSYCHOLOGICAL APPROACHES: PARENT EDUCATION [Mass Media / Group Discussion / Individual Guidance / Evaluation]*
PRIMARY PREVENTION IN THE SCHOOLS
● *EARLY IDENTIFICATION [The Preschool Period / The Elementary-School Period / Some Unresolved Problems]* ● *CURRICULUM APPROACHES [Incidental Instruction / Separate Courses / Units]* ● *THE ROLE OF STRESS: HARMFUL OR NEUTRAL? [Activities for Reducing Stress / Programs for Building Immunity to Stress]* ● *THE SUCCESSFUL SCHOOL PROGRAM [Preventing Stress and Strengthening Personality]*

It is customary to distinguish between three kinds or levels of prevention: primary, secondary, and tertiary. *Primary prevention* has as its objective the reduction of behavioral disorders; it aims to prevent various disorders from arising initially. Early identification of emotional disturbance represents one such strategy. In addition, this type of prevention involves the promotion of psychological robustness; that is, it attempts to strengthen personality development, for emotional well-being is more than the mere absence of pathology. Current curriculum approaches which strive to provide ego-enhancing experiences are illustrative of this phase of primary prevention. *Secondary prevention* involves the identification of vulnerable groups and is akin to the concept of treatment in that it aims to shorten the duration and diminish the impact of a given disorder through therapeutic interventions. Head Start programs constitute an example of attempts at secondary prevention. *Tertiary prevention* is similar to the concept of rehabilitation. The aim here is to assist the individual to live as useful a life as possible despite some degree of chronic impairment.

The ensuing discussion focuses for the most part on primary prevention. The chapter opens by establishing the need for preventive actions. Next, attention turns to some of the reasons why preventive programs have remained more at the conceptual level than at the action level. Discussion then centers around programs which have dealt with the biological, sociological, and psychological aspects of prevention. Finally, the chapter closes with a discussion of the role played by the school in primary prevention.

THE NEED FOR PREVENTIVE STRATEGIES

Three basic factors suggest the need for preventive action: (1) the scope of the mental-health problem; (2) the shortage of professional health specialists, generated in part by the clinic model of treatment; and (3) the dubious value of the majority of treatment approaches.

THE SCOPE OF THE PROBLEM

First, let us briefly review the incidence of maladjustment in youth. It is estimated that approximately 4-7 per cent of children have moderate to severe disturbances. The epidemiological data gathered by Bower (1960) indicated that 10 per cent of the public-school population have mental-health problems. Using this figure, Bower (1970) estimated that there are now 5.5 million youth, from kindergarten through college, with moderate to severe mental-health problems. As a conservative estimate, 300,000 youth under 18 years of age are seen annually in outpatient clinics for relatively less severe emotional disturbances, and an estimated additional 500,000 might be classified as manifesting psychotic or borderline behavior (National Association for Mental Health, 1966). Heightening the concern over this problem are the statistical projections which indicate that the rates are going to increase rather than decrease during the next decade (Rosen, Bahn, & Kramer, 1964).

THE SHORTAGE OF MANPOWER

The number of mental-health specialists has not kept pace with the rising number of cases. George Albee (1967), an authority on manpower needs in the mental-health fields, declares that the mental-health professionals are not going to be able to provide the services promised. He feels that practitioners have made irresponsible promises —to union workers, to the aged, to the poor, and to Congress. For example, if only 1 per cent of the United Auto Workers sought psychiatric service, there would be another 20,000 cases to treat annually. The Medicare bill not only promises such help to the elderly, but for all persons adjudged "medically indigent" and for their children. And with Kiddiecare programs in the offing, it is little wonder that Albee sees a day of reckoning before long.

Albee estimated that in 1965 there was need for an additional 2,500 psychologists. It should be noted that many trained psychologists assume positions in industry and universities. Because of the burgeoning college population, practically every Ph.D. psychologist produced in the next decade could be absorbed by college teaching vacancies. The picture is no more optimistic for the supply of psychiatrists and social workers. In 1965, the need was for an additional 2,200 psychiatrists and 5,200 social workers. Bower (1970) notes that there are only 300 members of the American Academy of Child Psychiatry and less than 50 being trained each year.

Note that the discussion pertains to *demand*—the number of professionals required to handle actual cases—and not *need*—the number required to perform an adequate job in the mental-health field. No one knows how many are *needed*, but it is known that the number is certainly much larger than the number of professionals *demanded*.

THE EXPENSE AND INADEQUACY OF TREATMENT

Not only have services been promised that cannot be delivered, but the services delivered are both expensive and inadequate. With respect to outpatient services, the lack of a centralized administration has resulted in the duplication of diagnostic and treatment services, with people being shunted from one community agency to another. The need for an administrative reorganization which meets the needs of the people rather than the needs of an antiquated organization is becoming increasingly apparent (Gardner, 1967). The costs incurred in the course of inpatient treatment are even higher in comparison to those associated with outpatient treatment. The cost of maintaining a single delinquent in a public training school is, for instance, $3,000 a year (Polk & Schafer, 1967), and private care units consisting of from 20 to 60 disturbed youngsters cost about $10,000 per child per year (Bower, 1970). The latest therapeutic bandwagon, the community mental-health center, is also tremendously expensive. In 1963, the Community Mental Health Act provided $150 million in grants from 1963 to 1967 for the construction of these centers. The projected operating costs of a given center for the first year is $500,000 (Bower, 1970). These costs are merely illustrative and do not speak to the cost of state and county mental hospitals, of outpatient treatment, and, most seriously, of wasted human resources.

The expense created by treatment of maladjusted youth might be tolerable—provided the services rendered were adequate. But this is not the case. Despite the existence of more than 2,000 outpatient clinics and 400 psychiatric units in general hospitals, the rates of mental disorders have remained unchanged or, perhaps, have increased. Just as the advent of the child-guidance movement in the early 1900's was hailed as a boon, so now the far-reaching benefits of the community health center are perhaps exaggerated. While a shift from the therapist's office to the community is needed, little benefit can be expected by simply transplanting present policies and practices to a new setting. As Cowen, Gardner, and Zax (1967) note:

Function, not locus, is the critical element, and the potential shift of our mental health operations to a community base should be a means rather than an end. Inherent in such a shift are the opportunities to study more relevant and meaningful questions, to extend the reach of mental health operations, to look at resources rather than deficits, and to develop specific mental health programs with greater social utility. Without recognition of the salience of these functions, there is the danger that the community approach will, in the final reckoning, offer little more than the oft-maligned "old wine in new bottles."

To be genuinely innovative, the workers in community mental-health centers must have knowledge of social processes and social organization (Reiff, 1966). Unfortunately, these centers are manned by the "old guard," who lack such knowhow. Since the old guard were trained primarily in therapy, the expectation may well be for "old wine in new bottles."

It should be apparent that unwarranted reliance has been on

treatment approaches, especially on psychotherapy. As noted in the section on the evaluation of therapy, the results have been disappointing despite the selection of the most suitable patients for treatment. Clearly, though there will always be a need for treatment interventions, there is no scientific basis for the assumption that traditional forms of treatment will provide an adequate solution to the nation's mental-health problems. Many workers now feel that the ounce of prevention could not conceivably be less effective than the pound of cure.

Medical science has accomplished much along the lines of mass prevention. Vaccines for polio, measles, and mumps are currently available. Yet, the behavioral sciences seem quite content to provide treatment on a one-to-one basis for psychological disturbances. The futility of this approach is well exemplified in Bower's (1964) relating an old Cornish custom for determining a man's sanity. According to this method, the suspect was given a scoop and asked to empty the water from a bucket placed under an open tap. If the man turned off the faucet, he was deemed rational and sane. If, on the other hand, he continued to scoop while leaving the water run, he was deemed insane. Reasoning analogously, it would appear that most mental-health workers might also be deemed irrational. Ingenuity has provided various curricula in bucket-scooping. It takes a psychiatrist approximately 12 years to become a fully trained bucket-scooper; a Ph.D. psychologist, about 8 years; and a social worker, about 6 years. As Bower queries, Is it not time to offer at least a 4-year curriculum in tap-turning?

DETERRENTS TO IMPLEMENTATION

The concept of prevention, as it receives increasing attention from certain mental-health professions, has, as Bower (1964) points out, taken on an air of magic. It has become a high-status term "that has had little action implementation in the field of mental and emotional disorders." Why has this concept not been more actively translated into action programs? What are the principal obstructions responsible for its remaining largely a theoretical construct? In addition to the general lack of useful knowledge about human behavior, deterrents to preventive programs have typically assumed one or more of the following forms (Bower, 1964).

1. The size and complexity of the problem have overwhelmed lay

groups and behavioral scientists alike. Since maladjustment arises from such varied sources as faulty parent-child relations, poverty, racial discrimination, constitutional factors, and school failure, many workers believe that anything short of a major societal overhaul would prove inconsequential. The problem is so vast that few know where to begin. The ensuing emotional response to the frustrations associated with prevention is one of despair. Consequently, few are inclined to make any full-hearted effort along this line.

2. A second resistance centers around the invasion-of-privacy issue. Always a cherished right, the freedom to live one's own life continues to be publicly reinforced. In certain states, for example, the schools need permission to administer personality tests to students. Now, to prevent maladjustment is to meddle in people's affairs. The crux of the difficulty lies in finding a way of intervention which is acceptable to the public. Traffic regulations and medical inoculations are accepted without much protest. Schools as a primary institution in society have an advantage in that they do have certain rights to interfere in the lives of their students. Moreover, there is a receptiveness on the part of most parents to such interventions. The schools must be careful, however, to restrict interference to their sanctioned function: the education of youth. Thus, schools must demonstrate that ancillary services (psychological evaluation, counseling, and the like) are necessary to the child's educational progress.

3. Another deterrent involves certain cultural values. Notable among these is the belief that by working hard, controlling impulses, and using intellect, a person will be successful and achieve virtue. Conversely, if he is not conscientious, follows the pleasure principle, and lets emotions override his better judgment, he will be unsuccessful, a failure, and regarded as evil. In short, the individual derives from life what he deserves.

4. Still another barrier to the development of prevention programs resides within the professional community itself. Unfortunately, the majority of mental-health professionals view their primary task as one of treatment, not of prevention. The preoccupation is more with mental *illness* than with mental *health*. Witness the fact that, until recently, there was no word in our language to describe ego-enhancing experiences *(strens)*. But there has long been a term *(trauma)* to indicate ego-debilitating experiences. An ever expanding segment of mental-health workers is becoming more prevention-oriented, but it

remains difficult to enlist the full-fledged support of those doing therapy on a one-to-one relationship. Preventive work is regarded as less concrete, less exciting, and less urgent than therapy, which is geared toward the immediate, the tangible, and the already overt disturbance (Cruickshank, 1963).

5. A final problem involves specifying and evaluating the goals of prevention. Is the goal that of promoting emotional robustness? Or is it that of reducing pathology; for example, delinquency? As Bower (1964) states:

If our prime intention is the promotion of emotional robustness and of the ability to cope with life rather than to defend against it, the goal needs to be given a base of health objectives that are specific, positive and (hopefully) measurable.

Difficult as the task may be, it is essential to establish both operational definitions of objectives and evaluative baselines if any programs are to be implemented and assessed. The day of the "soft sell" might well be on the way out for the mental-health fields; they will have to demonstrate their worth as helpers of humanity.

THE FOCI OF ATTACK

Since it is often impractical to deal with all of the complexities of the problem of prevention, various workers have concentrated their energies and competencies on more delimited aspects of the problem. For purposes of discussion, these efforts can be subsumed under three main headings: biological approaches, sociological approaches, and psychological approaches.

BIOLOGICAL APPROACHES

General Physical Robustness

Many authorities have emphasized the importance of an adequate physical constitution as a basis for sound mental health. Perhaps the first and most important influence is that of pregnancy and childbirth. Notable among the studies in this area are those of Pasamanick and Knobloch (1966; see also Knobloch and Pasamanick, 1966). These investigators, fully aware that many factors in addition to abnormalities of pregnancy and childbirth cause behavior disturbances, reported that inspection of the medical histories of children with behavior problems revealed more complications of pregnancy and more incidence of prematurity than existed in the matched controls. Such complications, especially evident for hyperactive, confused, and disorganized youngsters, also occurred more frequently in children having hearing defects, strabismus, school accidents, infantile autism, and delinquent symptoms.

One disconcerting fact concerning youngsters who suffer injury before or during birth is that a large proportion of them are born to mothers in the low socioeconomic strata. These mothers, in contrast to those who are more affluent, are more apt to have poor diets and to receive less careful medical care during pregnancy. That the diet factor can be critical is attested to by Knobloch and Pasamanick's (1966) finding that pregnancy abnormalities occur more often in mothers who are underweight at the beginning of pregnancy and who remain so during pregnancy. They also report that supplementing the mother's diet with vitamins and proteins can reduce the incidence of pregnancy problems. While this country as a whole enjoys the highest standard of living in the world, the nation is far from achieving the best record with respect to complications of pregnancy and birth. It may be necessary for health-department personnel to rent and operate buildings adjacent to laundromats so as to provide ready access to medical assistance for lower-class mothers. There seems little question but that promoting greater use of public-health services should reduce the amount of organically based pathology either via prevention or early indentification and treatment.

Genetic Aspects

In addition to the biological preventive measures of promoting physical health, attempts have been made to manipulate heredity in order to produce sound people from sound genes. In that some disorders are presumed or known to have a genetic basis, it is not unexpected to find that some workers have advocated eugenic measures. Foremost among these techniques have been sterilization, birth control, and therapeutic abortions. Certainly, few would question the need or desirability of a sound genetic base. Nevertheless, it would be premature and extremely questionable to apply genetic regulations or approaches on a wholesale basis in light of the present state of knowledge concerning the role of genetics in such disorders as schizophrenia, mental retardation, antisocial personalities, and neuroses. This caution is not to deny the value of genetic counseling in certain cases, however.

SOCIOLOGICAL APPROACHES

To a significant extent, modern mental-health concerns are intimately related to urbanization, technology, and contemporary civilization (Arnhoff, 1968). Indeed, as the mental-health fields become increasingly aware of the relationship between social structure and such social problems as violence, delinquency, poverty, and traditional mental disorder, the need for sociological intervention also becomes increasingly evident. Ivor Kraft's (1964) comments are noteworthy in this regard:

Over and over again, no matter how earnestly we may try to discuss prevention by confining it to the biological and psychological sectors, we are compelled to confront the sociological influences. Over and over again, in the studies, researches and reports on primary prevention, there loom in the background the mundane and inescapable conditions under which mothers, fathers, and children live out their lives. We confront problems of housing, jobs, travel, money, prejudice, the struggle for status and security. Over and over again, the ponderous and learned discussions on anxiety, guilt, shame, self-concept, aggression, negativism dissolve into the daily facts of daily living....

Our society is so constructed that it deliberately violates one of the basic insights about human nature.... This powerful insight asserts that it is the relationships which prevail among men as individuals and as members of a structured society that ultimately determine their basic states of mental health and spiritual well-being. It is possible to have a strong and healthy mind in a weak, even a tortured and devastated human body. The example of Helen Keller comes to mind. But to have strong and healthy *collectivities of minds* we must have healthy social relationships.

To have societies where creativity and vigorous altruism prevail, we must have a social structure which fosters altruism. To have free, strong and happy men and women, we cannot tolerate social conditions which breed inferiority, insecurity and systematic exploitation of certain segments of society by other segments....

The primary prevention of mental ill health does not have one precise locus. We cannot point to one action, one event, one mechanism, one area of intervention and say: this is the danger spot; this is where we do the preventing.

Indeed, in the final analysis we cannot prevent mental dysfunction in the way we speak of preventing typhus or polio, with inoculations or public health measures. There are no inoculations or public health measures that yield a healthy mind or a tranquil, loving soul. We prevent mental ill health through acts of universal promotion—through promoting social relationships and social structures which yield physical well-being, the general security and creative living patterns for all of mankind.

We shall be forever doomed to failure if we persist only in seeking to invent techniques of prevention, only in weaving subtle theories of human personality that will reveal the vulnerable crisis points, only in forwarding still newer and more fanciful fashions in psychotherapy. We are merely re-shuffling the deck; the cards remain the same. Until we learn to prevent as well in the social order, there will be no real primary prevention.

Social Engineering

To illustrate but one aspect of a total ecological orientation to behavior, let us consider briefly the population explosion. Calhoun (1967), who conducted the first major series of experiments in this area, found that by increasing population density among rats, he was able to produce social disorganization, rampant aggression, mater-nal deprivation, infanticide, deviant sexual behavior, and other socially destructive and irresponsible behaviors which could be termed "delin-quent." Before discounting the applicability of these findings among animals to humans, consider a pioneering study conducted in France (Chombart de Lauwe, 1959), in which the impact of housing space on workers' behavior was examined. In this investigation, a direct relationship was found between decreased living space and pathology. Physical and social pathology doubled once the available space fell below a specific range of square meters per person. Casual observa-tion of married students' housing accommodations also suggests the influence of overcrowding on adjustment. Though multiple factors are involved in these situations, it might well be that the stress associated with overcrowding produces adrenocortical changes that may lead to propensities for aggressiveness.

In light of the potential for the shaping of human behavior as a function of environmental forces, it is not surprising that attempts have been made to restructure the social and physical environment. Lazarus (1969) has labeled this solution a "social engineering" approach to mental health:

The questions professionals are trying to formulate have to do with social planning. For example, what are the resources available to members of the community for jobs, for functional education, for social interaction permitting self and social respect, for satisfactory race and ethnic relations, etc.? What are the key problems that the present community structure imposes on the people living in it? The implicit assumption that lies behind these questions is a restatement of old social psychological and developmental tradition, that people became neurotic, psychotic, criminal, alcoholic, suicidal, etc., because they must live lives deficient in the social conditions that nourish mental health. . . . If these social conditions can be improved early enough in the person's development, there is a better chance that he will grow into a socially healthy and effective individual.

Deterrents

Though sociological intervention is not yet a strong approach, resistances to such a movement are already evident. Many lay people fear that social engineering implies a costly welfare state. Support is also not strong among traditional mental-health professionals, who tend to feel threatened by the social-engineering approach. As Lazarus (1969) notes:

The most important force, however, which restrains the development of social-engineering programs for the community is uncertainty and ignorance about the community changes that would be desirable and feasible and about the results they would actually accomplish. Any plan would affect many people in a multitude of ways, and one cannot be sure either that the desired effects would be produced, or that other more undesirable effects would not be produced. Yet it is abundantly clear to increasing numbers of professional workers that the massive mental health problem cannot be solved or even dented by the traditional psychotherapeutic approach, and that engineered changes in the social conditions of life provide the ultimate answer.

PSYCHOLOGICAL APPROACHES: PARENT EDUCATION

Numerous studies have documented the need for healthy parent-child relationships. Because authorities have long recognized the significance of a family milieu which fosters growth, the psychological aspects of prevention have emphasized parent education as a preventive tool. The fundamental premise of parent education is based on the notion that childhood pathology is related to parental pathology and that alteration of undesirable parental influences can be beneficial to the child's emotional well-being. Parent education is by no means a recent intervention strategy, for man has been giving his fellow man advice on child rearing for hundreds of years. Today, the Child Study Association of America and the National Congress of Parents and Teachers represent the two major organizations concerned with parent education.

Parent educators come from diverse professional fields, such as child development, education, home economics, psychology, social work, pediatrics, and public nursing. Other caretakers include family physicians, clergymen, probation and parole officers, and public-school teachers. Most of these workers, unfortunately, receive very limited training in parent education, despite the fact that they are presumed to have competence in this field.

The basic aims of parent-education programs are to provide normative information about children, to offer recommendations on child-rearing practices, and to change parents' attitudes toward their children if indicated. The ultimate goal is not designed to modify parental attitudes and behaviors per se, but to promote the over-all development of children.

Three basic approaches to parent education have been identified by Brim (1959): (1) mass media, (2) group discussion, and (3) individual guidance.

Mass Media

The first approach, though making use of films, tape recordings, plays, and television, relies primarily on the printed word. More than ten years ago, Brim estimated that about 25 million pamphlets are distributed annually. Brim also includes a single-lecture technique in the category of mass media, for example, a meeting of the local Parent-Teachers' Association. There seems little doubt that this approach does succeed in reaching a large segment of the population. It may well be, however, that those parents most in need of such exposure do not receive it, while those who do not need it eagerly seek it. This situation might well be analogous to the Sunday sermon; that is, those who need it most are at home, not at church.

Group Discussion

The group-discussion approach varies with the nature of the group and the qualifications of the leader. At the extreme, these meetings sometimes border on group psychotherapy. Expectant mothers and parents of preschool children are perhaps the most common participants in group discussions. It is becoming increasingly popular, however, to offer group guidance to parents of handicapped youth. By sharing their joys and frustrations, by offering one another emotional support, by realizing that their situation is not unique, and by relating practical ways of helping their children, the parents (under the direction of an experienced professional) find renewed strength to cope with the daily demands of life with a handicapped child. Only those who have lived with an emotionally disturbed or mentally retarded or orthopedically handicapped child can fully appreciate the parental strains associated with the special child rearing such a child requires. Disbelief, bitterness, ambivalence, and uncertainty are common to all parents of handicapped youth (Kessler, 1966). Because people are more receptive to advice at the time of an emotionally upsetting incident, "crisis counseling" can be an effective technique.

Individual Guidance

Individual counseling of parents is frequently a common function of the clergyman, the pediatrician, and the teacher, for when confronted with a problem, the parent often turns to those personnel most immediately available in the community. Whereas most written material deals with the physical setting of the interview and the advance preparation of factual material about the child, little attention is directed to the *feelings* of the parent and the teacher as they anticipate the conference. The teacher as well as the parent may feel guilty over the child's failure and therefore behave defensively. Parents not uncommonly are afraid to speak openly with teachers for fear that (1) the teacher will be offended, thereby invoking his displeasure, (2) the teacher will not be interested or will not understand, and (3) the information will not be held in confidence or will become a permanent part of the child's cumulative folder.[1]

One recent approach which holds promise for individual counseling along the lines of parent education is that of behavior modification. In this approach, the parents are trained to identify and to respond systematically to target behaviors. The study by Hawkins and his associates (1966) is illustrative. The parent counseling in this investigation focused on the hyperactivity of a preschool child with borderline intelligence. The work was conducted in the home. There were five phases:

1. A baseline period, during which observations were made of mother-child interactions.

---

[1]Prospective and even seasoned teachers might well profit from reading Langdon and Stout (1954) on the emotional aspects of the teacher-parent relationship.

2. A first experimental period, during which the mother was given training in certain behavior-modification techniques.

3. A second baseline period, during which the mother was told to behave toward the child as she had previously.

4. A second experimental period similar to the first experimental period.

5. A followup, 24 days after the last experimental period.

One of the first steps in the behavior-therapy approach is the delineation of the specific disruptive target behaviors. In this case, the child's objectionable activities consisted in (1) biting his shirt or arm, (2) sticking out his tongue, (3) kicking or hitting himself, others, or objects, (4) using derogatory language, (5) removing or threatening to remove his clothes, (6) saying "No!" to requests made of him, (7) threatening to damage persons or objects, (8) throwing objects, and (9) pushing his sister.

After observing and recording the mother and child during the 16 baseline sessions (Phase 1), the investigators told the mother the nine objectionable target behaviors. She was shown three signals which were to be used by the experimenter to indicate how she should behave toward the boy (Phase 2). Upon Signal A, she was to tell him to stop whatever obnoxious behavior he happened to be engaging in at the time. Upon Signal B, she was to isolate him by placing him in his room and locking the door. Upon Signal C, she was to reward his behavior immediately through the use of praise, attention, and physical affection.

During this second phase, Signal A was given every time the child manifested one of the nine target behaviors. If he persisted, Signal B was given. When placed in the time-out room, he had to remain there for a minimum of five minutes and quiet down for a short period of time before being let out. The room was devoid of toys and other stimulating objects, so that placement there would not constitute a reward for misbehavior. Signal C was used whenever he showed desirable behaviors.

After 6 experimental sessions, the child's objectionable behaviors decreased to a stable level (see Figure 4). At this time, the mother was told to interact with him as she had prior to the training sessions (Phase 3). The experimenter observed the mother but did not cue her. After this second baseline period of 14 sessions, the second experi-

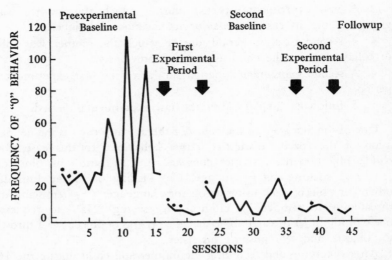

FIGURE 4. *Number of 10-second intervals, per 1-hour session, in which O (objectionable) behavior occurred. (Source:* R. Hawkins, R. Peterson, E. Schweid, & S. Bijou. Behavior therapy in the home: amelioration of problem parent-child relations with the parent in a therapeutic role. *J. exp. Child Psychol.,* 1966, **4**, 99-107.)

mental period of 6 sessions was begun. Finally, 24 days later, during which time the mother could use any techniques she chose, three post-treatment checks were made. As shown in Figure 4, the rate of objectionable behavior following parent training was about one-sixth of what it had been previously.

While the procedure described may be considered therapy and not prevention, the possible adaptation to prevention would seem quite promising. It has been demonstrated, for instance, that parents can benefit from observing (modeling) a behavior therapist at work with a child (Russo, 1964; Straughan, 1964). To date, regrettably, there has not been an attempt to implement a behaviorally oriented form of parent education. Though the example cited here involved the use of individual counseling, group-discussion techniques, coupled with the use of filmed observations of a behavior therapist at work on an actual case, are easily within the realm of possibility. Such a combined approach would have ready appeal to many parents because of its emphasis on practical aspects of child management.

Evaluation

One problem facing parent educators is the fact that the professional advice to parents on child-rearing practices changes with the times. Stendler (1950), for instance, after reviewing the articles on child rearing which appeared in three women's magazines between 1890 and 1950, described the period between 1890 and 1910 as one of "sweet permissiveness," during which "mother knew best." Between 1910 and 1930, rigid habit training was stressed; youngsters were not to be picked up when they cried for fear they would become spoiled. In 1948, feeding the baby on demand was in vogue, just the opposite of the 1920's, when rigid feeding schedules were in fashion. Today, mothers are encouraged to pick up their children, coo at them, cuddle them, and so on, to provide the stimulation necessary for proper development. Behavioral scientists do not have absolute truths; they merely establish temporary findings.

Frank's (1965) conclusion to his review of forty years of research also sounds a somber note:

No factors were found in the parent-child interaction of schizophrenics, neurotics, or those with behavior disorders which could Le identified as unique to them or which could distinguish one group from the other, or any of the groups from the families of the controls.

While such differences might exist, Frank's data certainly raise a question which proponents of parent programs must seriously consider.

Brim (1959) notes that evaluating the outcomes of parent education is not an easy process. Most research in this area has looked at the effects that such programs have had on the parents. Even with this relatively modest criterion, the results of parent programs must be regarded as inconclusive in light of the absence of reliable and valid measuring instruments and the lack of adequate control groups. It is recognized that the results of such programs should be assessed in terms of their effects on the children, but the methodological problems in such an assessment prove even more formidable. Take, for example, the matter of incidence. It is conceivable that an educational program for parents could reduce the actual incidence of emotional disturbance but produce an increase in recorded incidence because of such factors as the expanding definition of emotional disturbance, the increasing treatment facilities, and the growing concern about disturbed children. Brim (1959) also notes that parent programs could be improving the mental health of normal children; that is, healthy children might become psychologically more mature. Yet, such improvements might well go unnoticed.

PRIMARY PREVENTION IN THE SCHOOLS

Though no single institution appears to be adequate to the task of development and socialization, the school does have some advantages over other institutions. Briefly summarized, the school has access to large numbers of youths over long periods of time during the formative years. In addition, it has a culturally sanctioned right to "interfere" in other people's business, at least to the extent that the interference pertains to the child's educability. As psychology has become penetrated by public-health concepts and has advanced into community-action settings, mental-health specialists have become increasingly aware of the schools as a base of operation. Though there are many ways in which the educational process and mental health are interrelated, the current discussion will be limited to three aspects of the school's involvement in preventive efforts: (1) early identification, (2) curriculum approaches, and (3) the role of stress.[2]

EARLY IDENTIFICATION

The Preschool Period

Retrospective studies suggest the feasibility of identifying emotional disturbances at the preschool level. In one study, the investigators examined the histories of 60 youngsters seen at a child-guidance clinic and found that more than half of them had noticeable problems prior to school entrance (Oppenheimer & Mandel, 1959). Similarly, Bolton (1955) noted that 75 of 100 children seen at a clinic had manifested observable symptoms prior to kindergarten entrance. The difficulty of retrospective studies with respect to early identification and prediction is that they do not reveal how many youngsters in the general population had shown similar symptoms and yet later made an adequate adjustment to school (false positives) or how many who did not display observable symptoms grew up to be maladjusted (false negatives). Unfortunately, the retrospective research design cannot answer such vital concerns.

---

[2]For an extended discussion of the school's role in mental health, see Allinsmith and Goethals (1962), Bower and Hollister (1967), Clarizio (1969), and Rhodes (1968).

In another preschool study (Lindemann & Ross, 1955), which was a followup investigation, an attempt was made to predict kindergarten adjustment of 50 youngsters on the basis of parent interviews, systematic observation of the child, teacher ratings, teacher interviews, sociometric data, and the use of a standardized type of doll play. The play information was analyzed on the basis of four criteria: (1) the ease with which the child left the mother; (2) the extent to which the child controlled his emotions; (3) the amount of unusual behavior; and (4) the number of special demands made on the clinician. The investigators concluded that observation of the doll-play situation provided a relatively objective, economical, and valid indication of success in kindergarten.

The Elementary-School Period

Earlier discussion has already pointed out that elementary-school teachers are able to render reasonably reliable appraisals of a child's current personal adjustment. For instance, with respect to emotional disturbance, Lambert and Bower (1961) reported that 90 per cent of elementary-school pupils so labeled by teachers were also adjudged disturbed by experienced clinicians following individual assessment. Teacher ratings are also as reliable a technique as any available for the prediction of juvenile delinquency.

Programs of early identification and early secondary prevention have also been emphasized by Zax and Cowen (1967). On the basis of their research, these workers concluded that children likely to experience later emotional problems could be identified at the first-grade level. Two aspects of early secondary prevention were also examined. The first involved the use of teacher aides, who worked with problem children on a one-to-one basis. These aides were non-professional housewives who seemed well-adjusted and who enjoyed working with children. The second aspect of the secondary-prevention program involved the use of undergraduate volunteers to work with problem children on a one-to-one basis in a recreational setting two afternoons a week. It was felt that both programs were, for the most part, successful.

Some Unresolved Problems

Educators and mental-health specialists have often expressed a desire for earlier identification of emotional problems in children as a preventive step. Moreover, the research literature suggests that through a combination of approaches utilizing teacher judgment, peer perception, and self-rating, deviant youth can be identified during the early school years. Yet, several factors militate against the identification of problems in the early years of childhood (Bower, 1960):

1. Screening and diagnosing emotional problems during the preschool years and in kindergarten pose more difficulties than when attempted with somewhat older children. Even experienced teachers and clinicians, when dealing with individual children, have no reliable means for distinguishing between problems of a transitory nature and those indicative of later, more serious pathology. An extensive study involving more than 2,400 children in a southwest farming county in Minnesota demonstrated the difficulty associated with prediction of later individual adjustment (Anderson, 1959). In 1950, the subjects (who were in grades 4 through 12) were given a series of inventories dealing with such factors as family attitudes, social responsibility, and psychoneurotic symptoms. Teacher ratings on 20 personality characteristics were also obtained. Followup study conducted from 1954 to 1957 utilized personality inventories and teacher ratings. The major finding pertaining to prediction of individual behavior over a span of 5-7 years was essentially a negative one. In other words, it cannot be stated with certainty that a youngster who does poorly as measured by the available tests and rating scales will make a poor adjustment some years later. Changes within the person and changes in the demands made on him over time were regarded as two factors rendering prediction difficult. Curiously, it was easier to predict outstanding adjustment than poor adjustment. The present screening devices are not sufficiently discriminating to identify who will be emotionally disturbed in later life. As noted early in this book, it is not yet fully understood what kinds of disturbed youngsters grow up to be disturbed adults.

2. It is difficult to arouse parental concern when the child is young since the pathology is apt to express itself in a mild form. Likewise, teachers are often inclined to give the young pupil additional time in which to rally before requesting professional help. By the primary grades or early elementary-school years, however, teachers and parents become increasingly concerned about the child's maladjusted behavior and therefore seek assistance at that time.

3. It is often not until the middle elementary years that latent pathology becomes overt under the stresses and pressures for adjustment

to the academic and behavioral demands of the classroom. Torrance (1962) points to a number of cultural discontinuities which typically occur in the lives of middle-class pupils in the fourth grade. Classroom activities become more formal and organized, children are expected to sit in orderly rows in the classroom and are given less motoric freedom, and they are supposed to "get down to business."

4. Teachers and parents are quite able to tolerate the mild forms of overt pathology characteristic of young children, whereas they are less well equipped or prepared to cope with the acting-out behavior of older children.

5. As Bower (1960) notes, it is not known "how early is early" in the detection of childhood disorders. How soon must intervention procedures be implemented after the onset of a problem in order for the intervention to be economical and effective? For example, is identification at the third-grade level early enough for neurotic youth? for delinquent youth? for learning-disability cases? At present, the notion that early detection leads to efficient and effective treatment, though seemingly logical, remains an assumption rather than a fact. This idea raises a related point. If large numbers of maladjusted youngsters are identified, what is going to be done about them? Current treatment services are already overloaded. Few school administrators would care to have a large identifiable group of students whose educational and personal needs cannot be met. At the present time, there is no definite answer to such dilemmas.

6. Finally, many youngsters appear to "outgrow" their childhood disorders and enter successfully the mainstream of American adult life. What impact would the identification and labeling of such youngsters as "emotionally disturbed" have upon their later adjustment? Would the identification of these youngsters result in a self-fulfilling prophecy? Again, this is a difficult question to which there is no conclusive reply.

In summary, while the principle of early identification may in theory be a desirable one, it remains a very difficult practice to implement effectively and economically. The comments of Briggs and Wirt (1965) on the prediction of delinquent behavior also realistically depict some of the down-to-earth problems associated with prediction of deviant behavior in general:

Prediction involves attention to many factors that are largely utilitarian or functional. Examples of these points are the criterion of socially unacceptable delinquent behavior to be predicted, the cost of information relating to prediction, the use to be made of the prediction, acceptable rates of success, the cost of error in the prediction of a delinquent, and, finally, the costs of treatment and the availability of slots into which prospective treatment cases may be fitted. All prediction systems have left these factors unspecified, which leaves completely untold the value of such a system.

Hopefully, future research will provide answers to these pragmatic concerns.

CURRICULUM APPROACHES

Some workers believe that one of the most effective ways to promote the mental health of students entails the incorporation of psychological concepts into the curriculum. Such incorporation would not only insure a definite place for mental-health instruction, but also accomplish this instruction in a systematic manner. Curriculum approaches fall into one of three basic types (Kaplan, 1959): (1) incidental instruction, (2) separate courses, and (3) units. Each approach has advantages and disadvantages.

Incidental Instruction

Incidental instruction has in its favor the fact that instruction occurs at a time when problems are immediate and real, when motivation and interest are maximal. Drawbacks to this approach center around the need for teacher sensitivity and teacher sophistication in child developmental and mental health.

Separate Courses

Separate courses have also been used. Outstanding among these are the Bullis Project and Roen's behavioral-science curriculum. In the Bullis Project (described in Kaplan, 1959), the teacher is provided with a basic textbook containing lesson plans and stimulus stories. These stories, which center around emotional problems similar to those which preadolescents and early adolescents might be experiencing, are read to the class. After a discussion of the stories, the teacher summarizes the mental-health principles involved and the students record the conclusions in a daily log. Sample topics include "How Emotions Are Aroused," "Overcoming Personal Handicaps," and "Submitting to Authority." Kaplan (1959) contends that this approach is too didactic and moralistic. To the authors' knowledge, there has been no research evaluation of this approach.

More recently, Roen (1965, 1967) developed a behavioral-sciences course which he taught to fourth-graders. The class met for 40 minutes once a week over the school year. Roen reports that it was not difficult to recast concepts into terms the students could comprehend. A seminar entitled "Teaching the Behavioral Sciences to Children" was used to assist teachers. The course content included such topics as the influences of heredity and environment on development, Erikson's psychosocial stages of development, the self-concept, various learning-theory concepts, the concept of intelligence, institutional influences on development, and sociological analysis of the classroom. At the end of the course, each student was asked to write an autobiography discussing his uniqueness as a person and the particular forces producing that uniqueness. It is still too early to determine the effectiveness of this behavioral-science teaching program. Preliminary evaluation indicates, however, that these elementary-school students mastered the course content satisfactorily. Further, the children reportedly responded enthusiastically to the course and there were no complaints from adults in the community.

Units

The third approach, the use of mental-health units, is viewed by Kaplan (1959) as a compromise between the other two approaches. These units, which are built around problems at various stages of development, become an integral part of courses already in the curriculum and provide consistent and systematic mental-health instruction. The Ojemann Projects, which used special units in addition to revised basic text material, serve as an example of this approach.

Since 1941, Ojemann and his associates have developed and evaluated a curriculum approach to mental health which emphasizes a causal orientation to the social environment. By incorporating behavioral-science concepts into a curriculum which focuses on the causes or motivations of human behavior—as opposed to the surface or behavioral aspects—Ojemann hoped that the student would be better prepared to solve problems confronting him at the time and in the future. The basic rationale is that a person who becomes more fully aware and appreciative of the dynamics of human behavior in general and of his own in particular is better able to cope with personal and social crises.

A dynamic approach involves an awareness of the probabilistic nature of human behavior, an attitude of flexibility and tolerance, and an ability to view a given situation from another's perspective. A causal approach, in short, seeks to foster a greater sensitivity to interpersonal relationships so that more effective interaction with the environment is facilitated (see Table 18). Many adults are capable of solving impersonal problems but fail to "use their heads" in coping with personal and social anxieties. Ojemann (1967) contends, and we are inclined to concur, that a sensible arrangement would be to lay a foundation in the causal or motivational approach to behavior in children starting in kindergarten. Then, as the child passes into adulthood, he can add to this foundation and apply such a base to the study of marriage and family relationships, employer-employee interactions, and so forth. This approach not only enables the child to surmount current crises but establishes a foundation for the solution of crises in later development.

How does Ojemann hope to establish a causal approach? For one thing, he stresses the need to educate the teacher "to live a causal approach in the classroom." As a modeling procedure, daily associations with a teacher who handles situations in an understanding way can go far in developing a causal approach to life.

One teaching strategy used during the primary grades consists of narratives in which the surface and causal approaches are contrasted. In kindergarten and first grade, the teacher reads the narratives. In the later grades, the child reads them by himself. Each narrative depicts a situation in which a character in the story responds in a surface way initially, but in a causal way after he has thought-through the situation again. Realistic stories are used. To promote a more generalized approach, stories are described involving children older and younger than himself as well as those from different environments. Discussion focusing on the meaning and causes of the behavior in question follows each narrative.

At the elementary and secondary levels, the social sciences and English literature offer numerous opportunities to study the forces influencing the behavior of people. Even in areas such as math and science, the teacher can serve as a model for this type of approach.

Evaluations of this approach to date have been promising. The results of more than a dozen research studies indicate that an "appreciation of the dynamics of behavior is accompanied by significant changes in such dimensions as manifest anxiety, tendency to immediate

TABLE 18. THE SURFACE VERSUS THE CAUSAL APPROACH OF THE TEACHER TO CHILD BEHAVIOR [SURFACE VERSUS CAUSAL APPROACHES TO CHILDREN'S BEHAVIOR — LAFFERTY, DENNERLL, & RETTICH, 1964]

Surface	*Causal*
1. The teacher responds to the "what" of the situation in an emotional way.	1. The teacher responds to the "why" of the situation objectively.
2. The teacher does not appear to think of the causes of behavior when he:	2. The teacher appears to be thinking of the causes of behavior when he:
a. Responds to the action rather than to the reason for the action.	a. Runs over in his mind possible reasons for the action.
b. Labels behavior as "good," "bad," etc.	b. Seeks the meaning of the behavior and avoids snap judgments or hasty interpretations.
c. Makes generalizations to apply to every situation, e.g., "all boys are like that."	c. Searches for specific and concrete clues derived from details of the behavior.
d. Responds with a stock solution or rule of thumb procedure, e.g., lateness is punished by staying in after school.	d. Varies the method; uses a tentative approach, i.e., will try other ways of dealing with a situation if one does not work. In seeking a solution, takes into account motivating forces and particular method used.
3. The teacher does not take account of the multiplicity and complexity of causes.	3. The teacher thinks of alternative explanations for the behavior. The proposition that behavior has many causes may be elaborated as follows:
	a. The same cause may result in a variety of behaviors.
	b. A variety of causes may result in similar behavior.
4. The teacher fails to take into account the later effects of the techniques employed and assumes the effects.	4. The teacher checks for the effects of the method he employs and considers its effects before using it.
5. The "surface" approach is characterized by a rigidity of techniques — essentially static.	5. The "causal" approach is characterized by a flexibility, a tentativeness, a trying-out technique, which accommodates new information as it is accumulated — essentially dynamic.

Source: J. D. Lafferty, D. Dennerll, & P. Rettich. A creative school mental health program. *Nat. elem. Prin.,* 1964, 43, 28-35. Copyright 1964, Department of Elementary School Principals, National Education Association. All rights reserved.

arbitrary punitiveness, antidemocratic tendencies, conception of the teacher and tolerance of ambiguity" (Ojemann, 1967). There is some evidence, then, that education in the behavioral sciences can produce youngsters who are less anxiety-ridden, less arbitrary, and less authoritarian in handling personal problems.

Unfortunately, this curriculum has had very little impact on school procedures (Roen, 1967). Perhaps the reason is that effective use of this program demands specific training on the teacher's part. Then again, ever since the "Sputnik era" began, the emphasis in teacher-training institutions has been on cognitive development and not on cognitive-affective development. The trend today in education is not to view mental health as integral to a basic curriculum but as separate from cognitive development. As ego psychologists like Bower continue to point out the importance of ego or cognitive processes as basic to successful coping, this trend will hopefully be modified.

THE ROLE OF STRESS: HARMFUL OR NEUTRAL?

There are two divergent conceptions regarding the impact of stress on mental health. One, the traditional notion, views stress as something noxious and therefore to be averted. The other, which will be discussed later in this section, regards stress as a neutral force that can be used productively to build immunity to anxiety.

According to the traditional Freudian hypothesis, traumatic events during early life render the individual more susceptible to anxiety in adulthood. Proponents of the view which conceives of stress as undesirable typically oppose such practices as early reading, the use of grading in assessment, and the emphasis on academic excellence. They express concern over the price of competition, the frantic pace in education, and the emotional risks associated with increased demands for scholastic accomplishment. They raise such questions as: Does exposure to anxiety-producing situations endanger pupil mental health? What happens to students when they are prized more for academic achievement than for any other reason? What are the consequences of prolonged exposure to moderate stress?

What are some of the more common stresses in the educational setting? The post-Sputnik demands for increased intellectual competence have already been identified as one major source. Another common source of stress centers around the curriculum. Subsumed under the general heading of stress-inducing curricular experiences are grouping policies, promotional policies, and evaluational policies (Ringness, 1968). Inadequate provision for individual differences also constitutes a major shortcoming. For students exposed to a curriculum which does not match their abilities, interests, and cultural backgrounds, school soon becomes like a prison. Less obvious but nonetheless quite real and pervasive sources of frustration have been identified by Jackson (1968) from his observations of life in the classroom. He discusses four unpublicized features of school which can irritate students: delay, denial, interruption, and social distraction. Students seem to spend a surprising amount of time waiting—to sharpen pencils, to empty full bladders, to go to recess, to have teachers check papers, and so on. Denial is experienced when questions are ignored and requests refused. Classroom discontinuity stems from student misbehavior, outside visitors, bells ending classes, and other petty distractions and interruptions. It is difficult to determine the impact of these four hidden aspects of the school life. While the episodes, in and of themselves, appear trivial enough, their significance increases when they are considered cumulatively over a 12-year period.

Activities for Reducing Stress

A large number of options available to schools for reducing pupil stress has been listed by Lambert (1964). The stress-reducing activities suggested by Lambert fall into three basic categories: (1) modification or elimination, (2) isolation of vulnerable children from stress which cannot be modified, and (3) interception of problems at an early stage.

Specific activities for children who are subject to or threatened by stress that can possibly be modified or eliminated:

1. Find a temporary teacher for a short time.
2. Modify the pupil's daily schedule. Shorten the school day to a period of time in which he can function fairly well.
3. Experiment with finding a grade level where the child can expect to succeed, with both teacher and child understanding that successful learning for him would be to meet that level even though it may be far below grade. Carefully evaluate his needs with parents.
4. Place him in a smaller classroom group either within the class or in another class.
5. Have a home-school conference to help the parents understand the effects of excess pressures on the child.
6. See if welfare assistance is available to the family to cut down on economic stresses.

7. Lower, modify, or change curriculum demands.

8. Cut down the pressure on the family by reducing the number of care-taking workers who contact them. Decide on one person to be the coordinator of all counseling assistance.

9. If there is too much service to the child from too many sources, find a way to optimize and reduce contact.

10. Plan for reorganization of the classes into ungraded groups, with consultant help to teacher and administrative support.

11. Use brand-new teaching techniques for an area where a child has previously failed—for example, kinesthetic techniques in reading and spelling, programmed learning materials in some subject area, and counters in building arithmetic concepts.

12. Eliminate tests in classes containing children with serious emotional problems. The teacher should carefully supervise the learning program so that corrections of learning can be made as the child moves along.

13. Have a morning nutrition period to forestall hunger pangs that interfere with concentration on school work; during the period emphasize relaxation and teacher-pupil small talk.

Specific activities for children who need to be isolated from stress which cannot be modified:

1. Assign the child to a special class—based on specific learning needs—where he and other children in the class may have success.

2. Follow up on medical report to see if medication is needed; if so, check repeatedly to see if medication program is followed.

3. Use cubicles or "offices" in the classroom for a child who needs to have stimulation reduced; movable partitions make this possible.

4. Send a child to rest in the nurse's office when stress is excessive.

5. Provide a resource room in the school building where children can go to assist in activities that are not academic and not stress-producing.

6. Arrange for the child to attend school during periods where the stress is minimal; have him legally excluded from activities which are too stress-producing.

7. Ascertain whether foster-home placement is needed for a child in an especially disturbed family.

8. Find another class which would be less stressful and make a transfer.

9. Change the focus in curriculum planning. If, for example, arithmetic is the source of most stress, eliminate this from the pupil's requirements for a time.

10. Eliminate grading for the time being, substituting individual charts of the child's progress.

Interventions applicable for children who have already been hit by stress; the goal here is to intercept problems early, in an attempt to prevent further disorganization:

1. Routinely search out the children whose mothers will soon provide them

with siblings; find ways to assist their weathering the anticipated emotional situation.

2. Check pupil data regularly for children who may fail or have difficulty. Do not wait for referral; make regular contacts with schools and classrooms where such children are.

3. Check grade sheets at end of semester or school year and routinely evaluate all children who get failing marks.

4. Use remedial education wherever needed and as soon as the help is indicated.

5. Use medical and psychiatric referral to obtain additional information about a child's needs and to assist in outside intervention by other professional workers when it is indicated.

6. Have orientation programs for parents and children when the children are beginning in a new school or a new grade sequence.

7. Provide screening programs for locating children with potential physical, emotional, and social difficulties; follow up with adequate diagnosis and recommendations for specific interventions.

The contrasting philosophy, which views stress as a psychologically neutral force, contends that anxiety-producing experiences should be utilized to develop immunity to stress. There is a growing body of evidence indicating that some pain stimulation in early life might well have beneficial effects upon later adult adjustment. With respect to human subjects, Goertzel and Goertzel (1962) reported an interesting retrospective study of 400 eminent persons. Nearly 75 per cent of this group came from troubled or broken homes. Poverty, parental rejection and overprotection, and physical handicaps were among the conditions with which these children and their families had to contend. Almost half of the fathers experienced traumatic problems in their business and professional careers. Three-fifths of the fathers expressed dissatisfaction with school. Studies such as these suggest that the natural shocks of life can serve the purpose of growth and health.

Programs for Building Immunity to Stress

How can the schools use stressful experiences to promote healthy egos? As a starting point, Bower (1964) has delineated three potential programs for building immunity to stress.

1. *School-Entrance Stress.* The first program focuses on the crisis of school entrance. With the coming of school entrance, the child

undergoes a change in role. Now he must earn his place in the sun, for he is no longer accepted just because he is who he is. The school, he discovers, is different from his home, and the teacher has a different role from that of his mother. Further, the setting is more impersonal than the small-group settings he was used to during his preschool years. Research indicates that school entrance constitutes a growth-producing experience. Stendler and Young (1950) found, for example, that more than three-quarters of the mothers interviewed reported that their children had improved with respect to such traits as responsibility, helpfulness, good humor, and independence. Many youngsters recognize that going to school gives them a certain sense of status and prestige. Although these children give indications of increased self-importance upon entrance into school, they, as well as their parents, also become somewhat anxious. Mothers are concerned about how their children will fare. Youngsters also give evidence of adjustment difficulties. In one study, for instance, 80 per cent of the mothers interviewed reported that their children had problems of one kind or another during the primary grades (Moore, 1966). To use the stress of school entry positively, Bower (1964) suggests a specific program to be carried out by the schools:

One aspect of the program might be an assessment of each child prior to kindergarten entry or during his kindergarten experience, so that the school can plan more effective challenges for the child. In the preschool checkup the child may take the Stanford-Binet test, work with clay and fingerpaints, play in a play house and participate in some simple games with other children. The child's development and social history will be obtained from the parents by a school social worker. In the testing and play, the child's behavior and personality will be evaluated by observing the nature of separation from his parents, his affective control and spontaneity, any unusual behavior and the degree of dependency on the adult present. During games the child's ability to function with others will be observed: Can he abide by social rules such as taking turns; how does he deal with impulses and fantasies; is his curiosity acted upon or inhibited; to what extent can he tolerate frustration and tension; can he show joy or anger without losing control; and to what extent can he adapt to new games and new persons?

Both parents would probably be asked to attend one weekly two-hour meeting with seven other parents to keep in touch with their child's progress, his growing edges and his problems, if any. Children who might have some difficulty in school would be assessed individually for sensory, motor or emotional handicaps and appropriate adjustments made for them at school entrance. A school social worker would be assigned to those children or families who require additional help at this time, to work with them during the planning period.

A group meeting between parents and carefully selected teachers is also mentioned as a strategy for promoting harmonious school-home relations.[3]

2. *Onset-of-Puberty Stress.* The coming of puberty also marks a time of crisis. Youths must become reacquainted with their bodies and adjust to the rapid physical changes which have occurred. Too, they must learn new relationships with the opposite sex. Finally, they must strive to throw off parental restraints in their bid for independence. In brief, pubescents face an identity crisis which they must master to a reasonable degree. To cope with the crisis at this stage of development, Bower proposes the use of child-study classes at the junior-high level. Such a program might well entail two half-days of work each week in a child-care center sponsored by the school district for young children. These experiences would then be related to discussions of human behavior back in the social-studies class. One possible outcome is a fuller appreciation of the multiple motivations of behaviors. Learning to communicate and to share one's feelings are other possible values.

While many authorities, such as Freud, Erikson, and Havighurst, have pinpointed specific crisis points along the developmental trail which require resolution and deserve close attention, it is quite possible that personality development could be even more greatly enhanced through attention to mastery of the less celebrated or less obvious everyday crises which occur throughout the school years. For example, by simply helping the student to meet adequately the challenge of his daily arithmetic or English assignment, the teacher can foster personal maturity. In a society where status is accorded on the basis of effort and accomplishment, it is perhaps desirable that youth experience a sense of challenge and an ensuing sense of mastery. This proposal dictates an inevitable concern and provision for individual differences in student readiness.

3. *Games for Alleviating Stress.* The use of games is the third strategy cited by Bower. Games often provide us with an opportunity

---

[3]For an interesting preventive approach to developmental problems in elementary-school children, see Newton and Brown (1967).

to rehearse situations that may be anticipated as being troublesome to master in later life. Suchman's (1964) Inquiry Training Project, for example, is a game similar to "Twenty Questions" which is designed to promote problem-solving skills relating to scientific investigation. The use of games can promote personality and social growth as well as intellectual development. In playing games, the individual comes to abide by a set of rules, to expect penalties for rule infractions, to set goals, to experience a sense of accomplishment, to encounter failure, and to acquire the skills needed for cooperation. The use of games also provides the student with opportunities to integrate his intellectual self with his emotional self. Finally, games can be used to help motivate students who are having scholastic difficulty.

THE SUCCESSFUL SCHOOL PROGRAM

No attempt has been made to discuss school-based preventive stategies in a comprehensive manner. Instead, discussion has centered around some of the ideas stemming from mental-health professionals. It is recognized that a sound preventive program of mental health does not consist of a small number of specific intervention strategies. Rather, it must be part of the entire teaching-learning process, for the core of a good mental-health program is embodied in the way learning activities are guided. This viewpoint has been aptly expressed by Bower (1970):

Basically, the child's ability to deal with symbols, his ability to read with enjoyment, to communicate in speech and writing, to enjoy learning and working with others are the essential elements of a good mental health program in a school.

Thus the successful program has as its base teachers who are good teachers and a sound curriculum that is in tune with the range of competencies and values presented by the students.

The school cannot become a panacea for all of the ails afflicting youngsters, since many forces influencing psychological robustness are beyond the control of educational institutions as they are presently constituted. It would be extremely difficult for even the best school mental-health program to counteract the impact of such extraschool influences as geographical mobility, changing value systems in the culture at large, and undesirable child-rearing practices. Moreover, many of the formative influences may well have exacted their toll by the time youngsters enter school.[4]

Preventing Stress and Strengthening Personality

There are many ways in which the schools can foster positive mental health. Lambert's (1964) extensive list of interventions that prevent stress and build personality strength at the same time represents a germane conclusion to the section.

Interventions that build personality strengths by increasing psychological safety:

1. Make behavior prescriptions for a particular child. Ask him, for example, to be a "listener" for certain information in the class; ask him to act for one day as if "you are like Joe"; see if he can assist another child in some particular way; give him jobs which require self-control and assist him in understanding the responsibility involved.

2. If a child constantly wants to talk so that his hand is waving for teacher attention all the time, his chair can be placed directly in front of the teacher where she can see him at all times, but where she can see the rest of the class also.

3. Involve parents in what is expected of a child and keep them informed of his progress.

4. Where parents are hostile and blame the school, make contacts only when something positive can be said about the child.

5. Focus on curriculum content that is depersonalized such as science, nature studies, mathematics, and so on.

Interventions that assist in reinforcing personality strengths:

1. Find a new activity for a child, challenging enough that his success in it will help him feel his own ego strengths.

2. Find ways to let an insecure child know that he can trust you.

3. Help children through minor traumas by role playing.

4. Plan failure and success in ego-supportive situations.

5. Get children together in some type of nonacademic activity such as crafts, woodworking, music, arts, field trips, etc., to emphasize mutual interests and the development of special talents and skills.

---

[4]If the expectation is that the schools assume a greater preventive role by taking over some of the duties typically designated to the family (for example, early childhood education), then the educational setting must be radically transformed. As Rhodes (1968) notes, perhaps some merging of the child-forming institutions of the family and the school might accomplish the Herculean task associated with a preventive approach to developmental problems.

6. Assign adolescents to a group counseling setting where they can see others as human beings with problems similar to their own.

7. Find some way for the youngster who is poor at games to succeed in the eyes of his peers.

Interpersonal and group interventions that assist in relationship-building:

1. Establish a "mother" or "father" bank—adults in the school who can relate to a child who needs the extra support of either of these adult figures.

2. Find models for children—adequate masculine and feminine models and models of various types of acceptable behavior; especially aim at getting a child to try out options that may free inflexible, rigid behavior. Provide the behavior model that needs to be reinforced.

3. Build a relationship with a particular child by entering into the child's world for a time; find out what he thinks about and show him that you can accept him and his special ways of thinking.

4. Have birthday celebrations in which everyone in the class participates in some way (applicable to small classes, but difficult for large ones).

5. Use the physical education period as a way of observing peer relationships; provide a varied program, which will give children ample opportunities to find an activity in which they can succeed. Where there are poor peer relationships between members of the class, start with small game groups like 4-square and then move gradually on to larger team units.

6. Use a teacher other than the classroom teacher for an activity program that has less-defined rules than a classroom program. This lets the children see teachers in different roles and helps them recognize that behavior which is not acceptable in one situation may be acceptable in another.

7. Find some other adult besides the regular classroom teacher to whom the child can relate, e.g., an athletic coach, custodian, cook, bus driver, or another teacher.

8. Find reading materials which describe families differing in various ways from the troubled child's family; this may provide him with a new focus to better evaluate his own situation.

Interventions that have potential for motivation development:

1. Use confrontation routinely to let a child know that the role he is playing is perceived. At a grading period, for example, write 25 to 50 words for each child in the class, pointing up good and poorer qualities as a teacher sees them. This notation becomes the child's property and need not be shown to anyone—classmates or parents.

2. A cookbook might be used to teach the use of fractions; baseball cards for reading activities. Find what areas interest a child and teach him through that means until he can reach out to other areas; use the motor vehicle code, for example, to help adolescents learn to read to pass the examination for a driver's license.

3. Provide regular weekly tests to help a child keep track of his progress, and to help the teacher keep track of learning needs.

4. Remove demands for immediate achievement, then start with a single

learning area and focus attention on developing skills that will provide as much opportunity for success as possible.

Interventions that anticipate certain behaviors through guidance and corrective learning experiences:

1. Carefully define the classroom's place in the child's life and the teacher's expectancy for a particular child; after this definition the teacher should be consistent.

2. Introduce more competition as a child who has been in a special class gets ready to go back to a regular higher-level class. Too much reward at this point will keep children attending special programs too long.

3. Help pupils learn social skills by allowing them to plan a luncheon for parents, where they will perform in activities which they can do well, individually or in groups, or contribute to the success of the venture in various other ways.

4. Give every child a chance in turn to be captain of a team and help him understand what behavior is needed to do this job well.

5. Encourage a child to inhibit expression of hostility. Ask that he not tell you his dreams, or how he feels about other children.

6. Organize a child's day for him, working out with him his personal schedule so he will know what he will be doing at any particular time.

Interventions that assist in the management of group interaction:

1. A teacher who needs to spend time individually with certain children, and finds that other pupils resent this, should introduce some type of group activity and emphasize game rules and cooperation.

2. Vary the seating arrangements of the class where necessary to promote optimum contact with peers. On the other hand, in some instances "rigid" classroom seating may promote more consistent behavior of pupils until they are able to manage a more flexible room arrangement.

3. Minimize group contamination by careful seating arrangements. For instance, place a child who is poor at working alone amidst pupils who work well together; having no one with whom to engage in inappropriate activities, he may acquire the model of the workers.

4. Find "face-saving" devices for a child who is in trouble.

5. Never let a child's behavior cause him to be disgraced in front of his group; intervene long before the situation reaches this point.

6. Recognize individual differences in gregariousness; encourage social relationships to keep behavior options open, but remember that there is no perfect model of behavior for children of a given age.

SUMMARY

The emphasis in this chapter has been on primary prevention, especially as it relates to the schools. The need for preventive interventions are dictated by three factors: (1) the scope and complexities of the mental-health problem, (2) the continued shortage of mental-health specialists, and (3) the dubious outcomes of traditional treatment approaches. The concept of prevention is not easily implemented, however. Professional pessimism, the invasion-of-privacy issue, cultural values related to self-control and achievement, professional resistance, and difficulties in defining and evaluating objectives are foremost among the obstacles to the development of preventive programs. Current interventions have concentrated on biological, sociological, or psychological forces thought essential to sound mental health.

Schools are in a strategic position to undertake preventive actions because of their access to large numbers of youths over extended periods of time during the formative years and because of their culturally ordained prerogative to "meddle" in family affairs insofar as they are germane to the child's adjustment in school. Three aspects of the school's role in preventive efforts have been discussed: (1) the early identification of emotional disturbances, (2) various curriculum strategies, and (3) the use of stress. Several studies suggest the feasibility of detecting emotional disturbance in children early. There are difficulties, however, and these will require further research before the concept of early identification can be implemented effectively and economically on a routine basis. Specific curriculum approaches center around three basic approaches: (1) incidental instruction, (2) separate courses, and (3) units. The advantages and disadvantages of each have been noted, and examples given of some of the better-known programs. Divergent views on the role of stress have been presented. In general, it appears that stress which constitutes an appropriate challenge stimulates growth and maturity, while massive stress (with which the child does not successfully cope) is destructive and leads to unhealthy patterns of behavior.

SUGGESTED READINGS

American Educational Research Association. Mental and physical health. *Rev. educ. Res.,* 1968, **38** (5).

Clarizio, H. F. *Mental health and the educative process.* Chicago: Rand McNally, 1969.

Jones, R. M. *Fantasy and feeling in education.* New York: New York Univer. Press, 1968.

Torrance, E. P. *Constructive behavior: stress, personality, and mental health.* Belmont, Calif.: Wadsworth, 1965.

References   495

REFERENCES

Albee, G. The relation of conceptual models to manpower needs. In E. L.
Cowen, E. A. Gardner, & M. Zax (Eds.), *Emergent approaches to mental
health problems.* New York: Appleton-Century-Crofts, 1967. Pp. 63-73.

Allinsmith, W., & Goethals, G. *The role of the schools in mental health.* New
York: Basic Books, 1962.

Anderson, J. *A survey of children's adjustment over time: a report to the
people of Nobles County.* Minneapolis: Institute of Child Development
and Welfare, Univer. of Minnesota, 1959.

Arnhoff, F. N. Realities and mental health manpower. *Ment. Hyg.,* 1968, **52,**
181-189.

Bolton, A. A prophylactic approach to child psychiatry. *J. ment. Sci.,* 1955,
101, 696-703.

Bower, E. M. *The early identification of emotionally handicapped children in
school.* Springfield, Ill.: Thomas, 1960.

Bower, E. M. The modification, mediation and utilization of stress during the
school years. *Amer. J. Orthopsychiat.,* 1964, **34,** 667-674.

Bower, E. M. Mental Health. In R. Ebel (Ed.), *Encyclopedia of educational
research.* (4th ed.) New York: Macmillan, 1970. Pp. 811-828.

Bower, E. M., & Hollister, W. G. (Eds.) *Behavioral science frontiers in education.* New York: Wiley, 1967.

Briggs, P. F., & Wirt, R. D. Prediction. In H. C. Quay (Ed.), *Juvenile delinquency.* Princeton, N.J.: Van Nostrand, 1965. Pp. 170-208.

Brim, O. *Education for child rearing.* New York: Russell Sage Foundation,
1959.

Calhoun, J. B. Ecological factors in the development of behavioral anomalies.
In J. Zubin (Ed.), *Comparative psychopathology.* New York: Grune &
Stratton, 1967. Pp. 1-51.

Chombart de Lauwe, P. *Famille et habitation.* Paris: Editions de Centre
National de la Recherche Scientifique, 1959.

Clarizio, H. F. *Mental health and the educative process.* Chicago: Rand
McNally, 1969.

Cowen, E. L., Gardner, E. A., & Zax, M. (Eds.) *Emergent approaches to
mental health problems.* New York: Appleton-Century-Crofts, 1967.

Cruickshank, W. *Psychology of exceptional children and youth.* (2nd ed.)
Englewood Cliffs, N.J.: Prentice-Hall, 1963.

Frank, G. H. The role of the family in the development of psychopathology.
Psychol, Bull., 1965, **64,** 191-203.

Gardner, E. Psychological care for the poor: the need for new service patterns
with a proposal for meeting this need. In E. L. Cowen, E. A. Gardner, & M.
Zax (Eds.), *Emergent approaches to mental health problems.* New York:
Appleton-Century-Crofts, 1967. Pp. 185-213.

Goertzel, V., & Goertzel, M. *Cradles of eminence.* Boston: Little, Brown, 1962.

Hawkins, R., Peterson, R., Schweid, E., & Bijou, S. Behavior therapy in the
home: amelioration of problem parent-child relations with the parent in a
therapeutic role. *J. exp. Child Psychol.,* 1966, **4,** 99-107.

Jackson, P. *Life in classrooms.* New York: Holt, Rinehart & Winston, 1968.

Kaplan, L. *Mental health and human relations in education.* New York: Harper, 1959.

Kessler, J. W. *Psychopathology of childhood.* Englewood Cliffs, N.J.: Prentice-Hall, 1966.

Knobloch, H., & Pasamanick, B. Prospective studies on the epidemiology of reproductive casualty: methods, findings and some implications. *Merrill-Palmer Quart.,* 1966, **12**, 27-42.

Kraft, I. Preventing mental ill health in early childhood. *Ment. Hyg.,* 1964, **48**, 413-423.

Lafferty, J. D., Dennerll, D., & Rettich, P. A creative school mental health program. *Nat. elem. Prin.,* 1964, **43**, 28-35.

Lambert, N. *The protection and promotion of mental health in schools.* Washington, D.C.: Government Printing Office, 1964.

Lambert, N., & Bower, E. *Technical report on in-school screening of emotionally handicapped children.* Princeton, N.J.: Educational Testing Service, 1961.

Langdon, G., & Stout, I. *Teacher-parent interviews.* Englewood Cliffs, N.J.: Prentice-Hall, 1954.

Lazarus, R. S. *Patterns of adjustment and human effectiveness.* New York: McGraw-Hill, 1969.

Lindemann, E., & Ross, A. A follow-up study of a predictive test of social adaptation in preschool children. In G. Caplan (Ed.), *Emotional problems of early childhood.* New York: Basic Books, 1955. Pp. 79-93.

Moore, T. Difficulties of the ordinary child in adjusting to primary school. *J. Child Psychol. Psychiat.,* 1966, **7**, 17-38.

National Association for Mental Health. *Facts about mental illness.* New York: Author, 1966.

Newton, R., & Brown, R. A preventive approach to developmental problems in school children. In E. M. Bower & W. G. Hollister (Eds.), *Behavioral science frontiers in education.* New York: Wiley, 1967. Pp. 499-528.

Ojemann, R. Incorporating psychological concepts in the school curriculum. *J. Sch. Psychol.,* 1967, **5**, 195-204.

Oppenheimer, E., & Mandel, M. Behavior disturbances of school children in relation to the preschool period. *Amer. J. publ. Hlth,* 1959, **49**, 1537-1542.

Pasamanick, B., & Knobloch, H. Retrospective studies on the epidemiology of reproductive casualty: old and new. *Merrill-Palmer Quart.,* 1966, **12**, 7-23.

Polk, K., & Schafer, W. Delinquency and the schools. In Task Force on Juvenile Delinquency, *Juvenile delinquency and youth crime.* Washington, D.C.: Government Printing Office, 1967. Pp. 222-227.

Reiff, R. Mental health manpower and institutional change. *Amer. Psychologist,* 1966, **21**, 540-548.

Rhodes, W. Utilization of mental health professionals in the school. In American Educational Research Association, Mental and physical health. *Rev. educ. Res.,* 1968, **38** (5).

Ringness, T. *Mental health in the schools.* New York: Random House, 1968.

Roen, S. R. The behavioral sciences in the primary grades. *Amer. Psychologist,* 1965, **20**, 430-432.

Roen, S. Primary prevention in the classroom through a teaching program in the behavioral sciences. In E. L. Cowen, E. A. Gardner, & M. Zax (Eds.), *Emergent approaches to mental health problems.* New York: Appleton-Century-Crofts, 1967. Pp. 252-270.

Rosen, B. M., Bahn, A. K., & Kramer, M. Demographic and diagnostic characteristics of psychiatric clinic outpatients in the U.S.A., 1961. *Amer. J. Orthopsychiat.,* 1964, **34**, 455-468.

Russo, S. Adaptations in behavioral therapy with children. *Behav. Res. Ther.,* 1964, **2**, 43-47.

Stendler, C. Sixty years of child training practices: revolution in the nursery. *J. Pediat.,* 1950, **36**, 122-134.

Stendler, C., & Young, N. The impact of beginning first grade upon socialization as reported by mothers. *Child Develpm.,* 1950, **21**, 241-260.

Straughan, J. Treatment with child and mother in playroom. *Behav. Res. Ther.,* 1964, **2**, 37-41.

Suchman, J. R. The child and the inquiry process. In H. Passow & R. Leeper (Eds.), *Intellectual development: another look.* Washington, D.C.: Association for Supervision and Curriculum Development, 1964. Pp. 59-77.

Torrance, E. *Guiding creative talent.* Englewood Cliffs, N.J.: Prentice-Hall, 1962.

Zax, M., & Cowen, E. Early identification and prevention of emotional disturbance in a public school. In E. L. Cowen, E. A. Gardner, & M. Zax (Eds.), *Emergent approaches to mental health problems.* New York: Appleton-Century-Crofts, 1967. Pp. 331-351.

Periodicals Abbreviated in thé Text

Amer. educ. Res. J.	*American Educational Research Journal*
Amer. J. ment. Defic.	*American Journal of Mental Deficiency*
Amer. J. Orthopsychiat.	*American Journal of Orthopsychiatry*
Amer. J. Psychiat.	*American Journal of Psychiatry*
Amer. J. publ. Hlth	*American Journal of Public Health*
Amer. J. Sociol.	*American Journal of Sociology*
Amer. Psychologist	*American Psychologist*
Amer. sociol. Rev.	*American Sociological Review*
Ann. Amer. Acad. polit. soc. Sci.	*Annals of the American Academy of Political and Social Sciences*
Annu. Rev. Psychol.	*Annual Review of Psychology*
Arch. gen. Psychiat.	*Archives of General Psychiatry*
Arch. Neurol. Psychiat.	*Archives of Neurology and Psychiatry*
Behav. Res. Ther.	*Behavior Research and Therapy*
Brit. J. Psychiat.	*British Journal of Psychiatry*
Brit. J. Psychol.	*British Journal of Psychology*
Chicago Sch. J.	*Chicago School Journal*
Child Develpm.	*Child Development*
Childh. Educ.	*Childhood Education*
Crime & Delinq.	*Crime and Delinquency*
Educ. psychol. Measmt	*Educational and Psychological Measurement*
Educ. Res. Bull.	*Educational Research Bulletin*
Elem. Sch. J.	*Elementary School Journal*
Except. Child.	*Exceptional Children*
Fam. Process	*Family Process*
Fed. Probation	*Federal Probation*
Genet. Psychol. Monogr.	*Genetic Psychology Monographs*
Hlth, Educ. Welfare Indic.	*Health, Education and Welfare Indicators*

Integr. Educ.	*Integrated Education*
Int. J. Psychother.	*International Journal of Psychotherapy*
J. abnorm. Psychol.	*Journal of Abnormal Psychology*
J. abnorm. soc. Psychol.	*Journal of Abnormal and Social Psychology*
J. Amer. Acad. Child Psychiat.	*Journal of the American Academy of Child Psychiatry*
J. Amer. psychoanal. Assn	*Journal of the American Psychoanalytic Association*
J. Child Psychol. Psychiat.	*Journal of Child Psychology and Psychiatry*
J. clin. Psychol.	*Journal of Clinical Psychology*
J. consult. Clin. Psychol.	*Journal of Consulting and Clinical Psychology*
J. consult. Psychol.	*Journal of Consulting Psychology*
J. crim. Law, Criminol. Police Sci.	*Journal of Criminal Law, Criminology, and Police Science*
J. Educ.	*Journal of Education*
J. educ. Psychol.	*Journal of Educational Psychology*
J. educ. Res.	*Journal of Educational Research*
J. exp. Anal. Behav.	*Journal of Experimental Analysis of Behavior*
J. exp. Child Psychol.	*Journal of Experimental Child Psychology*
J. exp. Educ.	*Journal of Experimental Education*
J. exp. Psychol.	*Journal of Experimental Psychology*
J. exp. Res. Pers.	*Journal of Experimental Research in Personality*
J. genet. Psychol.	*Journal of Genetic Psychology*
J. ment. Sci.	*Journal of Mental Sciences*
J. Negro Educ.	*Journal of Negro Education*
J. nerv. ment. Dis.	*Journal of Nervous and Mental Disorders*
J. Offender Ther.	*Journal of Offender Therapy*
J. Pediat.	*Journal of Pediatrics*
J. Pers. soc. Psychol.	*Journal of Personality and Social Psychology*
J. psychiat. soc. Wk	*Journal of Psychiatric Social Work*
J. Psychol.	*Journal of Psychology*
J. Sch. Psychol.	*Journal of School Psychology*
J. soc. Issues	*Journal of Social Issues*
J. soc. Psychol.	*Journal of Social Psychology*
J. spec. Educ.	*Journal of Special Education*
J. Tchr Educ.	*Journal of Teacher Education*
Ment. Hyg.	*Mental Hygiene*
Ment. Retard.	*Mental Retardation*
Merrill-Palmer Quart.	*Merrill-Palmer Quarterly of Behavior and Development*
Milbank mem. Fund Quart.	*Milbank Memorial Fund Quarterly*
Monogr. Soc. Res. Child Develpm.	*Monographs of the Society for Research on Child Development*

Nat. elem. Prin.	*National Elementary Principal*
Nerv. Child	*Nervous Child*
Percept. mot. Skills	*Perceptual and Motor Skills*
Proc. Amer. Assn ment. Defic.	*Proceedings of the American Association on Mental Deficiency*
Proc. Child Res. Clin.	*Proceedings of the Child Research Clinic, Woods Schools*
Progr. Psychother.	*Progress in Psychotherapy*
Psychiat. Quart.	*Psychiatric Quarterly*
Psychiat.	*Psychiatry*
Psychol. Bull.	*Psychological Bulletin*
Psychol. Monogr.	*Psychological Monographs*
Psychol. Rec.	*Psychological Record*
Psychol. Rep.	*Psychological Reports*
Psychosom. Med.	*Psychosomatic Medicine*
Publ. Hlth Rep.	*Public Health Reports*
Quart. J. Child Behav.	*Quarterly Journal of Child Behavior*
Reading Tchr	*Reading Teacher*
Rev. educ. Res.	*Review of Educational Research*
Sat. Rev.	*Saturday Review*
Sci. Amer.	*Scientific American*
Soc. Forces	*Social Forces*
Soc. Prob.	*Social Problems*
Soc. Sci. Rev.	*Social Science Review*
Soc. Wk	*Social Work*
Sociol. Quart.	*Sociological Quarterly*
Sociol. soc. Res.	*Sociology and Social Research*
S. Afr. med. J.	*South African Medical Journal*
Tchrs Coll. Bull.	*Teachers College Bulletin, Indiana University of Pennsylvania*
Tchrs Coll. Rec.	*Teachers College Record*
Train. Sch. Bull.	*Training School Bulletin*
Univer. Mich. Sch. Educ. Bull.	*University of Michigan School of Education Bulletin*
Welfare Rev.	*Welfare in Review*
Yearb. nat. Soc. Stud. Educ.	*Yearbook of the National Society for the Study of Education*

INDEX OF NAMES

INDEX OF TOPICS